Pain in Children

Pain in Children

A Practical Guide for Primary Care

Edited by

Gary A. Walco, PhD

Director, The David Center for Children's Pain and Palliative Care,
Hackensack University Medical Center, Hackensack, NJ
Professor of Pediatrics, University of Medicine and Dentistry of New Jersey,
New Jersey Medical School, Newark, NJ

Kenneth R. Goldschneider, MD, FAAP

Director, Division of Pain Management, Department of Anesthesia,
Cincinnati Children's Hospital Medical Center,
Associate Professor of Clinical Anesthesia and Pediatrics,
University of Cincinnati College of Medicine, Cincinnati, OH

Foreword by

Charles B. Berde, MD, PhD

Professor, Departments of Anesthesia and Pediatrics, Harvard Medical School;
Director, Pain Treatment Service, Department of Anesthesia,
Children's Hospital Boston, Boston, MA

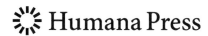 Humana Press

Editors
Gary A. Walco
The David Center for Children's Pain and
    Palliative Care
Hackensack University Medical Center
Hackensack, NJ

Kenneth R. Goldschneider
Division of Pain Management
Department of Anesthesia
Cincinnati Children's Hospital Medical Center
Cincinnati, OH

ISBN: 978-1-934115-31-2   e-ISBN: 978-1-59745-476-6
DOI: 10.1007/978-1-59745-476-6

Library of Congress Control Number: 2008920316

© 2008 Humana Press, a part of Springer Science+Business Media, LLC
All rights reserved. This work may not be translated or copied in whole or in part without the written permission of the publisher
(Humana Press, 999 Riverview Drive, Suite 208, Totowa, NJ 07512 USA), except for brief excerpts in connection with reviews or
scholarly analysis. Use in connection with any form of information storage and retrieval, electronic adaptation, computer software,
or by similar or dissimilar methodology now known or hereafter developed is forbidden.
The use in this publication of trade names, trademarks, service marks, and similar terms, even if they are not identified as such, is not
to be taken as an expression of opinion as to whether or not they are subject to proprietary rights.
While the advice and information in this book are believed to be true and accurate at the date of going to press, neither the authors nor
the editors nor the publisher can accept any legal responsibility for any errors or omissions that may be made. The publisher makes
no warranty, express or implied, with respect to the material contained herein.

Cover illustration: "Caring for Each Other," by Evelyn Berde.

Printed on acid-free paper

9 8 7 6 5 4 3 2 1

springer.com

To my father, Jerald, whose guiding spirit is a source of motivation every single day.
-GAW

To Jennifer, Jaye, and Benjamin, for whom my love is an 11/10: You inspire me to live, love, and be my best.
-KRG

Foreword

Pain in Children: A Practical Guide for Primary Care, edited by Drs. Walco and Goldschneider, provides a road map for general pediatricians, family practice physicians, pediatric nurses and nurse practitioners, child psychologists, pediatric subspecialists, and a range of other clinicians who care for infants, children, and adolescents to manage pain, suffering, and a range of distressing symptoms in everyday practice. It is a pleasure to add a foreword to a wise and practical book edited by two friends and colleagues. Although the work was all his, I take some personal pride in seeing Dr. Goldschneider, a former fellow from our program, join the ranks of book editors.

The reader will find several themes running through the chapters of this book.

1. Pain often, but not always, signals impending or actual harm.

The neural mechanisms that encode pain perception and that shape our responses to pain develop early in life—pain shapes how we learn and develop. Pain reports, pain behaviors, and physiologic responses may help pediatricians make a diagnosis in many situations. When interacting with a child in pain, we need to think in both mechanistic and biopsychosocial terms.

2. Assessing and treating pain, distress, suffering, and a range of symptoms is part of the job when you care for children.

During the past 25 years, clinical specialists in pain management and multidisciplinary pediatric pain clinics have emerged (Chapter 14). Nevertheless, most children with acute or chronic pain do not require a specialist for assessment and management. A major message of this book (included in virtually every chapter) is that all pediatric clinicians need to learn how to assess and manage pain for the wide range of situations that they face in daily practice.

3. Pain can be measured and assessed in a majority of situations (See Chapter 3).

Pain assessment should be multidimensional. It is not as simple as measuring heart rate or blood pressure. It often involves gathering information from multiple sources: patients' or caregivers' reports, behavioral observations, physiologic measurements, considering the context (medical, psychosocial, cultural), and gauging responses to therapeutic trials. Each of these sources of information, taken in isolation, can be erroneous. Combining this information is better, but still can be imperfect. Apparent discrepancies between different sources of information should prompt clinicians to slow down and think. Patient reports are the first-line source of information, whenever available, and most patients and their parents are accurate, truthful reporters. Nevertheless, a child who reports 10/10 pain, but jumps up on the exam table, smiles, and moves around easily is somehow different from a child who reports 10/10 pain, but who grimaces and tightens his or her muscles with slight movements, or who looks like the character in Munch's famous painting, "The Scream."

4. Assessment of pain is important; assessment of functionality is equally important.

In considering adults with low back pain, clinicians would be remiss if they did not ask questions about the patient's ability to walk, perform daily self-care, go to work, and function socially. Similarly, the interview would be incomplete without questions about injuries, legal claims, and workmen's compensation claims.

For the busy physician, seeing a child with recurrent headaches, abdominal pains, chest or limb pains, along with the standard medical history and physical exam, one should never omit asking about school attendance and performance, and participation in activities in and outside of the home. Chapter 13 provides wonderful guidance for engaging parents in understanding the relationship between pain and daily functioning, and how to prevent or reverse pain-related disability.

5. No single type of intervention works for every clinical situation.

As highlighted in Chapter 6, pediatricians need to apply a range of different interventions in different situations. The selection of interventions must be individualized and based on medical diagnosis, mechanisms of generation and perpetuation of pain, and the child's unique biopsychosocial situation. For example, rest or immobilization of a painful extremity may be the right thing to do in the short-term for a child who has sustained a fracture; it might be exactly the wrong thing to do for a child with complex regional pain syndrome (reflex sympathetic dystrophy).

6. We know more now than we did 25 years ago about what treatments are effective and safe, and we do a somewhat better job now than we did then.

Chapters 6 through 16 will show the reader that we know a fair amount about the clinical effectiveness of medications, cognitive-behavioral interventions, and physical therapeutic interventions for a variety of acute and chronic pain in infants, children, and adolescents. Surveys from the 1970s and early 1980s reported that children undergoing surgery often received inadequate postoperative analgesia and, in some cases, inadequate anesthesia during surgery. More recent surveys indicate that this situation has improved substantially. Children now receive anesthesia for surgery in almost all cases in developed countries. Analgesics are administered more effectively, and most pediatric tertiary centers have evolved more systematic approaches to treating acute pain in recent years.

Similarly, treatment of cancer pain appears to have improved over time, although surveys of parents' recollections published as recently as 2001 [1] would suggest that we still fail to provide adequate treatment of pain and dyspnea, and that other symptoms, such as fatigue, often receive little treatment. Recent data suggest that coordinated team approaches to palliative care can improve many aspects of symptom management, at least for children with cancer.

As experience in pediatric palliative care grows, it has become increasingly clear that models developed for children with cancer may need to be adapted for children with neurologic diseases. At the hospital where I practice, referrals for children with neurologic diseases now outnumber those with cancer. Further research is needed to delineate how best to improve symptom management and supportive care for these children and their families. As outlined in Chapter 22, general pediatricians have a vital role to play in caring for children and families who are facing life-limiting conditions.

Evidence that supports cognitive-behavioral treatment for a number of types of chronic pain in children and adolescents continues to grow (See Chapters 10 and 15, and sections of many other chapters). A primary barrier to wider implementation of cognitive-behavioral interventions, at least in the United States, is the failure of third-party payers to reimburse for these services, despite the robust evidence supporting their cost-effectiveness. Pediatricians, family practice doctors, pediatric nurses, and others need to learn and practice these techniques, while recognizing that some situations still require the more specific expertise of pediatric psychologists.

7. Pendulums swing forward and backward.

Two current examples of pendulum swings that are relevant to pediatric pain management concern the use of opioids in treating acute and chronic pain, and use of general anesthesia for newborns and very young infants.

a. Opioids

Prior to the 1980s, opioids were, by most accounts, clearly underused for postoperative pain and cancer pain in children, and were rarely prescribed for children with a variety of forms of chronic non-cancer pain. In the 1980s and 1990s, there appears to have been a worldwide increase in prescribing opioids for children following surgery and with cancer, and also wider use of opioids for treating chronic non-cancer pain. In the past 5 to 7 years, there has been a tendency to reduce opioid prescriptions based on the following viewpoints:

i. Opioids are effective and generally safe for postoperative pain, but they inevitably incur a significant frequency of annoying side effects, including nausea, itching, ileus, urinary retention, etc. As detailed in Chapters 8, 11, and 12, a major evolution in postoperative analgesia for children, as championed previously for adults by Kehlet and coworkers in Denmark [2], and by several groups in North America, is to optimize non-opioid analgesic approaches, including acetaminophen, NSAIDs, infiltration of operative sites with long-acting local anesthetics, peripheral nerve blocks, and neuraxial regional anesthesia. Opioids are increasingly used for many types of surgery as rescue analgesics in conjunction with these non-opioid approaches.

ii. Opioid tolerance is a major problem with long-term use, as commonly recognized in NICUs, PICUs, and in use for chronic pain. Animal and human studies by Palmer and coworkers indicate that this propensity to opioid tolerance is one of the downsides of the greater neuroplasticity in younger subjects, as compared to older subjects [3, 4]. Tolerance develops faster in infant humans and animals compared to young adult humans and animals who, in turn, develop tolerance faster than older adult humans and animals. Current research focuses on opioid sparing and tolerance-preventive approaches in these settings as well.

iii. In long-term prescribing of opioids to adults with chronic non-cancer pain, initial reports in the early 1980s (e.g., a widely quoted paper by Portenoy and Foley [5]) claimed good safety, good effectiveness, relatively slow dose escalation, and relatively low abuse potential. The growing literature in adults suggests that this assessment may have been overly optimistic. True drug-seeking behavior occurs in only a minority of patients with chronic pain. However, it is difficult to tell which patients are which. Of equal importance is the observation that, in controlled trials of adults with chronic non-cancer pain, opioids, on average, produce only very modest reductions in pain scores over time. However, these studies have shown essentially no improvement in mean scores for a variety of measures of functional rehabilitation or quality of life.

Few data are available on the outcomes of chronic opioid prescribing for children and adolescents with chronic pain associated with non-life-shortening conditions; these data are sorely needed. In our clinic, opioids are used on a long-term basis for a small number of children with non-life-shortening conditions associated with severe chronic pain, but great efforts are made to optimize all non-opioid approaches whenever possible.

iv. As noted above, even among children with advanced cancer, where evidence suggests that opioids are effective at relieving pain and dyspnea in most cases, a growing literature indicates that fatigue, somnolence, and mental clouding all cause suffering and reduced quality of life, and that opioids appear to be significant contributors to these symptoms. This does not mean that we should abandon opioids as first-line medications for treatment of pain, dyspnea, and other distress in children with cancer—only that we need to do a better job of treating opioid side effects in general and, in particular, treating the related symptoms of fatigue, somnolence, and mental clouding.

b. General anesthesia

Case series from the 1950s and 1960s documented high rates of cardiac arrest and perioperative death in neonates and infants undergoing surgery. Through the 1970s and 1980s, there was a rapidly growing body of knowledge on anesthetic pharmacology in neonates and infants, and a growing understanding of how to provide anesthesia safely even for sick infants undergoing complex procedures. Subsequently, we saw a substantial decline in the frequency of cardiac arrests and deaths in neonates and infants, although overall these events continue to occur more frequently in these age groups compared to older children, even when accounting for preexisting illness or complexity of surgical procedures. Through the 1980s we learned that even critically ill neonates could tolerate several types of general anesthesia and, in fact, adequate depth of general anesthesia appeared to improve several measures of postoperative morbidity and mortality.

What has recently thrown a "monkey wrench" into the use of general anesthesia for neonates and younger infants has been several animal studies examining effects of general anesthetics and sedatives on programmed neuronal cell death in the brains of infant animals at specific developmental stages. These data suggest that providing general anesthesia to human infants, at least for prolonged periods of exposure, and providing prolonged dosing of sedatives (e.g., midazolam, diazepam, lorazepam, phenobarbital) in newborn intensive care may be causing clinically significant brain injury. As expected, these studies have generated extensive controversy. Critics note that hours of anesthetic exposure in a newborn rat corresponds to weeks of anesthetic exposure for an infant human. They also note that anesthesiologists and neonatologists provide more intensive physiological support than most of the investigators who work on infant rats. Although methodologically hampered, available outcome studies indicate that a vast majority of children who underwent surgery as infants under general anesthesia are neurologically normal. The developmental effects of general anesthesia and sedation are a "hot topic" in pediatric anesthesia research. The attendant controversy may find its way into the primary care provider's office during preoperative visits, or concerns about postmorbid development expressed by parents of formerly critically ill patients.

8. We cannot make the world a painless place.

The title of the final chapter of this book, "What to Do When There Is Nothing to Do," is partly ironic and partly straight-up. Human existence includes experiencing pain, and while some interventions work for many patients for many situations, we cannot relieve all pain, distress, and suffering. If pediatricians and others caring for children read this book, they will do a better job of administering tablets, elixirs, injections, topical creams, physical interventions, and behavioral interventions in their daily practice. In a majority of situations, they can help the child to feel less physical pain and distress.

But our job does not end there. Even in those situations where pain, distress, and suffering cannot be fixed by a pill or an injection, we can help with anticipatory guidance, an explanation, comfort, and support. Support and guidance can sometimes be hard (e.g., "I know that your headaches are very painful, but I want you to understand that it won't do you harm to go to school tomorrow, and in the longer run, you will feel better by working with us in finding ways to stay in school even when it hurts…."). So, there is never "nothing to do."

To paraphrase Benjamin Spock's famous opening line: "You already know more than you think about assessing and managing pain." *Pain in Children: A Practical Guide for Primary Care* will make you feel more confident in approaching these challenging situations in everyday pediatric practice.

Charles B. Berde, MD, PhD

References

1. Wolfe J, Grier HE, Klar N, Levin SB, Ellenbogen JM, Salem-Schatz S, Emanuel EJ, Weeks JC. Symptoms and suffering at the end of life in children with cancer. N Engl J Med 2000;342:326–333.

2. Kehlet H. Acute pain control and accelerated postoperative surgical recovery. Surg Clin North Am 1999;79:431–443.

3. Wang Y, Mitchell J, Moriyama K, Kim KJ, Sharma M, Xie GX, Palmer PP. Age-dependent morphine tolerance development in the rat. Anesth Analg 2005;100:1733–1739.

4. Buntin-Mushock C, Phillip L, Moriyama K, Palmer PP. Age-dependent opioid escalation in chronic pain patients. Anesth Analg 2005;100:1740–1745.

5. Portenoy RK, Foley KM. Chronic use of opioid analgesics in non-malignant pain: report of 38 cases. Pain 1986;25:171–186.

Preface

There is some very good news in the world of pediatric medicine. Advances over the past two decades have enabled us to revolutionize the manner in which we can assess and manage children's pain. Thirty years ago it was thought that young children did not experience pain and, therefore, it was not necessary to treat it. Today, professionals from a variety of disciplines have contributed data that have revolutionized our perspectives. Technological advances now enable us to treat acute pain in fetuses, premature neonates, infants, toddlers, children, and adolescents with increasing precision and efficacy. Research highlighting the context of chronic pain has moved us away from a mind–body dichotomy and toward an integrated, holistic perspective that leads to substantial improvement in children's adaptive functioning, as well as subjective discomfort.

The less-than-wonderful news, however, is that primary care practitioners, those on the front lines in providing pediatric care, have not had easy access to much of this information. As a result, there is a gap between the attention to comfort and distress one finds in a tertiary care children's hospital, where relatively few children receive their care, and the general practitioner's office, where many more millions of children are seen each year.

Pain in Children: A Practical Guide for Primary Care is intended to close that gap. The target audience is anyone who provides medical care to children. This includes primary care pediatricians, family practice physicians, pediatric nurses, physician assistants, and pediatric and other subspecialists who see children. We have been privileged to assemble a "Who's Who" of pediatric pain specialists to write in their fields of specialty with the intent of communicating with you, the primary practitioner, about how to recognize, conceptualize and intervene on an array of common concerns, including when to refer to a specialized pediatric pain service.

Each chapter provides an overview of the problem, followed by a "hands-on" description of relevant assessment and intervention strategies. The role of the primary care practitioner is highlighted, both as a frontline resource and as a consumer of specialized pediatric pain treatment services. Each chapter ends with a summary and specific bullet points highlighting the most central elements, making for quick and easy reference. As a practical guide, this book is designed so that readers are free to direct their attention to individual chapters of interest without requiring knowledge of the preceding chapters. As a reference, the book chapters refer to key articles, website URLs, and books for further focused and practical investigation.

The text is divided into five major sections. The first section, General Considerations, provides an overview of the context of pain in development; pain assessment in infants, children, and adolescents; pain in children with developmental disabilities; and novel strategies to help manage pain more remotely, such as over the telephone or through the Internet. The second section, Acute Pain Management, addresses acute pain management, including common pain problems seen in the office, topical anesthetics and office-based procedures, analgesic medications for infants and children, pain treatment for trauma and in the emergency room, preparing children for invasive procedures and surgery, and postoperative pain management in the hospital and at home. The third section, Recurrent and Chronic Pain Management, addresses general issues in recurrent and chronic pain concerns in children. This includes how to talk to parents about recurrent and chronic pain, as well as interdisciplinary approaches, psychological interventions, and complementary and alternative medicine paradigms for chronic pain. The fourth section, Common Recurrent and Chronic Pain Problems in Primary Care, focuses on specific pain problems, including chronic abdominal pain, headaches, musculoskeletal and back pain, sickle cell disease, and pelvic pain. The last section, Special Topics, is reserved for special areas of interest to the primary care practitioner, including pediatric

palliative care, processes of drug approval labeling for children, and the pediatrician and family practice physician as advocate for better pain management in children.

It is our hope that *Pain in Children: A Practical Guide for Primary Care* will be useful in improving the care of infants, children, and adolescents across settings. Reducing or eliminating needless suffering would be wonderful for care providers, parents and, of course, our pediatric patients. As highlighted in some of the chapters, it may also reduce the risk of pain problems in the future.

Gary A. Walco, PhD
Kenneth R. Goldschneider, MD, FAAP

Acknowledgements

Undertaking an effort such as this requires the input and collaboration of many talented individuals. We are extremely indebted to our esteemed colleagues and friends who contributed chapters to this text. The depth of your insights and your passion in communicating your messages were obvious and we are proud to be part of such a gifted professional community.

I (GAW) am grateful to the professional and support staff in the David Center for Children's Pain and Palliative Care and Hackensack University Medical Center, especially Susan Cohen and Tommysena Smith-Fields, who offer so much on so many fronts. I deeply appreciate the backing of the Healing Heart Foundation and Lisa Nehmer, its executive director. I am also so fortunate to have the unending professional and loving support of my wife, Jayne, and the work becomes so much more meaningful because of Jeremy, Daniel, and Emily.

For me (KRG), Michelle Tate and Richard Goins at the Cincinnati Children Hospital Division of Pain Management provided both administrative and moral support, for which I am much obliged. Special thanks for their clinical work and advocacy go to our advanced practice nurses: Suzanne Black, Keeley Harding, Lori McKenna, Nora Paulford-Lecher, Debbie Wolf, and to Debby Palmisano, MSW. Throughout the whole process, my family cheered and believed; dedicating the book to them just seems inadequate to express my gratitude and appreciation.

Thanks go to the staff at Humana Press, especially Amy Thau for her "save the day" editorial skills, and Richard Lansing for working with us from inception to completion. It is amazing what can emerge from sharing a cab to the airport!

Finally, we thank Evelyn Berde for creating such a beautiful painting for the front cover.

GAW
KRG

Contents

I. General Considerations

II. Acute Pain Management

V. Special Topics

Contributors

Debbie Avant, RPh
Regulatory Project Manager, Food and Drug
Administration, Center for Drug Evaluation
and Research, Office of New Drugs-Immediate
Office Pediatric and Maternal Health Staff,
Beltsville, MD

Carl L. von Baeyer, PhD, RD Psych
Professor of Psychology and Associate Member
in Pediatrics, University of Saskatchewan,
Saskatoon, Saskatchewan, Canada

Charles B. Berde, MD, PhD
Professor, Departments of Anesthesia
and Pediatrics, Harvard Medical School;
Director, Pain Treatment Service, Department
of Anesthesia, Children's Hospital Boston,
Boston, MA

Ronald L. Blount, PhD
Professor, Department of Psychology,
University of Georgia, Athens, GA

Mark A. Connelly, PhD
Assistant Professor, Department of Pediatrics,
University of Missouri-Kansas City School
of Medicine; Co-Director, Integrative Pain
Management Clinic, Children's Mercy Hospitals
and Clinics, Kansas City, MO

Kenneth D. Craig, PhD
Department of Psychology, University of British
Columbia; Senior Investigator, Canadian Institutes
of Health Research Vancouver, British Columbia,
Canada

Carlton Dampier, MD
Professor and Associate Chair of Pediatrics
for Research, Drexel University College
of Medicine; Chief of Hematology and Director
of the Marian Anderson Comprehensive Sickle
Cell Center, St. Christopher's Hospital
for Children, Philadelphia, PA

Subhadra Evans, PhD
Project Coordinator, Pediatric Pain Program,
Mattel Children's Hospital at UCLA,
David Geffen School of Medicine
at UCLA, Los Angeles, CA

Paula A. Forgeron, RN, MN
Clinical Nurse Specialist, Pediatric Pain
Management, IWK Health Centre;
Interdisciplinary PhD student, Dalhousie
University, CIHR PhD, Fellowship Trainee,
Halifax, Nova Scotia, Canada

Artee Gandhi, MD
Attending Physician, Anesthesia and Pain
Management, St. Joseph Medical Center,
Kansas City, MO

Kenneth R. Goldschneider, MD, FAAP
Director, Division of Pain Management,
Department of Anesthesia, Cincinnati Children's
Hospital Medical Center; Associate Professor of
Clinical Anesthesia and Pediatrics,
University of Cincinnati College of Medicine,
Cincinnati, OH

Christine D. Greco, MD, FAAP
Director, Acute Pain Services, Department
of Anesthesiology, Perioperative
and Pain Medicine, Children's Hospital Boston;
Instructor in Anesthesia, Harvard Medical School,
Boston, MA

Zeev N. Kain, MD, MBA
Executive Vice-Chair and Professor
of Anesthesiology, Pediatrics and Child
Psychiatry; Executive Director, Center for
Advancement of Perioperative Health, Yale
University School of Medicine,
New Haven, CT

Susmita Kashikar-Zuck, PhD
Associate Professor of Pediatrics and Clinical
Anesthesia, Division of Behavioral Medicine
and Clinical Psychology, Department of Pediatrics,
Cincinnati Children's Hospital Medical Center,
University of Cincinnati College of Medicine,
Cincinnati, OH

Michael K. Kim, MD, FAAP
Associate Professor of Pediatrics, Medical College
of Wisconsin, Milwaukee, WI

Christine T. Korol, PhD
Psychologist, Pediatric Complex Pain Clinic
and Burn Unit, Alberta Children's Hospital,
Calgary, Alberta, Canada

Elliot J. Krane, MD
Professor of Anesthesia and Pediatrics, Stanford
University School of Medicine; Director, Pediatric
Pain Management Center, Lucile Packard
Children's Hospital at Stanford, Palo Alto, CA

Alyssa A. Lebel, MD
Associate Director, Pain Treatment Service,
Department of Anesthesiology, Perioperative
and Pain Medicine, and Pediatrics, Neurology
Division, Children's Hospital Boston; Assistant
Professor of Anesthesia and Neurology, Harvard
Medical School, Boston, MA

Anne M. Lynch, PhD
Assistant Professor of Pediatrics and Clinical
Anesthesia, Division of Behavioral Medicine
and Clinical Psychology, Department of Pediatrics,
Cincinnati Children's Hospital Medical Center,
University of Cincinnati College of Medicine,
Cincinnati, OH

Jill E. MacLaren, PhD
Postdoctoral Fellow, Center for Advancement
of Perioperative Health, Department
of Anesthesiology, Yale University School
of Medicine, New Haven, CT

Megan L. McCormick, BA
Clinical Psychology Graduate Student, Department
of Psychology, University of Georgia, Athens, GA

Patrick J. McGrath, OC, PhD, FRSC
CIHR Distinguished Scientist, Canada Research
Chair; Vice President, Research, IWK
Health Centre; Professor of Psychology, Pediatrics
and Psychiatry, Dalhousie University,
Halifax, Nova Scotia, Canada

Mark J. Meyer, MD
Assistant Professor, Clinical Anesthesia
and Pediatrics, Division of Pain Management,
Department of Anesthesia, Cincinnati Children's
Hospital Medical Center, Cincinnati, OH

Tim F. Oberlander, MD, FRCPC
R. Howard Webster Professorship in Early Child
Development, Associate Professor, Pediatrics,
Division of Developmental Pediatrics,
Complex Pain Service, British Columbia
Children's Hospital, University of British
Columbia, Vancouver, British Columbia, Canada

Tonya M. Palermo, PhD
Associate Professor, Anesthesiology
and Peri-Operative Medicine and Psychiatry,
Oregon Health and Science University,
Portland, OR

R.J. Ramamurthi, MD
Clinical Assistant Professor of Anesthesia, Stanford
University School of Medicine, Palo Alto, CA

William J. Rodriguez, MD, PhD
Pediatric Science Coordinator, Food and Drug
Administration, Office of the Commissioner,
Office of Pediatric Therapeutics; Professor Emeritus
of Pediatrics, Children's National Medical Center,
George Washington University School of Medicine
and Health Sciences, Washington, DC

John Barns Rose, MD
Associate Professor of Anesthesiology
and Pediatrics, University of Pennsylvania
School of Medicine; Clinical Director,
Pain Management Service, Department of

Anesthesiology and Critical Care Medicine,
Children's Hospital of Philadelphia,
Philadelphia, PA

Hari Cheryl Sachs, MD
Medical Officer, Food and Drug Administration,
Center for Drug Evaluation and Research, Office
of New Drugs-Immediate Office, Pediatric
and Maternal Health Staff; Professor of Pediatrics,
Children's National Medical Center, George
Washington University School of Medicine
and Health Sciences, Washington, DC

Carol Schadelbauer
Vice President and Director, Burness Health
and Science Advocacy Institute, Burness
Communications, Bethesda, MD

Laura E. Schanberg, MD
Associate Professor, Duke University School
of Medicine; Co-Chief, Pediatric Rheumatology,
Medical Director, Pediatric Pain Evaluation Clinic,
Duke Children's Services, Duke University
Medical Center, Durham, NC

Lisa Scharff, PhD
Assistant Professor of Psychiatry,
Harvard Medical School, Children's Hospital
Boston, Boston, MA

Neil L. Schechter, MD
Professor of Pediatrics, Head, Division
of Developmental and Behavioral Pediatrics,
University of Connecticut School of Medicine;
Director, Pain Relief Program, Connecticut
Children's Medical Center, Hartford, CT

Navil F. Sethna, MB, ChB
Senior Associate in Anesthesiology and Associate
Director of Pain Treatment Service, Department
of Anesthesiology, Perioperative and Pain
Medicine, Children's Hospital Boston; Associate
Professor of Anesthesia, Harvard Medical School,
Boston, MA

Harold (Hal) Siden, MD, MSc, FRCPC
Medical Director, Canuck Place Children's Hospice;
Clinical Associate Professor, Paediatrics,
British Columbia Children's Hospital,
University of British Columbia, Vancouver,
British Columbia, Canada

Laura E. Simons, PhD
Research Assistant Professor, Department
of Psychology, Boston University,
Boston, MA

Gary A. Walco, PhD
Director, The David Center for Children's Pain
and Palliative Care, Hackensack University
Medical Center, Hackensack, NJ; Professor of
Pediatrics, University of Medicine and Dentistry
of New Jersey, New Jersey Medical School,
Newark, NJ

Norbert J. Weidner, MD
Associate Professor, Clinical Anesthesia
and Pediatrics, Medical Director, Pediatric
Palliative and Comfort Care Team, Division of
Pain Management, Department of Anesthesia,
Cincinnati Children's Hospital Medical Center,
Cincinnati, OH

Steven J. Weisman, MD
Jane B. Pettit Chair in Pain Management, Children's
Hospital of Wisconsin; Professor of Anesthesiology
and Pediatrics, Medical College of Wisconsin,
Milwaukee, WI

Robert T. Wilder, MD, PhD
Associate Professor of Anesthesiology; Director,
Pediatric Pain Service, Mayo Clinic, Rochester, MN

Lonnie K. Zeltzer, MD
Professor of Pediatrics, Anesthesiology,
Psychiatry and Biobehavioral Sciences; Director,
Pediatric Pain Program, Mattel Children's
Hospital at UCLA, David Geffen School
of Medicine at UCLA, Los Angeles, CA

William T. Zempsky, MD
Associate Director, Pain Relief Program,
Connecticut Children's Medical Center; Associate
Professor of Pediatrics and Emergency Medicine,
University of Connecticut School of Medicine,
Hartford, CT

Part I
General Considerations

1
Pain and the Primary Pediatric Practitioner

Gary A. Walco

Abstract: Over the past two decades there have been major strides made in our understanding of the mechanisms, assessment and management of pain in children. By and large, however, mainstream primary pediatric care has not kept pace with many of these advances. After a brief review of the growth of the field, this chapter discusses the ethics of pain management in children. We begin with the notion that pain is harmful to children and thus failure to adequately treat pain without sufficient justification may violate the basic ethical principle of "do no harm."

Insight into the development of pain networks is provided, followed by a discussion of individual differences in pain response. This includes the influence of genetic factors and temperament, after which some of the findings on the consequences of untreated pain in the young are discussed.

Key words: Pediatric pain, primary care, ethics, neurodevelopment, individual differences.

Introduction

A 4-year-old boy goes to the same day surgery center for a tonsillectomy. Three days later the mother calls you, the primary care provider, saying that her son is still in severe pain. The otolaryngologist has made it clear that the acute postoperative pain period has passed and tells her to continue the codeine preparation as needed. Why has the acute pain persisted? Is this normal? What else might be done to help this child? What is your role?

A 12-year-old girl has been in your office frequently complaining of severe abdominal pain. You sent her for a consult with the pediatric gastroenterologist who did a full workup, including endoscopy and colonoscopy. The concluding diagnosis is mild gastritis and functional abdominal pain. She continues to be miserable, is missing a great deal of school, and often goes to the emergency department because her pain gets so severe. The gastroenterologist suggested that the family seek psychological services, but they have not followed through because "the pain is not all in her head." What is your next step?

A 9-year-old boy severely sprained his ankle in a soccer game. Over-the-counter analgesics, such as ibuprofen, are not managing his pain and so you consider prescribing a more potent analgesic, such as an opioid derivative. However, his parents raise concerns about side effects and possible addiction, making it clear that they would prefer not to use such drugs and that "since he is an athlete he can tough it out." What is your course of action?

These represent just a few scenarios that may be encountered by pediatricians, family practice physicians, and other general care providers. Although pain is one of the most common complaints that bring patients in to see their doctors, it is not a topic on which most practitioners are well-studied. By and large, pain management in children is learned on the fly. There are few courses dedicated to the assessment and treatment of pain in medical school, and during residency there may be various opportunities to learn about pain, but rarely is the approach systematic or consistent. As a result, pain in the young is often inadequately assessed and undertreated.

The good news is that the field of pediatric pain management has progressed tremendously in the last three decades. The First International Symposium on Pediatric Pain took place in Seattle, Washington in 1988. Individuals representing a number of professional disciplines—pediatricians, anesthesiologists, psychologists, nurses, rehabilitation specialists, developmental physiologists, pharmacists—met and realized they had very similar views and common areas of interest. That collaborative spirit and cross-fertilization of ideas has remained the hallmark of the endeavor and proudly permeates the chapters that follow.

The field of study has continued to grow and thrive. The International Association for the Study of Pain (IASP) formed a special interest group on pain in childhood and the international symposia continue to be held every three years. The American Pain Society likewise has a special interest group that has been active, including the formation of a task force to author the American Academy of Pediatrics policy statement on the assessment and management of pain in infants, children and adolescents [1]. The AAP has also authored statements on palliative care and chronic abdominal pain [2, 3]. Of course various other professional organizations focused on the care of infants and children have paid increasing attention to the issue as well.

Most children's hospitals have some recognizable pain service. This may range from model programs with multidisciplinary teams that comprehensively address acute and chronic pain problems, to services that are substantially more limited in scope (e.g., acute postoperative pain). In addition to providing clinical care, these groups are responsible for a good deal of the translational and clinical research that has been generated, and some of the larger programs offer postgraduate training programs in pediatric pain management across disciplines. An impressive innovation is Pain in Child Health (PICH), a project sponsored by the Canadian Institutes of Health Research to provide a training consortium for the development of young independent investigators in the field.

The growth of the area of study may be measured to some degree by scientific contributions in the literature. A Medline® search entering the broad topic of "pain" and limiting results to include populations between the ages of 0 and 18 years demonstrated a steady increase over time, as shown in Table 1-1.

Entering the same broad search term of pain, 233 out of the 24,885 papers published between 1949 and the present in Pediatrics, the official journal of the American Academy of Pediatrics, were on the topic. Similarly, in American Family Physician, the journal of the American Academy of Family Physicians, out of 8,920 papers published between 1969 and today, 174 were on pain, only 24 of which included all children between the ages of 0 and 18 years.

So, although scholarly work on the assessment and management of pain has expanded dramatically over the past two decades, the literature published in the two journals most read by general pediatricians and family practice physicians—those on the front line in treating infants and children—is lacking both in relative and absolute terms. The intent of this text is to help fill that void. We offer a series of chapters, each written by top experts in their respective fields, that explain pain problems and issues related to pain, providing overviews for the primary care practitioner. It is not intended to address issues comprehensively, preparing one to be an expert in the field, but rather to provide the information needed to improve skills of differential diagnosis, to invoke treatments for common pain problems, and to know when to refer for additional expertise. For example, the reader will not be able to perform various regional blocks after reading this text, but will understand the issues confronted by the pediatric anesthesiologists with that expertise and therefore be able to better interface with them in the care of patients.

The remainder of this chapter will round out a broad introduction, focusing on some central issues regarding pediatric pain. Included will be brief discussions of the ethics of pain management in children, the development of pain systems, individual differences in pain responses, including the role of genetics and temperament, and the consequences of untreated pain in children.

TABLE 1-1. Number of publications on pain in children over time.

Time Period	Number of publications
1953–1970	728
1971–1980	1,815
1981–1990	2,888
1991–2000	3,917
2000–2007*	3,973

*Through September 2007.

1. Managing Pain in Children: Your Ethical Obligation

A paper published in the *New England Journal of Medicine* in 1994 summarized the ethical challenge of managing pain in children [4]. A fundamental principle of responsible medical care is not "do not hurt," but "do no harm." Harm occurs when the amount of hurt or suffering is greater than necessary to achieve the intended benefit. Since pain is harmful to patients, and caregivers are categorically committed to preventing harm to their patients, not using all the available means of relieving pain must be justified.

A comparative justification focuses on the benefits and risks of unrelieved pain against those of pain relief. A responsible conclusion may be that the harm of unrelieved pain is less severe than the harm of pain relief. In arriving at such a conclusion, one must consider the physiologic state of the child, the disease causing the discomfort and the analgesics themselves, as well as how an analgesic will be administered and its potential side effects and long-term consequences. One must be evidence-based in these appraisals, adequately assessing the pain and relying on available data about the treatments under consideration.

Pain may be useful in monitoring an illness or indicating the ineffectiveness or limits of treatment. One must, therefore, weigh the benefit of immediate relief against that of long-term recovery. As defined above, the default position is to provide full treatment of pain in children unless otherwise justified by defined therapeutic benefits. In such circumstances three specific tests should be applied. First, is the pain useful as a means to achieve an important goal? Second, is the pain necessary or are there other less hurtful means of achieving that goal? Third, is the pain at the lowest possible level?

Character development is based on a moral view that champions traits such as courage, self-discipline, independence, and self-sacrifice. Although encouraging such virtues is generally positive, imposing the burden of character development on a child already encumbered by sickness and suffering reflects a lack of compassion and is ethically indefensible. When the total eradication of pain is not possible (as in the case of chronic pain associated with chronic illness), strengthening the child's capacity to cope with the pain is beneficial and may be justifiable. However, to withhold analgesics from a suffering child in the hope of influencing character development ignores the child's real present need for pain relief.

In sum, as concluded in the original paper [4], "All health professionals should provide care that reflects the technological growth of the field. The assessment and treatment of pain in children are important parts of pediatric practice, and failure to provide adequate control of pain amounts to substandard and unethical medical practice."

2. Development of Pain Systems

Understanding of the ontogeny of the pediatric pain experience has increased significantly over the past two decades. Accumulating evidence has demonstrated that pain is perceived earlier in life than had previously been believed. For example, a little over 30 years ago it was thought that infants did not feel pain or if they did there was no lasting memory of it. Today it is clear that very premature neonates experience pain and the "lower limit" of ages at which pain systems are intact continues to be revised [5]. More recent data on fetal pain further supports the view that pain systems develop and function very early in the gestational period, certainly by 23 weeks gestation, if not much earlier [5].

Nociception is the excitation of peripheral afferent neurons in response to a noxious stimulus. Axons of these peripheral sensory nerves terminate at synapses in the dorsal horn of the spinal cord. Reflex arcs in the spinal cord lead to reflexive responses, such as withdrawal from the stimulus. In addition, neurons ascend through the spinal cord to the brain, and it is only once higher centers are stimulated that one perceives pain. Thus, nociception is merely sensory excitation; pain is the subjective perception and the usual focus of concern.

Animal models show that sensory nerve fibers involved in nociception grow out of the dorsal root ganglia during the prenatal period and eventually innervate the skin in a proximodistal manner [6]. The outgrowth of sensory neurons from the dorsal root ganglia to the periphery occurs with larger diameter A fibers forming a cutaneous nerve plexus first, after which comes the formation of C fibers. In addition, centrally directed dorsal root fibers reach the lumbar cord, again with A fibers penetrating the gray matter first, followed by the C fibers. From the outset these fibers terminate in a somatotopically precise manner and shortly thereafter reflex arcs begin to develop. Descending fibers from the brain stem that modulate excitation and inhibition are the last element to appear, often well past the 40-week gestational age mark [7].

Considering all of these concepts together, it is clear that even very premature infants experience pain, that the "loudest" part of pain networks develops first (A-δ fibers) and the descending mechanisms to modulate that pain appear last. Thus, the need for attention to pain begins with even the very youngest of children; of note, fetal surgery, the practice of which is limited to a few centers, often includes opioid treatment during the process of surgery [8].

3. Individual Differences in Pain Response

As is the case with so many developmental phenomena, pain responses are determined by genetic factors that interact with environmental events. Research on inherited elements related to the pain response fall into two major related categories, the genetics of pain and temperament. These endowments predispose utilization of related coping strategies in response to various life experiences and stressors and, over time, response styles emerge which may be predictive of adjustment to painful situations.

3.1. Genetics of Pain Response

In a review of the role of genetics in pain responsiveness, Mogil et al. [9] contended that it is unlikely that a simple genetic basis will be found to account for individual variability in pain response. Very few genetic mutations or polymorphisms have been identified that account for specific pathological pain states in humans (e.g., congenital insensitivity to pain, familial hemiplegic migraine). Most information on the genetics of pain has come from studies involving animal models (typically mice) and has focused on differences in nociception and analgesia sensitivity. Although some principles may apply, the genetics of pain in humans appears far more complex than in other species. It is reasonable to expect in addition to animal research, further studies of pharmacogenetics (specific genetic variations that give rise to differing responses to drugs) and pharmacogenomics (the broader study of the entire human genome's response to drugs as they move through the system) will advance our knowledge of pain mechanisms and optimal matches to treatment modalities.

For example, in a recent study of two different topical anesthetic agents used during insertion of an intravenous catheter, based on ratings of pain intensity, child participants were divided into low pain and high pain phenotypes [10]. Analyses revealed that children in the high pain group were younger, more active, and scored higher for both state and trait anxiety. In addition, alleles in three candidate genes in a pain pathway influenced by topical anesthetics (endothelin-1 [EDN1], endothelin receptor A [EDNRA] and endothelin receptor B [EDNRB]) were examined and the presence of the EDNRA gene–TT genotype was found to be significantly more prevalent in the high pain group. The ultimate goal of such research is to match analgesic or anesthetic agents to specific patient characteristics, including their genotypes.

3.2. Temperament

Although further research is needed, it appears that the relationship between pain responsiveness and temperamental variables related to pain reactivity is strong. Temperament refers to unique genetically-based behavioral traits that appear early in life [11]. Studies have shown the relationship between procedural pain response and temperamental factors such as distractibility, intensity, sensory threshold, mood, activity levels, and persistence [12, 13]. Pain responses to immunizations have been shown to correlate with temperaments characterized as low in adjustment (negative mood, unadaptable, withdrawn) [14].

There is also evidence that the relationship between temperament and pain experiences is long-lasting. For example, Conte et al. [15] compared temperament and pain reactivity in adolescents with fibromyalgia, arthritis, or healthy controls. Children and adolescents with fibromyalgia demonstrated more temperamental instability (lower mood, irregularity of daily habits, lower task orientation, and higher distractibility), as well as higher perceptual sensitivity, more symptom reporting, and greater total pain sensitivity. Thus, the predispositions associated with certain temperamental styles may affect responses to acute painful stimuli, as well as long-term chronic pain problems.

4. Consequences of Untreated Pain in the Young

There are several short- and long-term consequences of tissue damage during early periods of rapid nervous system development. With injury there is significant C fiber activation over a prolonged period of time, and these fibers are further sensitized by inflammatory chemicals. Repetitive stimulation evokes a "wind-up" in which response amplitude increases with each subsequent stimulus. Thus, such injury results not only in an immediate nociceptive response, but hyperalgesia (an increased response to a stimulus that is normally painful) and allodynia (pain due to a stimulus that usually does not evoke pain) are likely to occur [7].

Although many nervous system responses may resolve after the injury has healed, tissue damage during certain critical periods of development may have a more lasting effect, even into adulthood [6, 7]. An array of possible mechanisms exist, including alterations in synaptic connectivity and signaling, changes in the balance of inhibition versus excitation, and increased terminal density in the injured area due to increased concentrations in nerve growth factor. While this remains an emerging area of study in rodent models, analogous hyperalgesic effects have been shown in human studies as well [7].

Studies of children beyond the neonatal period raise some interesting concerns. In a study of 4- to 6-month-old boys undergoing routine vaccinations, it was observed that boys who were circumcised demonstrated significantly higher pain scores and duration of crying than boys who were uncircumcised [16]. Furthermore, among the circumcised group, those provided with a topical anesthetic for that procedure demonstrated an attenuated pain response to vaccination. Thus, it is possible that untreated pain at one point in time, especially a vulnerable period in development, will have effects on subsequent pain responses, even weeks to months later.

Finally, growing up with recurrent or chronic pain appears to sensitize children to subsequent pain experiences. Threshold pain levels of direct pressure and circumferential pressure were examined in children with juvenile arthritis (a chronic illness in which chronic pain is a feature), sickle cell disease (a chronic illness in which chronic and recurrent pain is a feature), asthma (a chronic illness in which pain is not a feature) and healthy controls. Although one might suspect that those who live with pain may become a bit "immune" to it and have higher thresholds, the opposite was found—children with arthritis and sickle cell disease demonstrated lower pain thresholds [17]. Thus, pain seems to beget more pain rather than dampen the response.

The development of pain systems in humans and factors that affect individual differences in pain responses is an area of research that is expanding geometrically. By focusing on genetic bases, temperament, and the impact of various pain experiences, increasing variance will be accounted for. Many of these issues will be explored in more depth in later chapters.

Take-Home Points

- It is the ethical obligation of care providers to reduce needless suffering in children to the degree possible, unless it is sufficiently justified to do otherwise.
- Insight into the development of pain systems in humans helps us to better understand the necessity of attending to pain, even in the very youngest neonates.
- Genetic endowment and factors related to temperament underlie significant elements of pain responses as we develop, including response to analgesic medications.
- Untreated pain in young children may have profound effects, both in the short-term and potentially lasting for years, even into adulthood.

References

1. American Academy of Pediatrics Committee on Psychosocial Aspects of Child and Family Health, American Pain Society Task Force on Pain in Infants, Children, and Adolescents. Policy statement: The assessment and management of acute pain in infants, children and adolescents. Pediatrics 2001;108:793–797.

2. American Academy of Pediatrics Subcommittee on Abdominal Pain. Chronic abdominal pain in children. Pediatrics 2005;115:812–815.

3. American Academy of Pediatrics Committee on Bioethics and Committee on Hospital Care. Palliative care for children. Pediatrics 2000;106:351–357.

4. Walco GA, Cassidy RC, Schechter NL. Pain, hurt, and harm: The ethical issue of pediatric pain control. N Engl J Med 1994;331:541–544.

5. Anand KJS, Aranda JV, Berde CB, Buckman S, Capparelli EV, Carlo W, Hummel P, Johnston CC, Lantos J, Tutag-Lehr V, Lynn AM, Maxwell LG, Oberlander T, Raju TNK, Soriano SG, Taddio A, Walco GA. Summary proceedings from the neonatal pain-control group. Pediatrics 2006;117:S9–22.

6. Fitzgerald M, Howard RF. The neurobiologic basis of pediatric pain. In: Schechter NL, Berde CB, Yaster M, editors. Pain in Infants, Children, and Adolescents, 2nd ed. Philadelphia: Lippincott, Williams & Wilkins, 2002:19–42.

7. Fitzgerald M. The development of nociceptive circuits. Nature Rev Neurosci 2005;6:507–520.

8. Lee SJ, Ralston HJP, Drey EA, Partridge JC, Rosen MA. Fetal pain. A systematic multidisciplinary review of the evidence. JAMA 2005;294:947–954.

9. Mogil JS, Yu L, Basbaum AI. Pain genes?: natural variation and transgenic mutants. Annu Rev Neurosci 2000;23:777–811.

10. Kleiber C, Schutte DL, McCarthy AM, Floria-Santos M, Murray JC, Hanrahan K. Predictors of topical anesthetic effectiveness in children. J Pain 2007;8:168–174.

11. Wachs TD. Contributions of temperament to buffering and sensitization processes in children's development. Ann NY Acad Sci 2006;1094:28–39.

12. Bournaki MC. Correlates of pain-related responses to venipunctures in school-age children. Nurs Res 1997;46:147–154.

13. Broome ME, Rehwaldt M, Fogg L. Relationships between cognitive behavioral techniques, temperament, observed distress, and pain reports in children and adolescents during lumbar puncture. J Pediatr Nurs 1998;13:48–54.

14. Rocha EM, Prkachin KM, Beaumont SL, Hardy CL, Zumbo BD. Pain reactivity and somatization in kindergarten-age children. J Pediatr Psychol 2003;28:47–57.

15. Conte PM, Walco GA, Kimura Y. Temperament and stress response in children with primary juvenile fibromyalgia syndrome. Arthritis Rheum 2003;48:2923–2930.

16. Taddio A, Katz J, Ilersich AL, Koren G. Effect of neonatal circumcision on pain response during subsequent routine vaccination. Lancet 1997;349:599–603.

17. Walco GA, Dampier CD, Hartstein G, Djordjevic D, Miller L. The relationship between recurrent clinical pain and pain threshold in children. In: Tyler DC, Krane EJ, editors. Advances in Pain Research and Therapy: vol. 15. Pediatric Pain. New York: Raven Press, 1990:333–340.

2
Developmental Issues in Understanding, Assessing, and Managing Pediatric Pain

Kenneth D. Craig and Christine T. Korol

Abstract: Infants, children, and adolescents presenting with pain differ dramatically in physical, cognitive, emotional, behavioral, and social characteristics. This chapter presents an overview of basic concepts that should be understood in the delivery of developmentally appropriate care and addresses their relevance to pain assessment and management. The developmental issues concern variations in maturation and growth in perception and central processing of nociceptive information, and its expression in the actions of the child, as well as consideration of how pain affects different spheres of activity at different ages.

Key words: Pediatric pain, long-term outcome, developmental biology, development.

Introduction

Infants, children, and adolescents presenting with pain differ dramatically in physical, cognitive, emotional, behavioral, and social characteristics. Pediatric practitioners deliver services to patients as remarkably different as very low birth weight, pre-term newborns and precocious, socially competent teenagers. The considerable variations among children over the course of development necessitate use of different assessment instruments and pain management strategies. Competent adults often intuitively understand and adapt caregiving to children of varying ages, but an emerging literature on child development, including consideration of variations in children's pain, permits matching professional practice to unique needs of children. This chapter presents an overview of basic concepts that should be understood in the delivery of developmentally appropriate care and addresses their relevance to pain assessment and management. The developmental issues concern variations in maturation and growth in perception and central processing of nociceptive information, and its expression in the actions of the child, as well as consideration of how pain affects different spheres of activity at different ages.

Misconceptions and myths about children's pain and its control have been accepted by lay people and practitioners alike. However this intuitive, often misinformed approach (see Table 2-1) makes it important to develop a systematic, empirically based understanding of children's pain. The errors relate to misguided assumptions about both biological maturation and psychological functioning of children of differing ages. In some instances, these led to devastating neglect of infants and children, encouraging failure to recognize and assess pain in the first instance and ensuring underestimation and inadequate management thereafter. Fortunately, these beliefs and practices have yielded to a better understanding as rigorous scientific methodology has evaluated the propositions and there has been widespread, but not complete, abandonment of these and other erroneous beliefs.

Because caregiver misconceptions about pain can be detrimental to proper assessment and treatment, it is important to include the social contexts in which pain is experienced and managed when conceptualizing developmental issues related to pain. The social communication model of pain [1, 2] provides a framework for integrating issues concerning both

G.A. Walco and K.R. Goldschneider (eds.), *Pain in Children: A Practical Guide for Primary Care.*
© Humana Press, a part of Springer Science + Business Media, 2008

TABLE 2-1. Discredited beliefs concerning developmental variations in children's pain.

1. The nature of pain in infants, children and adolescents:
    The brain of the preterm neonate is insufficiently mature to experience pain
    Newborns are incapable of experiencing pain
    Infants and young children do not remember pain; it has no lasting impact
    Children are not as sensitive to pain as adults
    Adolescents are biologically disposed to be healthy and cope readily with pain
    Sex differences are unimportant as they only reflect boys' tendencies to be stoical
    Children who are in pain are not interested in playing
2. How one should undertake assessment:
    Pain is private and subjective and not accessible to measurement
    Self-report is the only valid approach to pain assessment
    Pain is a sensory experience requiring only blocking of sensory pathways to the brain
    Children are often devious and should be distrusted
    Reports of pain require evidence of tissue damage or physiological arousal to be credible
3. Management of pain in infants, children and adolescents:
    Children can be treated as if they were little adults
    Controlling pain is more dangerous than allowing it to run its course
    If children really were in pain, they would readily accept medication and care
    Medication will have a negative impact on physical development

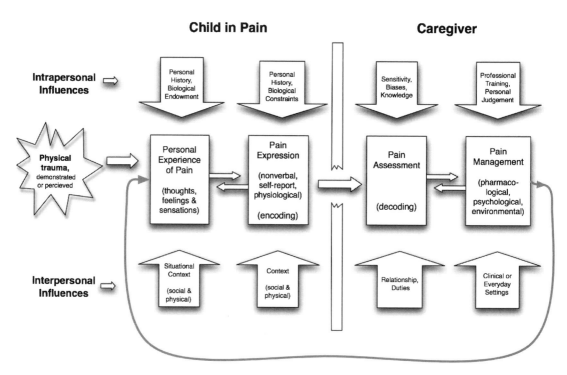

FIGURE 2-1. The social communications model of pain integrates features of both the child in pain and caregivers' reactions as developmentally-appropriate care is the responsibility of the latter

children and their caregivers, as addressed below (see Fig. 2-1). This formulation considers causes of pain relating to biological endowment and personal experiences, as well as the immediate physical and social context. More important, it addresses how pain is expressed by children and how observers make judgments and make treatment decisions. Caregivers' decisions are often key determinants of subsequent pain and its consequences for the child. The challenges of pain assessment and management are considerable, with caregivers often becoming frustrated or dismissing the concerns of children and their parents when the children or the parents appear unrealistic or overly somatically focused. Recognizing psychological and social factors in controlling children's pain is important if we are to avoid the failure to treat pain as a result of judgments that pain is inconsistent with medical pathology or that children are misrepresenting or exaggerating what is really happening.

1. The Child in Pain

Fundamental to understanding age-related variations in pain experience and expression is recognition that changes associated with age reflect both biological growth and the formative impact of personal life experiences. They are intimately intertwined. Age provides a valid, but rough proxy for both biological maturation and the accumulation of life experience. Biological maturation has a predetermined quality, with variation reflecting genetic differences, but gene expression will also be influenced by nutrition, disease, stress, and life experience. It is wrong to assume pain and other traits are exclusively hardwired, as biological systems are malleable and plastic, allowing experience to affect the individual child. Biological systems change with experience, and humans in particular are programmed to change or benefit from their personal history of experiences of pain, even during infancy [3]. This includes biological dispositions transformed by familial and cultural socialization, and the acquisition of skills that determine how one should experience and respond before, during, and following painful events [4]. Substantial variability in both biology and the individual's history of experiences further complicates their interaction, as experience is processed by biological systems differing in receptivity and maturity to ongoing life challenges.

2. The Role of the Caregiver

Caregivers must recognize the distinction between pain expression and experience. Different biological systems control each, although they are intimately related. Understanding and controlling painful experience may be the ultimate objective, but only through expression can caregivers understand the experience and evaluate efforts at control. The overt manifestations of pain transform developmentally and vary widely, depending upon the person and circumstances. The evolution of biological systems enabled infants and children to protect themselves by communicating distress at the same time caregivers acquired a capacity to recognize and assess pain. Crying and facial expression illustrate primary protective tools in newborns that engage the attention of adults. Infants can do little else. Using language to express painful distress and engage others illustrates emergent expressive capabilities in older children, adolescents, and adults.

A broad and sometimes confusing range of information contributes to caregiver judgments, including crying and other paralinguistic vocalizations, self-reports, nonverbal behavioral expression, physiological indices, evidence of tissue stress, damage, or disease, contextual factors, including presence and magnitude of injurious, toxic or dangerous events [5], general knowledge of the child's health and temperament, appreciation of transitory states (e.g., hunger, fatigue, sleep and wakefulness states), and information concerning medical treatment, such as analgesics or surgery. The availability and importance of these considerations for those who must identify and assess a child's pain will vary with the child's age. Given a long history of tendencies to neglect, discount, underestimate, and inadequately control pain in children [6, 7], it is incumbent upon practitioners to understand the developmental transformations in the various sources of information.

3. Domains of Development

Somewhat arbitrary categories of developmental change were selected for consideration in this chapter. Transformations in physical growth, cognitive capabilities, emotional processes, behavioral competence, and social interaction receive separate attention, even though all categories implicate the others. For example, physical growth constrains behavioral expression, and thoughts are invariably related to mood states and emotions. In the following sections we briefly consider each of these developmental domains, prior to examining them as they relate to different epochs of development.

3.1. Physical Growth

The most conspicuous changes throughout childhood are in body growth, physical appearance, and motor and perceptual competencies. In healthy children, perceptual and motor competence become progressively better attuned to finely coordinated interaction with physical and social environments. Pain, particularly chronic pain, and the stress associated with it can have a cascading detrimental impact on motor and perceptual competencies that is not seen in adults, because adults largely have mastered the developmental challenges prior to the onset of pain. Children need to manipulate and explore their physical surroundings to acquire competence in most spheres of life activity. Children in pain become inactive and vulnerable to deconditioning and loss of muscle tone that affects the ability to benefit from exploratory activities or to learn motor skills. Less obvious would be the impact of pain-related stress on physical growth and behavioral and hormonal reactivity [8, 9].

3.2. Cognitive Capabilities

With time, children become able to process information they need to effectively engage with their social and physical environments. A developmental progression is seen in problem solving, judgment, and memory, although there are substantial individual differences. In a parallel manner, pain reactivity becomes less reflexive and children become more capable of deliberative behavior, learning to suppress immediate reactivity or to accelerate the display of distress when appropriate. In consequence, self-management skills supplant inherent homeostatic regulatory systems, and children begin to exercise skill in coping with painful events. Pain can interfere with the normal developmental progression in children experiencing acute and chronic pain by affecting communication, daily living skills, socialization, and motor skills [10].

Evidence supports the proposition that the experience of pain transforms as cognitive advances allow greater differentiation of internal and external experiences, and children come to understand the nature of painful events. In contrast to older children, newborns do not attach meaning to experiences and do not understand temporal features of painful experiences (e.g., that pain is transitory).

However, a primal capacity for consciousness, including sensory and emotional awareness, is now recognized in the neonate [11].

Language development parallels cognitive maturation. Language is important because it both organizes perception and permits detailed accounts of subjective experiences. Increased competence in the use of language to communicate painful distress indicates a progression from a relatively reflexive language (e.g., "ow," "ouch") first evident at about 14 to 16 months, to the use of culture specific words (e.g., "hurt") at about 36 months, and culminating in the use of sophisticated words, such as "pain," and more descriptive language at about 6 years [12]. This process enables children to engage others who may assist them when in pain and to use talk to benefit from treatment. Children with intellectual disabilities, cognitive impairments, or communication limitations are handicapped in this respect [10].

Gaffney and Dunne's studies [13, 14] of children's definitions, descriptions, and understanding of the causes of pain led to the conclusion that three stages can be identified. Young children through to about 7 years of age focus primarily on physical features of pain. Children between 8 and 10 years used physical analogies to describe pain and demonstrate a developing awareness of the psychological concomitants of pain, such as recognizing that pain affected one's mood. Older children, 11 to 14 years of age, use both physical and psychological terms to characterize pain, and recognize that one can address pain actively, perhaps by reacting stoically.

Elsewhere, McGrath and Craig [15] have summarized children's understanding of pain in the context of how they appreciate health and illness in general (See Table 2-2). Three stages are apparent. Between 2 and 7 years of age, children perceive their world concretely in terms of what they are able to touch, see or manipulate. Experience is temporally immediate and less dependent upon explanation or what children are told. Concrete, logical thinking is evident between 7 and 9 years of age, with children capable of understanding relationships between pain, other symptoms, and disease, but without clear understanding of the causation of pain. They come to appreciate that difficult procedures may be needed to monitor or treat disease. At roughly 11 years of age, adolescents begin to understand formal logical explanations, and begin to comprehend more coherent

TABLE 2-2. Developmental sequence of how children understand pain (updated from McGrath and Craig, 1989).

Age	Understanding
0–3 months	No apparent understanding of pain, but prototypical sensory and emotional perceptual awareness; memory for pain available shortly after birth
3–6 months	Immediate pain response of infancy supplemented by increased emotional differentiation
6–18 months	Children develop clear fear of pain situations. Words to describe pain more reflexive ("ouch," "owie") and available at 14 months. Somatic localization becomes evident
Up to 6 years	Prelogical thinking characterized by concrete understanding, egocentrism, and transductive logic. Meaningful description of pain and pain language ("hurt," "pain")
7–10 years	Concrete operational thinking characterized by child being able to distinguish self from environment. Beginning capacity for behavioral coping strategies (use of hypnosis, relaxation, guided imagery training)
11+ years	Formal logical thinking, characterized by abstract thinking and introspection. Increased use of cognitive coping skills

and sophisticated models of the complex interactions between experience and physiological mechanisms of health and illness. The understanding may not be complete, as must be the case with illnesses whose origins are poorly understood (typically abdominal pain, headache, growing pain, etc.), but this does not differentiate them from adults. There is great variability among individuals in acquiring these levels of understanding and clinicians tend to overestimate a child's capacity for coherent and logical understanding. The stress of pain or illness is also likely to make the challenge more confusing. Nevertheless, school-aged children become open to learning about the nature of pain, its impact upon them, and how they can cope with it [16], and can benefit from such instruction. This is consistent with their emerging capacity to benefit from cognitive/behavioral therapy. Most children will volunteer coping strategies they use spontaneously, but they need to be encouraged to use them systematically and consistently [17]. A broad range of coping skills can be effectively taught to children, particularly when the therapist is present and prompts them during painful procedures. Teaching coping skills benefits the patient by reducing passivity, depression, and distress [18]. See Chapter 15 for details.

3.3. Emotional Processing

Newborns are capable of emotional processing of pain and other experiences, but emotions are relatively undifferentiated early in life and appear in the form of negative and positive states. The development of emotional expression continues through toddlerhood, with children's emotions differentiating over time. In the second year of life one can observe a range of the universal emotional states, *viz.*, fear, anger, disgust, sadness, happiness, surprise. Early in life children learn a great fear of needle injections, with the fear embedded in a complex of thoughts and feelings of anger and sometimes disgust. Failure to address this can lead to a lifetime of avoiding required health care. It is not uncommon for children, and adults, to fear medical procedures more than lethal injuries and diseases.

As the child enters toddlerhood the self-conscious emotional states that involve other people, including shame, embarrassment, guilt, and pride, become evident. The presence of these emotions adds a new layer of complexity to the assessment of pain as children demonstrate the beginnings of altering their own social communications out of awareness of how they will be perceived by others and the desire to present themselves in a positive light. During childhood, a capacity for self-regulating emotions is acquired, as tolerance for emotional distress and coping capacities emerge. In addition, while infants are remarkably attuned to the emotions of their parents and caregivers, children become more capable of reading the emotions of others [19]. While somatic features of emotional states, particularly stress, probably are evident to all children, we see that somatically focused children are more likely to misinterpret those physical sensations as pathology rather than as normal expressions of emotion.

Children in pain suffer particularly strong emotions. Anxiety and depression are elevated in children with chronic and recurrent pain [20], although most children with chronic or recurrent pain do not have clinical levels of anxiety or depression [21].

Nevertheless, children with chronic pain can become enmeshed in vicious circles of emotional distress (primarily depression), interpersonal conflict and avoidance, reduced physical activity, and declining engagement with normal activities such as school [22]. Chronic pain tends to persist for children, and the frequency of pain episodes increases with age [23]. If depressed, they may withdraw from school and contact with friends, thereby missing out on important developmental experiences. The intimate relationship among pain, thoughts, and feelings is well illustrated by findings using the Pain Catastrophizing Scale for Children [24] which indicates that children who think the worst when confronted with pain (i.e., they have mental scripts that magnify the seriousness of the pain, ruminate upon it, and believe they are helpless in controlling pain) tend to be more emotionally distressed, report higher levels of pain, and are more dependent upon care provided by others [25].

3.4. Behavioral Competence

It is convenient to differentiate between immediate behavioral reactions, which tend to be relatively reflexive or involuntary, and intentional behavior used to control the social and physical environment [26]. The former provide the means for assessing pain in infants and young children, as well as those with cognitive impairment. At the most primitive level would be reflex arcs [27], but facial activity, crying, and protective escape are at play in newborns. A developmental progression can be observed, with older children becoming better able to exercise protective, voluntary actions necessary to avoid or escape painful situations. This instrumental behavior continues to be accompanied by nonverbal, relatively automatic reactions. Therefore, nonverbal assessment remains an important practice from infancy through adolescence [28]. One can also distinguish different types of communicative acts. Crying and facial activity reflecting pain fall in the category of automatic behaviors, even though there are some features of voluntary control, whereas language reflects higher level, purposeful action.

3.5. Social Interaction

Humans are inherently social animals with care from others essential to survival from birth [29]

and for normal development thereafter. It has been demonstrated that the role of touch and physical contact foster healthy development during infancy [30], and the stimulation provided by physical contact (kangaroo care) has been demonstrated to be analgesic for full-term [31] and preterm newborns [32, 33]. Infants avidly attend to the actions of others, and facial displays in particular command their attention. Early vocalizations and facial displays signaling pain can be seen as evolved adaptive behaviors available at birth for commanding the attention of others [34].

Infants and children become increasingly socially competent, with socialization being the process whereby specific skills and practices attuned to the child's family and culture are taught and acquired through direct instruction and observational learning [35]. Pain behavior transforms from spontaneous, reflexive reactions to include purposive actions highly sensitive to social settings. Countless personal and observed experiences with pain provide salient opportunities to learn family and cultural beliefs and attitudes concerning how one should experience and cope with pain, both in terms of self-control and how to maximize the benefit of care from others. Children who do not cope well may have been exposed to adverse or incompetent coping models. Families who do not cope well with chronic illness or are already heavily engaged with the health service delivery system or are over involved in their child's life pose particular challenges to clinicians [36]. Disentangling this variability from cultural influences that may encourage ready expression of pain or stoical forbearance is a challenge for clinicians [4]. Parents deserve special attention, as they must assume responsibility for their children's well-being and physical safety, and typically structure their children's lives to ensure a slow but steady progression from close supervision and physical guidance to independent self-control. The task is challenging as parents recognize some risk is necessary, yet they do not want to expose their children to excess danger. Some parents are overly cautious and readily alarmed, engaging in catastrophizing concerning their children's well-being [37]. Parents who misinterpret headache, abdominal pain, or limb pain as diagnostic of cancer, for example, can potentially do harm to their children.

Throughout childhood, children also begin to develop a sense of themselves in relation to others.

Self-esteem and self-confidence are developed over time through social skills, such as learning to make friends in early childhood, learning to share and help others, managing conflict, and even through awkward attempts at dating in adolescence. Negotiating one's way through the minefield of interpersonal relationships is difficult at the best of times and rarely does one make it to young adulthood without their share of hurt feelings, embarrassment, or drama. However, for most children, there are enough positive social experiences to help them develop a balanced and healthy sense of their own self-worth. Unless they are extremely socially adept, children who have chronic pain have a much more difficult time developing and maintaining certain types of social relationships.

The source and nature of pain is often invisible; children must be able to communicate their needs effectively to those around them, but credibility is always a challenge. Young friends, unfortunately, are not always willing to change recreational plans if a child has a flare-up of pain. A common complaint among children attending pain clinics is that friends begin to get frustrated because they must cancel or change plans so frequently due to pain. Or worse yet, they find that they have to drop out of an athletic pursuit altogether due to their injury or pain, and lose their entire social network. They may be able to arrange a few visits here and there, but many children find that friends begin to fall away as they become more functionally limited by their pain. As children become less involved with school, spend more time at the hospital or in therapy, they not only lose close friendships, but begin to miss out on day-to-day social interactions that would help them develop a variety of important social skills. In addition, they may encounter more hostility, as teachers, friends, health care professionals, and even family members become angry and frustrated, thinking they are exaggerating their pain or that it may not even be real.

4. Stages of Development

In the following sections we differentiate among conventional developmental stages, recognizing that these several categories are arbitrary, since, for the most part, development is continuous, but not uniform, across physical, psychological, behavioral, and social trajectories. Within any age group there is substantial developmental variation in these characteristics, with some children delayed and others precocious, necessitating attention to the specifics of development in these children.

4.1. Newborns

At this stage of development, prominence of sensory qualities and emotional distress and the absence of a capacity for cognitive appraisal and control would leave very young children particularly vulnerable to distress. The newborn typically reacts vigorously to painful distress. Research is unequivocal that even extremely premature neonates are able to cry, wince, and grimace, and that a variety of physiological parameters (e.g., heart rate, oxygen saturation) change in response to pain. These responses may be muted or subtle in the sick or extremely premature neonate, and some neonates remain very passive during invasive procedures. Nevertheless, even in the absence of a pain response, one should assume that tissue damaging procedures or illnesses that ordinarily would be painful are painful. It is noteworthy that while painful reactions are relatively undifferentiated and not well localized somatically in the newborn [38], they display relatively stereotyped patterns of pain behavior. Early pain experience is now recognized as having an impact on subsequent development and may alter life trajectories. This contributes to an emerging literature demonstrating that infants exposed to intensive care or multiple episodes of pain and stress have long-term behavioral, physiological, and endocrine sequelae [39].

4.2. Infants

Rapid changes take place in the first year of life, reflecting increasing competence in motoric, affective, cognitive, and social self-regulation. Through this span of time, pain is an important and influential feature of life. There is a higher probability of certain painful events, including teething, earaches, reflux, and immunizations. Individual differences in reactivity become apparent even at this young age. At about 6 to 8 months of age, improved cognitive competence becomes evident as children learn to anticipate painful events. They display anticipatory distress, exercise effort to avoid procedures, and display anger. Behavioral reactions remain vigorous, although diminishing somewhat in vigor throughout infancy as vocalizations come to control the reactions of caregivers, suggesting that pain is more severe in the earlier months of life than later in infancy [15, 40]. Nevertheless, the stereotyped reaction patterns observed in the neonate remain relatively stable [41]. We are beginning to see that immediate facial display, body activity, and crying in response to needle injections did not differ across the first 18 months of life, even though the children clearly were different across this span of life [42]. While it may be difficult to differentiate painful distress from other sources of distress in children, *viz.*, hunger, fatigue, fear, anger, and irritability, particularly when the source has not been observed or cannot be discovered, it is important to not discount a child's reaction as non-painful until there is some certainty as to another source.

Adult perceptions of pain in infants are strikingly variable. For example, when judging videotaped reactions to immunization injections in a group of infants ranging between 2 and 12 months of age, people who were not health care professionals, but were parents (of other children), systematically judged the pain to be substantially more severe than did a group of pediatricians, with nurses' judgments intermediate to these two groups [34]. It is also noteworthy that the capacity for the conscious experience of pain was judged by all groups to increase with age through the first year, in contrast to the usual observation that pain seems to diminish throughout the first year of life [43]. Parents are often the best source of information about pain in this age group as they are the most sensitive to changes in the child's behavior or appearance. As cognitive skills and emotional modulation emerge in the child, the parents potentially become appropriate targets for intervention.

4.3. Toddlers

The increased mobility of toddlers makes them vulnerable to experience painful events, compared to infants. It is easier to localize the pain (they will point to it) and may even solicit help from caregivers (e.g., asking mommy to kiss it better). Nonverbal cues (e.g., facial grimaces, protective behavior) remain more important than language for identifying and understanding a child's pain at this age.

Accompanying development of normal language, they begin to use pain language more often when interacting with others, perhaps role-playing painful predicaments during play, manipulating parents by dissembling pain when playing with siblings, or commanding attention from parents by pretending to be in pain. Social referencing becomes more important, as they will look to their mother or other caregivers when in pain. These transformations imply an increasing ability to understand and attach meaning to the painful experience. This should not be interpreted as suggesting emotional distress diminishes at this age. Indeed, emotional turmoil and demands for parental attention tend to accelerate. Demonstrations of pain empathy for others might also be present [44]. They may bring their own mommy to care for others when the latter are in painful distress. Distraction has been shown to be a powerful tool with children at this age; TV can be a powerful analgesic. Children in pain will continue to play, with younger children doing this more promptly than older children [45], suggesting that play serves as a coping strategy in its own right.

4.4. Preschoolers

The preschooler's world begins to be more interpersonal. While they may deny pain to avoid intramuscular injections, it is easier to gain their compliance by reasoning with them and offering rewards when they exercise self-control. They begin to understand explanations for sources of pain and appreciate the role of medications and other remedies in alleviating pain and other illness. One may successfully begin to tell stories in a soothing voice or to teach hypnosis at this age. Adult support remains very important. They begin to be more responsive to "metacognitive" strategies, for example, "Let's watch TV to take your mind off your discomfort" or "My tummy is sore because I ate too much candy." The simpler self-report scales (the poker chip tool, faces scales) begin to be useful, but make sure the child understands these before using them.

While socialization in how one should experience and express pain appears continuous throughout early childhood, parental strategies designed to provide explicit instruction become more evident and potent at this age [46]. Socialization takes the form of direct instruction and observational learning. Parents' importance to children is evident in the debate concerning whether they should be present during painful medical procedures. While parental presence is often a comfort to children, some patients will show greater pain or distress behaviors when their parents are present. The children may feel more open to express themselves when parents are present than when they are alone with clinicians, who are relative strangers. Perhaps most important is identifying and working with parents who are likely to become highly distressed as the potential for emotional contagion with their children is considerable (see Chapter 10 for further discussion). Most parents are aware of the impact their demeanor will have on their child and are open to suggestions about how they may teach the child better coping strategies. Generally, teaching parents to use distraction and positive coping statements will help the child cope with procedurally related distress. Critical comments or apologies such as, "It's not so bad; your brother would be able to get through this," or "I'm so sorry you have to go through this" tend to have an adverse effect [47]. Similarly, parents of children with chronic pain who discourage coping behaviors when a child is complaining about pain have the impact of encouraging off-task behavior and inadequate coping [48].

4.5. Elementary School-Aged Children

Pain produced by minor invasive medical procedures (e.g., immunization injections, venipuncture) tends to diminish in severity after the age of 6, as indicated by both self-report [49] and behavioral measures [50]. In contrast, recurrent abdominal pain and growing pains become the prominent pain problems. Self-report begins to have greater reliability and validity at this age [51]. Children become more capable of articulated statements concerning the nature (location and severity) and sources of pain, but remain less capable of using affective and qualitative descriptors of pain. Most of the self-report tools are likely to become useful. During the course of an interview, structured interviews and simpler questionnaires can be used (e.g. Beck Youth Inventories, PedsQL). At this age, they may become skilled verbally and nonverbally in suppressing pain expression (e.g., to avoid

embarrassment with peers) or to dissemble pain (e.g., to get attention) [52]. One can begin to teach specific coping strategies, such as self-hypnosis, relaxation, pacing, cognitive restructuring, and other approaches to self-management of pain. They typically enjoy these "tricks" for controlling pain. Nevertheless, one should not assume these children will understand explanations in the way that is intended. One must work carefully with the children to ensure they understand explanations and expectations, preferably using the child's idiosyncratic language. Some children equate pain with punishment and they must come to understand that this is not the case.

4.6. Adolescence

The journey towards independence from parents becomes accelerated and there is increased dependence upon peers and adolescent culture. Chronic pain at this age is associated with high levels of disability, depression, and anxiety, and parents report high levels of depression, anxiety, and parenting stress [53]. The nature of painful conditions tends to change, with gender differences in pain becoming more conspicuous with pubescence. Females generally become more expressive of pain [54]. Further, Western society fosters suppression of pain expression in boys, yet tolerates it to a greater degree in girls. Adolescents' personal perspectives on pain and other dilemmas become very important in both assessment and treatment. They can become blasé in their pain presentation, reporting severe pain, but not complaining a lot. Early adolescent difficulties with compliance and desires to not be different from peers must be respected. Sexual intimacy may become important in their lives, and privacy and confidentiality must be respected. Older adolescents may no longer be preoccupied with school issues, with vocational issues becoming their focus. Failure to respect their independence can lead to hostility and impulsivity. Feelings of depression and being overwhelmed may make it difficult for the older adolescent to fully participate in the development of their pain management program. Nevertheless, they tend to become more serious around 16 or 17 years and appear more capable of investing personal energy and being proactive in addressing persistent pain. They recognize that health care professionals and parents have minimal ability to provide further care and want to exercise more personal care. Older adolescents can be taught more abstract strategies, such as acceptance of pain and mindfulness strategies [55, 56].

Take-Home Points

- There is a complex interplay in the expression and experience of a child's pain among noxious input, the child's developmental level, previous experience with pain, and familial and cultural expectations.
- Awareness of common misconceptions about pain in childhood will help to avoid inaccurate judgments and inadequate treatment of pain (see Table 2-1).
- Caregiver judgments of pain depend on their knowledge of various pain indicators (e.g., self report, facial expression, crying, physiological parameters), familiarity with the child's temperament, and the nature and severity of the child's medical condition, as well as the training and experience of the caregiver.
- Pain can negatively affect the physical development of children when it prevents them from exploring their environment or causes them to become deconditioned. Social development suffers when pain leads to missed social opportunities—including school absence, withdrawal from athletic pursuits, and reduced peer interactions.
- The capacity to process emotional aspects of pain is present even in the smallest newborn baby, albeit emotions are not well differentiated. Emotional development continues throughout toddlerhood and fear, anger, stress, and sadness may accompany painful events. The self-conscious emotions (e.g., shame, guilt, embarrassment, pride) appear early in life and mark the beginning of the child altering his or her pain expression to fit social considerations.
- Children learn how to respond to and cope with pain from their parents. The child's social context is one primary reason why treatment should include, whenever possible, all the important stakeholders in the child's life.

References

1. Craig KD, Lilley CM, Gilbert CA. Social barriers to optimal pain management in infants and children. Clin J Pain 1996;12:232–242.

2. Craig KD, Korol CT, Pillai RR. Challenges of judging pain in vulnerable infants. Clin Perinatol 2002;29:445–458.

3. Taddio A, Katz J, Ilersich AL, Koren G. Effect of neonatal circumcision on pain response during subsequent routine vaccination. Lancet 1997;349:599–603.

4. Craig KD, Pillai RR. Social influences, ethnicity, and culture. In: Finley GA, McGrath PJ, editors. The Context of Pediatric Pain: Biology, Family, Society, and Culture. Seattle: IASP Press, 2003:159–182.

5. Hadjistavropoulos HD, Craig KD, Grunau RE, Whitfield MF. Judging pain in infants: Behavioral, contextual, and developmental determinants. Pain 1997;73:319–324.

6. Anand KJS, McGrath PJ. Pain in Neonates. Amsterdam: Elsevier, 1993.

7. Walco GA, Cassidy RC, Schechter NL. The ethics of pain control in infants and children. N Engl J Med 1994;331:541–544.

8. Fitzgerald M. Painful beginnings. Pain 2004;110:508–509.

9. Grunau RE, Holsti L, Haley DW, Oberlander T, Weinberg J, Solimano A, Whitfield MF, Fitzgerald C, Yu W. Neonatal procedural pain exposure predicts lower cortisol and behavioral reaction in preterm infants in the NICU. Pain 2005;113:293–300.

10. Breau LM, Camfield CS, McGrath PJ, Finley GA. Pain's impact on adaptive functioning. J Intellectual Disabil Res 2007;51:125–134.

11. Anand KJS, Craig KD. Editorial: New perspectives on the definition of pain. Pain 1996;67:3–6.

12. Stanford EA, Chambers CT, Craig KD. A normative analysis of the development of pain-related vocabulary in children. Pain 2005;114:278–284.

13. Gaffney A, Dunne EA. Developmental aspects of children's definition of pain. Pain 1986;26:105–117.

14. Gaffney A, Dunne EA. Children's understanding of the causality of pain. Pain 1987;29:91–104.

15. McGrath PJ, Craig KD. Developmental and psychological factors in children's pain. Pediatr Clin North Am 1989;36:823–836.

16. Claar RL, Walker LS, Smith CA. The influence of appraisals in understanding children's experiences with medical procedures. J Pediatr Psychol 2002;27:553–563.

17. Bennett-Branson SM, Craig KD. Postoperative pain in children: Developmental and family influences on spontaneous coping strategies. Can J Behav Sci 1993;25:355–383.

18. Walker LS, Smith CA, Garber J, Claar RL. Testing a model of pain appraisal and coping in children with chronic abdominal pain. Health Psychol 2005;24:364–374.

19. Deyo K, Prkachin KM, Mercer SR. Development of sensitivity to facial expressions of pain. Pain 2004;107:16–21.

20. Palermo TM. Impact of recurrent and chronic pain on child and family daily functioning: A critical review of the literature. J Dev Behav Pediatr 2000;21:58–69.

21. Larsson BS. Somatic complaints and their relationship to depressive symptoms in Swedish adolescents. J Child Psychol Psychiat 1991;32:821–832.

22. Kashikar-Zuck S, Vaught MH, Goldschneider KR, Graham TB, Miller JC. Depression, coping, and functional disability in juvenile primary fibromyalgia syndrome. J Pain 2002;3:412–419.

23. Martin AL, McGrath PA, Brown SC, Katz J. Children with chronic pain: Impact of sex and age on long-term outcomes. Pain 2007;128:13–19.

24. Crombez G, Bijttebier P, Eccleston C, Mascagni T, Mertens G, Goubert L, et al. The child version of the Pain Catastrophizing Scale (PCS-C): A preliminary validation. Pain 2003;104:639–646.

25. Vervoort T, Craig KD, Goubert L, Dehoorne J, Joos R, Matthys D, Buysse A, Crombez G. Expressive dimensions of pain catastrophizing: A comparative analysis of school children and children with clinical pain. Pain 2008;134:59–69.

26. Hadjistavropoulos T, Craig KD. A theoretical framework for understanding self-report and observational measures of pain: A communications model. Behav Res Ther 2002;40:551–570.

27. Andrews KA, Fitzgerald M. Flexion reflex responses in biceps femoris and tibialis anterior in human neonates. Early Hum Dev 2000;57:105–110.

28. von Baeyer CL, Spagrud LJ. Systematic review of observational (behavioral) measures of pain for children and adolescents aged 3 to 18 years. Pain 2006;127:140–150.

29. Johnston CC, Aita M, Campbell-Yeo M, Duhn L, Latimer M, McNaughton K. The social and environmental context in which pain is experienced in neonates. In: Anand KJS, Stevens BJ, McGrath PJ, editors. Pain in Neonates, 3rd ed. Amsterdam: Elsevier, 2007.

30. Field TM. Touch therapy effects on development. Int J Behav Dev 1998;22:779–797.

31. Gray L, Watt L, Blass EM. Skin-to-skin contact is analgesic in healthy newborns. Pediatrics 2000;105:e14.

32. Johnston CC, Stevens B, Pinelli J, Gibbins S, Filion F, Jack A, Steele S, Boyer K, Veilleux A. Kangaroo Care is effective in diminishing pain response in preterm neonates. Arch Pediatr Adolesc Med 2003;157:1084–1088.

33. Ludington-Hoe SM, Hosseini R, Torowizc DL. Skin-to-skin contact (Kangaroo Care) analgesia for preterm infant heelstick. AACN Clinical Issues 2005;16:373–387.

34. Pillai Riddell RR, Craig KD. Judgments of infant pain: The impact of caregiver identity and infant age. J Pediatr Psychol 2007;32:501–511.

35. Hermann C. Modeling, social learning of pain. In: Schmidt RF, Willis WD, editors. The Encyclopedia of Pain. Berlin: Springer, 2006.

36. Chambers CT. The role of the family factors in pediatric pain. In: McGrath PJ, Finley GA, editors. Pediatric Pain: Biological and Social Context. Seattle: IASP Press, 2003:99–130.

37. Goubert L, Eccleston C, Vervoort T, Jordan A, Crombez G. Parental catastrophizing about their child's pain. The parent version of the Pain Catastrophizing Scale (PCS-P): A preliminary validation. Pain 2006;123:254–263.

38. Craig KD, McMahon RJ, Morison JD, Zaskow C. Developmental changes in infant pain expression during immunization injections. Soc Sci Med 1984;19:1331–1332.

39. Grunau RVE, Holsti L, Peters JWB. Long-term consequences of pain in human neonates. Sem Fetal Neonatal Med 2006;11:268–275.

40. Anand KJS, Hickey PR. Pain and its effects in the human neonate and fetus. N Engl J Med 1987;317:1321–1329.

41. Johnston CC, Stevens B, Craig KD, Grunau RVE. Developmental changes in pain expression in premature, full-term, two- and four-month-old infants. Pain 1993;52:201–208.

42. Nader R, Korol CT, Craig KD. Constancy and change in pain expression during the first year of life: Facial activity, body movement and cry, in preparation.

43. Pillai Riddell RR, Badali MA, Craig KD. Parental judgments of infant pain: Importance of perceived cognitive abilities, behavioral cues and contextual cues. Pain Research and Management 2004;9:73–80.

44. Goubert L, Craig KD, Vervoort T, Morley S, Sullivan MJL, Williams A, Cano A, Crombez G. Facing others in pain: the effects of empathy. Pain 2005;118:286–288.

45. Leikin L, Firestone P, McGrath PJ. Physical symptom reporting in Type A and Type B children. J Consult Clin Psychol 1988;56:721–726.

46. Palermo TM, Chambers CT. Pediatric and family factors in pediatric chronic pain and disability: An integrative approach. Pain 2005;119:1–4.

47. Chambers CT, Craig KD, Bennett SM. The impact of maternal behavior on children's pain experiences: An experimental analysis. J Pediatr Psychol 2002;27:293–301.

48. Reid GJ, McGrath PJ, Lang BA. Parent-child interactions among children with juvenile fibromyalgia, arthritis, and health controls. Pain 2005;113:201–210.

49. Goodenough B, Thomas W, Champion GD, Perrott D, Taplin JE, von Baeyer CL, Ziegler JG. Unraveling age effects and sex differences in needle pain: Ratings of sensory intensity and unpleasantness of venipuncture pain by children and their parents. Pain 1999;80:179–190.

50. Fowler-Kerry S, Lander J. Assessment of sex differences in children's and adolescents' self-reported pain from venipuncture. J Pediat Psychol 1991;16:783–793.

51. Stinson JN, Kavanagh T, Yamada J, Gill N, Stevens B. Systematic review of the psychometric properties, interpretability and feasibility of self-report pain intensity measures for use in clinical trials in children and adolescents. Pain 2006;125:143–157.

52. Larochette AC, Chambers CT, Craig KD. Genuine, suppressed and faked facial expressions of pain in children. Pain 2006;126:64–71.

53. Eccleston C, Crombez G, Scotford A, Clinch J, Connell H. Adolescent chronic pain: patterns and predictors of emotional distress in adolescents with chronic pain and their parents. Pain 2004;108:221–229.

54. Perquin CW, Hazebroek Kampscheur, AAJM, Hunfeld JAM, et al. Pain in children and adolescents: a common experience. Pain 2000;87:51–58.

55. McCracken LM, Carson JW, Eccleston C, Keefe FJ. Acceptance and change in the context of chronic pain. Pain 2004;109:4–7.

56. Eccleston C, Malleson PM, Clinch J, Connell H, Sourbut C. Chronic pain in adolescents: evaluation of a programme of inter-disciplinary cognitive behaviour therapy (ICBT). Arch Dis Child 2003;88:881–885.

3
Measurement and Assessment of Pediatric Pain in Primary Care

Carl L. von Baeyer

Abstract: Regularly measuring pain improves pain management. If a child is old enough (4 years and older) and calm enough to understand a self-report scale, then this should be the primary source to measure pain over time. Quick and simple self-report tools include faces scales and numerical rating scales, which produce scores on the widely accepted 0 to 10 metric. For infants and younger children, and in situations where self-report is considered unavailable or unreliable, quick observational tools can be used. Specific tools and approaches are recommended here for use in primary care with various populations, and some complexities of interpretation are discussed. Pain intensity scores can be used to guide analgesic dosage and timing, and to communicate with other health care providers about what makes the pain better or worse.

Key words: Pain scale, pain measurement, pain assessment, child, pediatric, self-report, observation.

1. Measurement of Pain: Why and How?

Pain is better managed when it is regularly measured and assessed [1, 2]. Pain scores can and should be regularly charted to determine the pain relieving treatments' effectiveness and, if necessary, guide practitioners in further intervention. Routinely recording pain scores as "The Fifth Vital Sign" has been advocated by the American Pain Society and the American Academy of Pediatrics [3]. Regular measurement is helpful, both for acute pain (injury- or disease-related,

procedural and postoperative pain), and for recurrent or chronic pain, although different measures are needed in different contexts and at different ages.

Measuring pain means assigning a number to express its intensity. By convention, such scores, whether based on self-report or observation, are usually on a 0 to 10 scale [4], where 0 is no pain and 10 is loosely defined as the most pain. This is obviously an oversimplification, like describing music only in terms of its loudness. Other aspects of pain that need to be assessed are the location, sensory qualities, triggering and maintaining factors, and emotional and social aspects of the experience of pain.

2. Pain Measurement in Primary Care Versus Specialized Settings

In research and in specialized pain care, many complex and time-consuming measures of pain are used [5, 6]. Primary care physicians rarely have time to learn and apply all of these tools. In the following sections, the state-of-the-art in pain measurement is described for the purpose of explaining general principles. After that, brief and simple pain measurement methods are suggested.

3. How Pain is Measured

The first step in initial assessment of most pain problems—to establish the clinical context for specific measures of pain intensity—is an interview with the patient and parent. Where is the pain located?

G.A. Walco and K.R. Goldschneider (eds.), *Pain in Children: A Practical Guide for Primary Care.*
© Humana Press, a part of Springer Science + Business Media, 2008

What sensory qualities does it have? What makes it worse? What makes it better? When and how did it start? These matters are not readily quantified in numbers, but they set the stage for measuring pain intensity. It is essential to establish rapport with the child and parent at this stage; pain symptoms can be understood largely as a communication process [7].

There are three general modalities used to measure pain intensity: by self-report [5, 8], observational [6, 9] and physiological [10] methods. These three sources of information, however, often do not correlate highly with each other [11, 12].

Because pain is primarily a subjective experience [13], **self-report is recommended as the primary source for pain measures whenever possible**. Tools for obtaining self-report include numerical scales, visual analog scales, and faces scales. Self-report measures can be used with children who are old enough to understand and use simple scales (usually 4 years and up), are not overly distressed, do not have impaired cognitive or communicative abilities, and whose self-report ratings are not considered exaggerated or minimized due to cognitive, emotional, or situational factors [6].

When self-report measures are considered to be unavailable or unreliable, then observational measures can be used. These are based on parents' or clinicians' observations of the child's facial expression, physical movement, vocal behavior such as moaning or crying, and social responsiveness [6]. It is important to note that well-validated observational scales exist only for acute pain, not chronic or recurrent pain, because the overt behavioral signs of pain such as grimaces tend to diminish when pain lasts hours or longer.

In some cases neither self-report nor observational measures of pain can be readily used, as may occur with sedated or ventilated patients in critical care. In such cases, physiological measures such as blood pressure, heart rate or respiration rate may be used, although their validity as indices of pain experience is questionable [9, 14].

4. Interpretation and Use of Pain Scores

Pain scores are more valid and useful in intra-individual comparisons (tracking pain over time within individuals) rather than interindividual (com-

paring scores across different patients). In other words, comparing pain scores across children generally does not contribute to understanding because different children understand and utilize pain scales differently. A child who reports pain intensity of 10/10 may or may not be experiencing more pain and distress than a child whose score is just 6/10. On the other hand, a reduction in pain score over time is meaningful for both of those patients.

A change in pain of more than one point (out of 10) is considered to be clinically significant [15, 16]. Some algorithms treat a pain score of 4/10 sustained for more than an hour as the threshold for stepping up pain relieving treatment (adding nonpharmacological modalities, increasing the analgesic dosage, reducing the interval, or selecting a more powerful analgesic). On the other hand, because scores differ in meaning (hence, need to treat) from one patient to the next, blanket algorithms may not be appropriate. Anything beyond a minimal score should trigger a clinician to more closely monitor a patient who may require additional treatment.

The concordance between pain scores based on different sources is usually low to moderate. Therefore, there are often disagreements between scores provided by children, parents, and clinicians, and between self-report versus observational scores. In such cases, the scores can be considered to reflect different perspectives on the pain experience [12, 17]. Such differences can be very informative and they should not be interpreted as indicating that any of the informants is necessarily unreliable.

Children often show fear-related distress before an impending painful event such as a needle, and this behavior may be indistinguishable from pain after the event. Both distress and pain are important to assess, prevent, and relieve.

Communication about pain among parents, nurses and physicians is fostered by use of mutually agreed upon pain scales, and by sharing information about children's pain scores.

5. Neonates, Infants, and Toddlers up to 2 Years

The days of assuming that babies cannot experience or remember pain are past; there is now evidence of neural and behavioral responses to painful stimulation, positive response to analgesia, and long-term memory for pain occurring in infants (see [18, 19, 20] for examples).

Since infants are unable to provide verbal self-report, pain measurement relies on noticing and interpreting their behavior and their physiological response to pain. The best-studied and most reliable indices of pain in infants are specific facial expressions. These include eyes squeezed shut, brows lowered and furrowed, nasal roots widened, deepened nasolabial furrow, a square mouth, and a taut, cupped tongue [1, 21].

Crying is non-specific and may signal other sources of distress besides pain. However, when an infant produces a high-pitched, intense or harsh cry, it alerts the caregiver or clinician, who is then in a position to assess the child's facial expression for the above cues indicating pain [21–23].

In fact, the state-of-the-art in pain measurement in infants has advanced far beyond what is achievable in a primary care setting. Over a dozen scales have been designed to measure pain in infants [1, 24–26], and many putative physiological signs of pain in infants are under investigation. However, these measures used in research and specialty care settings require time, training, and sophisticated physiological monitoring equipment. Instead, an informed observational pain rating can be made by the primary care physician based on the child's facial actions, which provide the best information, as well as rigidity, guarding, and respiration.

6. Preschool-Age Children (3 to 5 Years)

Some normally developing preschool-age children can understand and apply simple self-report scales, while others cannot. The choice of scale and the way

the scale is explained to the child are important. The scale should be explained at a time when the child is not highly distressed. Faces scales that are suitable for older preschool-age children are discussed in the next section. To find out whether a particular child understands the scale or not, the clinician can ask hypothetical questions about no pain and high pain situations that are familiar to the child.

For toddlers and preschoolers who do not understand how to provide a quantified self-report on a faces scale (most children under 4 years, and many 4- and 5-year-olds), observational methods are needed. A recommended scale for this purpose is the FLACC [27]. The acronym stands for Face, Legs, Arms, Cry and Consolability, with each item assigned 0 to 2 points to yield a sum score on a 0 to 10 scale. This instrument is also suitable for older children where a corroborating observational pain measure is needed. It takes a few minutes for the clinician to learn how to use the scale which can then be administered in less than a minute. It is available online (see Table 3-1).

7. School-Age Children (6 to 12 Years)

Many good self-report tools are available for school-age children [8]. For those aged 8 and up, the simplest scale to administer (because no equipment is needed), and probably the most widely used self-report measure of all, is the verbal numerical rating scale (NRS-11). Instructions are something like, "Tell me a number from 0 to 10 to show much it hurts. Zero is no pain, and 10 is the most pain." To use this scale, children need to know not only how to count, but also how to

TABLE 3-1. Simple, validated pain scales suitable for use in primary care. World Wide Web references are current as of February 2007.

Self-report scales
- Age 4 up: *Faces Pain Scale – Revised* [30]
  - *www.painsourcebook.ca* (with instructions in many languages)
- Age 8 up: *Numerical Rating Scale* – No printed tool needed (see text)

Observational scales
- Age 2 up: *FLACC Scale (Face, Legs, Arms, Cry, Consolability)* [27]
  - *childcancerpain.org/print.cfm?content=assess08*
  - *www.aboutkidshealth.ca/clinicalAreas.asp?pageContent=PN-nh2-03a*
- Children with communication impairment: *Non-Communicating Children's Pain Checklist – Revised (NCCPC)* [32]
  - *www.aboutkidshealth.ca/PDF/AKH_Breau_everyday.pdf*

estimate quantity using numbers, so the numerical rating scale is not suitable for most children aged 7 or younger. Children often report numbers outside the suggested range, such as 20 out of 10, and these can generally be understood as an effort to convey the severity of the child's distress. It is not fruitful to ask the patient to reframe their answer to suit the scale; rather, use the original number as a starting point and monitor progress, using the patient's interpretation of the scale. There has been almost no pediatric research on this scale despite its very wide usage with children and adults.

For children aged 4 through adolescence, faces scales have been well-validated. One faces scale, the Oucher, uses a vertical array of six color photographs of children showing a range of pain expressions; versions are available for both sexes and various ethnic groups [28, 29]. Others, such as the Faces Pain Scale – Revised [30], use line drawings (*www.painsourcebook.ca*—see Table 3-1) which can be photocopied inexpensively and easily disposed of, thus requiring no cleaning for infection control. The child's task is simply to point to the face that shows how much she or he hurts; the child does not need to speak. Faces scales are generally scored 0 to 10 in increments of two.

Many forms of visual analog scales are available. These employ a line, usually 10 to 20 cm in length, with one end labeled "No pain" and the other end labeled "Worst pain." The child's task is to make a mark or to move a plastic slider to indicate the point along the line corresponding to the child's pain.

To complement or replace self-report scores where necessary, observational scales can be used and the FLACC, discussed above, is recommended.

For measurement of long-term chronic or recurrent pain, no validated observational methods exist, so the clinician must rely on self-report together with informal observations by parents and possibly teachers. However, the child can be asked (with parental support) to keep a pain diary for 2 or 3 weeks where the child can record episodes of pain, together with intensity ratings and notes about possible triggering events (foods, activities), as well as what was done to relieve the pain.

Parents' observations at home of children's postoperative pain, as well as children's self-reports, can be obtained by telephone using a numerical rating scale. It is worthwhile to ask for these ratings, given the widespread tendency for children to be undermedicated for pain at home following surgery [31].

8. Adolescents

Adolescents with normal cognitive development do well with a numerical scale such as NRS-11, discussed above. In general, their ability to use self-report scales is the same as that of adults.

9. Children with Developmental Disabilities

Chapter 4 reviews special considerations in assessing pain in children with developmental disabilities. It may be difficult to obtain their self-report, and their behavioral expression of pain may be idiosyncratic. Tools such as the Non-Communicating Children's Pain Checklist [32, 33] can be applied by parents and clinicians, and can be of great help in monitoring and managing pain in this population.

10. Children in Critical Care

Special challenges in pain measurement occur with children who are unable to provide a self-report because they are seriously injured, sedated, intubated, and/or paralyzed. Specialized pain measures in such cases are based on physical movement, muscle tone, facial tension, and cardiovascular variables [34].

11. Four Brief Case Examples

The following vignettes are intended to illustrate applications of simple, rapid pain measurement in various clinical situations.

11.1. Self-Report Numerical Pain Scores in a Headache Diary

A 12-year-old boy reports headaches of three months' duration, with no obvious signs of any organic cause. To identify stress and dietary triggers and diurnal and weekly patterns, the physician asks him to keep a 2-week diary showing pain scores before school, after school, and at bedtime, on a 0 to 10 numerical scale of intensity. The diary also contains notes on activities and foods consumed at those times when pain scores exceed a baseline level.

11.2. Self-Report Faces Pain Scores in Repeated Injections

A 6-year-old girl must have frequent injections of growth hormone, which distress her greatly. As part of a "Better Needles Plan" involving education, distraction, and reward for good coping, the pediatrician asks her to record a score using the Faces Pain Scale – Revised after each injection. Variables such as time of day, injection site, and type of distraction used can be controlled to maintain the lowest possible pain ratings. Coping may be promoted by the girl's recognition that her pain ratings are lower when distraction and reward for coping are used.

11.3. Observation by Parents to Control Post-Tonsillectomy Pain at Home

The parents of a 4-year-old are instructed while still in the day surgery unit to record pain behaviors and estimates of pain intensity on a 0 to 10 observational scale, so that they can report to the surgeon or pediatrician from home by phone in case of high pain levels or other adverse incidents.

11.4. Physician's Use of a Global Numerical Rating Scale in a Busy Infant Ward

In a situation where no structured and validated pain scales are available, even a simple observer estimate can be better than nothing. The physician records pain scores (on a 0 to 10 scale) informally based on observation of the specific pain cues in the baby's facial expression (see section 5 of this chapter), guarding, crying, response to contact, and other behavior. These allow monitoring of the child's response to analgesic treatment. Moreover, nurses may use an exact description of the baby's behavior to communicate a need for increased analgesics: "He has a high-pitched cry, furrowed brow, and open square mouth when his dressing is changed."

Take-Home Points

Most busy primary care physicians do not have time to investigate, acquire, learn, and apply the complex pain scales used in research and in specialty pain services. Instead, the following quick approach is suggested. While simple and practical, it is based on extensive reviews of this domain, to which the reader is referred for further detail [5, 6, 35].

- Pain scores should be recorded using a consistent tool whenever pain is the focus of treatment or is an important symptom or complaint of the patient.
- If a child is old enough (4 years of age or older) and calm enough to understand a self-report scale, then this should be the primary source of pain measures and should be repeated over time.
- If the child is 8 years of age or older and has normal cognitive development, use the Numerical Rating Scale (NRS-11) where 0 is no pain and 10 is the most pain. Scores over 10 on this scale can be accepted without comment; they usually represent the child's effort to convey the seriousness of the pain problem.
- If the child is 4 to 8 years of age, consider the use of a faces scale (see Table 3-1; www.painsourcebook.ca). Children this age can also show where their pain is located using crayons on a body outline.
- Most children under 4 years of age cannot provide a meaningful self-report of pain intensity, so observational tools are needed. The FLACC is recommended for many situations.
- If neither self-report nor observational validated tools are available, an informal global observational rating (0 to 10) provides at least a basis for comparison over time.
- If you think a procedure would hurt you, it hurts and scares a child more. Context variables such as what kind of procedure it is can be taken into account, along with observed behavior in recording a pain score.

- Record pain scores along with the scale or source, the time frame, and the scale denominator (e.g., self-reported worst pain in past day, 6/10; mother's rating of usual pain over the past week, 4/10).
- Use pain scores to guide analgesia dosage and timing, and to communicate with other health care providers about what makes the pain better or worse.

Acknowledgments. The author thanks the following (in alphabetic order) for their helpful comments on an earlier version of this chapter: K. Baerg, C.T. Chambers, T. Jaaniste, C.C. Johnston, D. Lake, T. Palermo, J. Rozdilsky, S. Seshia, and F. Visram. Opinions expressed and any errors should be attributed solely to the author.

References

1. Franck LS, Greenberg CS, Stevens B. Pain assessment in infants and children. Pediatr Clin North Am 2000;47:487–512.
2. Treadwell M, Franck L, Vichinsky E. Using quality improvement strategies to enhance pediatric pain assessment. Int J Qual Health Care 2002;14:39–47.
3. American Academy of Pediatrics. The assessment and management of acute pain in infants, children, and adolescents. Policy statement by Committee on Psychosocial Aspects of Child and Family Health, Task Force on Pain in Infants Children and Adolescents. Pediatrics 2001;108:793–797.
4. von Baeyer CL, Hicks CL. Support for a common metric for pediatric pain intensity scales. Pain Res Manage 2000;5:157–160.
5. Stinson JN, Kavanagh T, Yamada J, Gill N, Stevens B. Systematic review of the psychometric properties, interpretability and feasibility of self-report pain intensity measures for use in clinical trials in children and adolescents. Pain 2006;125:143–157.
6. von Baeyer CL, Spagrud LJ. Systematic review of observational (behavioral) measures of pain for children and adolescents aged 3 to 18 years. Pain 2007;127:140–150.
7. Hadjistavropoulos T, Craig KD. A theoretical framework for understanding self-report and observational measures of pain: a communications model. Behav Res Ther 2002;40:551–570.
8. Champion G, Goodenough B, von Baeyer CL, Thomas W. Measurement of pain by self-report. In: Finley G, McGrath P, editors. Measurement of pain in infants and children. Seattle: IASP Press, 1998:123–160.

9. McGrath P. Behavioral measures of pain. In: Finley G, McGrath P, editors. Measurement of pain in infants and children. Seattle: IASP Press, 1998:83–101.
10. Sweet SD, McGrath PJ. Physiological measures of pain. In: Finley G, McGrath P, editors. Measurement of pain in infants and children. Seattle: IASP Press, 1998:59–81.
11. Beyer JE, McGrath PJ, Berde CB. Discordance between self-report and behavioral pain measures in children aged 3-7 years after surgery. J Pain Symptom Manage 1990;5:350–356.
12. Chambers CT, Reid GJ, Craig KD, McGrath PJ, Finley GA. Agreement between child and parent reports of pain. Clin J Pain 1998;14:336–342.
13. Merskey H, Bogduk N, editors. Classification of Chronic Pain: Descriptions of Chronic Pain Syndromes and Definitions of Pain Terms. 2nd ed. Seattle: IASP Press, 1994.
14. Marco CA, Plewa MC, Buderer N, Hymel G, Cooper J. Self-reported pain scores in the emergency department: lack of association with vital signs. Acad Emerg Med 2006;13:974–979.
15. Kelly A. Setting the benchmark for research in the management of acute pain in emergency departments. Emerg Med 2001;13:57–60.
16. Kelly A. The minimum clinically significant difference in visual analogue scale pain score does not differ with severity of pain. Emerg Med J 2001;18:205–207.
17. Manne SL, Jacobsen PB, Redd WH. Assessment of acute pediatric pain: Do child self-report, parent ratings, and nurse ratings measure the same phenomenon? Pain 1992;48:45–52.
18. Slater R, Cantarella A, Gallella S, et al. Cortical pain responses in human infants. J Neurosci 2006;26:3662–3666.
19. Anand KJ, Johnston CC, Oberlander TF, Taddio A, Lehr VT, Walco GA. Analgesia and local anesthesia during invasive procedures in the neonate. Clin Ther 2005;27:844–876.
20. Taddio A, Katz J, Ilersich AL, Koren G. Effect of neonatal circumcision on pain response during subsequent routine vaccination. Lancet 1997;349:599–603.
21. Grunau RV, Craig KD. Pain expression in neonates: facial action and cry. Pain 1987;28:395–410.
22. Craig K. The facial display of pain. In: Finley G, McGrath P, editors. Measurement of pain in infants and children. Seattle: IASP Press, 1998:103–121.
23. Craig KD, Grunau RV, Aquan-Assee J. Judgment of pain in newborns: Facial activity and cry as determinants. Can J Behav Sci 1988;20:442–451.
24. McNair C, Ballantyne M, Dionne K, Stephens D, Stevens B. Postoperative pain assessment in the neonatal intensive care unit. Arch Dis Child Fetal Neonatal Ed 2004;89:F537–F541.

25. Stevens B, Johnston C, Petryshen P, Taddio A. Premature Infant Pain Profile: Development and initial validation. Clin J Pain 1996;12:13–22.
26. Ballantyne M, Stevens B, McAllister M, Dionne K, Jack A. Validation of the premature infant pain profile in the clinical setting. Clin J Pain 1999;15: 297–303.
27. Merkel SI, Voepel-Lewis T, Shayevitz JR, Malviya S. The FLACC: A behavioral scale for scoring postoperative pain in young children. Pediatr Nurs 1997;23: 293–297.
28. Beyer JE, Denyes MJ, Villarruel AM. The creation, validation, and continuing development of the Oucher: A measure of pain intensity in children. J Pediatr Nurs 1992;7:335–346.
29. Beyer JE, Knott CB. Construct validity estimation for the African-American and Hispanic versions of the Oucher Scale. J Pediatr Nurs 1998;13:20–31.
30. Hicks CL, von Baeyer CL, Spafford PA, van Korlaar I, Goodenough B. The Faces Pain Scale-Revised: Toward a common metric in pediatric pain measurement. Pain 2001;93:173–183.
31. Gauthier JC, Finley GA, McGrath PJ. Children's self-report of postoperative pain intensity and treatment threshold: determining the adequacy of medication. Clin J Pain 1998;14:116–120.
32. Breau L, McGrath P, Camfield C, Finley GA. Psychometric properties of the Non-Communicating Children's Pain Checklist-Revised. Pain 2002;99: 349–357.
33. Breau LM, Finley GA, McGrath PJ, Camfield CS. Validation of the Non-communicating Children's Pain Checklist-Postoperative Version. Anesthesiol 2002;96:528–535.
34. Ambuel B, Hamlett KW, Marx CM, Blumer JL. Assessing distress in pediatric intensive care environments: the COMFORT scale. J Pediatr Psychol 1992;17:95–109.
35. von Baeyer CL. Children's self-reports of pain intensity: scale selection, limitations and interpretation. Pain Res Manage 2006;11:157–162.

4

Pain Management for Children with a Developmental Disability in a Primary Care Setting

Harold (Hal) Siden and Tim F. Oberlander

Abstract: Pain in children with developmental disabilities is common, but the expression of that pain is frequently ambiguous and thus clinical decision making becomes highly subjective and challenging. New assessment tools and specific management techniques have become available and can be used in a wide variety of clinical settings. Nevertheless, even with improved knowledge of pain, the underlying conditions, and clinical pharmacology, our ability to understand and manage pain in children with developmental disabilities remains a significant challenge. Use of a coordinated pain management approach that includes effective communication between the child, family, and allied health care professionals is essential.

Key words: Assessment, developmental disability, significant neurological impairment, cerebral palsy, head injury, chronic pain, pediatric pain.

Introduction

Inherent to the health and well-being of children with developmental disabilities is the timely and appropriate management of pain. However, the presentation of pain can be confusing, as it is frequently confounded by the individual's functional disabilities, undercurrent illnesses, side effects of medications, as well as the underlying neurological condition itself. When the expression of pain is ambiguous, decision making becomes highly subjective and both the assessment and management of pain present tremendous challenges.

Until recently, pain in children and youths with developmental disabilities received very little scientific attention. They have been systematically excluded from mainstream research, leading to under-recognition of their pain and hence, under-treatment. This has now started to change. The International Association for the Study of Pain (IASP) defines pain as "*an unpleasant sensory and emotional experience associated with actual or potential tissue damage, or described in terms of such damage*" [1]. Because the emphasis on self-report assumes a capacity for verbal communication, the IASP has clarified the definition of pain to recognize that "*the inability to communicate in no way negates the possibility that an individual is experiencing pain and is in need of appropriate pain relieving treatment*" [2]. Our goal is to recognize and measure features of the individual's behavioral and physiologic repertoire that are indices or expressions of pain.

This chapter will illustrate, using a clinical vignette, approaches to the assessment and management of pain in a child with a developmental disability presenting in an everyday setting. The reader is directed to other sources for a detailed and broad discussion of pain assessment, epidemiology, and ethical issues related to management in this setting [3].

1. What is a Developmental Disability and Where is the Pain?

Gena is a 12-year-old girl with multiple developmental disabilities associated with central nervous system impairment. She has multiple cognitive, language,

G.A. Walco and K.R. Goldschneider (eds.), *Pain in Children: A Practical Guide for Primary Care.*
© Humana Press, a part of Springer Science + Business Media, 2008

and motor impairments (cerebral palsy), is fed via a gastrostomy tube (G-tube), has infrequent seizures, and has been treated for gastroesophageal reflux. She also has a ventriculoperitoneal shunt for hydrocephalus and is thought to have recurrent head pain, which has been treated unsuccessfully with nonsteroidal anti-inflammatory medications. Gena's other medications include phenobarbital, ranitidine, and lactulose, with glycerin suppositories, phosphate enemas, acetaminophen, and lorazepam given as needed. Her parents and caregivers rely on a variety of nonspecific verbal and hand and head movements to understand her communication of pleasure or discomfort. She was brought to her pediatrician's office by her mother because of a gradual, but noticeable increased generalized arousal and irritability, thought to reflect a painful condition.

2. What Is an SNI and How Can it Lead to Painful Conditions?

A significant neurological impairment (SNI), whether from multifactorial causes (e.g., genetic/metabolic disorders, multi-organ syndromes, traumatic brain injury), or disorders of unknown origin, can be associated with multiple sources of acute and chronic pain. The term "developmental disability" is used to describe clinical conditions with diverse etiologies, anatomic lesions, and functional limitations and thus precise relationships between specific neural substrates and the functioning of the pain system are difficult to articulate. Clinical assessment thus focuses on pain and arousal behavior in the context of the functional impairments that arise from a spectrum of cognitive, motor, and communication limitations.

Beyond the everyday pain associated with bumps and scrapes of childhood, neurologic impairment increases the risk for multiple pain experiences. The activities of daily living for a child with a disability may involve the use of assistive devices for positioning and mobility (walkers, seating systems, manual and power wheelchairs, etc.) and brings with it new and different sources of pain. Dislocated hips, pressure sores from skin breakdown, and repetitive use injuries do occur and must be considered in the distressed child. Splinting and casting may be required for the prevention and treatment of contractures and can be associated with pain. For some, eating and swallowing are difficult and special feeding

techniques or enterostomy feeds are required. Feeding tubes can result in gastric distention, tugging or pulling of the tube, or skin breakdown at the tube site and are a potential cause of pain on an everyday basis. Constipation is a common source of discomfort. Even communication (either verbal or through the use of a mechanical device), though not typically thought of as painful, has been reported by adolescents using such devices as a source of discomfort.

The majority of children with a significant neurological impairment experience motor changes characterized by increased tone, spasms, increased deep tendon reflexes, and clonus, coupled with weakness and loss of dexterity (cerebral palsy). Spasticity and spasms can cause significant discomfort through waking and sleeping hours. Treatment of spasticity frequently involves invasive procedures; high tone/spasticity may be treated through surgical intervention (selective dorsal rhizotomy) or by surgical implantation of an intrathecal baclofen pump, while pharmacologic management of tone may include intramuscular injection of botulinum toxin A. Noninvasive therapies can also contribute heavily to frequent pain. In one study, parents of patients with cerebral palsy reported that assisted stretching was the most painful activity of daily living [4].

Although the nociceptive pain of surgery is obvious, there are times when repeated surgery, or direct trauma to a nerve results in long-lasting pain. Neuropathic pain can be difficult to identify and treat, but should be considered in SNI patients with prolonged pain after an intervention. Another source of pain is central in origin, where the pain afferents appear to be activated

TABLE 4-1. Factors to consider in assessment of pain in children with a developmental disability.

- What is the underlying neurological condition/process (how might this influence the pain system?)
- Developmental level
- Usual behavioral and health condition: baseline condition and everyday function
- Usual means of communication
- Caregivers' views and understanding of what is happening
- Role of intercurrent illness
- Differential diagnosis: what else is going on?

without ongoing input either from tissue damage or peripheral nerve injury. The major evidence for such an entity comes from the observation of pain behavior in children with advancing neurodegenerative diseases such as Krabbe's disease, children with SNI such as Gena, adults with thalamic strokes and Alzheimer's disease [5,6], but the pain mechanisms associated with these conditions remain to be demonstrated. The nosology regarding pain is not uniform; some authors may use the term neuropathic to specifically address pain secondary to peripheral nerve injury only, while others may include any pain not due to nociceptive or inflammatory causes, such as the central pain described.

3. Pain Expression in SNI

With the altered behavior, Gena's mother reported that her daughter feels "upset," shouts, and screams because of her "pain." Her condition has led to altered sleep behavior, poor school attendance, and more limited social contact. Her mother is very concerned that her behaviors represent an underlying painful condition. She has been to many clinicians and her condition and the role of pain is not well understood by her family or physicians.

Expression of distress among children like Gena is frequently ambiguous and its recognition by caregivers becomes highly subjective. Even when pain-specific behaviors are present, such behaviors seem altered, blunted (see Table 4-1) or can be confused with other sources of generalized arousal.

Gena's mother reported that a substantial increase in her irritability began 1 to 2 weeks prior to the clinic visit, initially with crying episodes at school. The child's in-class special education assistant reported that the crying started around 1 p.m. following a midday feeding and a rest out of her wheelchair. There were no apparent problems with the gastrostomy, and the child was repositioned in her chair, but the crying persisted. The school contacted the family to take the child home. By the time the mother had arrived at school, the crying had abated, although the child "did not seem herself." This happened repeatedly and over the proceeding weeks she was frequently sent home early from school, not able to participate in her regular social and recreational activities, leading to further social isolation and unhappiness. This was very frustrating for her and her family.

4. Pain Assessment

In the absence of easily recognized verbal or motor-dependent forms of communication, it remains uncertain if the pain experience itself is different, or whether only the expressive manifestations are altered (see Table 4-1). Effective assessment of pain is an essential step towards establishing a diagnosis, selecting an appropriate treatment plan, assessing treatment efficacy, and ultimately relieving pain. Pain assessment in children without disabilities needs to be calibrated to age-specific language and cognitive skills. Over the past three decades, a multitude of scales to assess self-report, behavioral elements, and physiologic indicators of pain has been validated for children of different ages. However, even adjusting for developmental level, these scales are not readily applicable to children with developmental disabilities. For example, over the course of normal development affect differentiates; over time emotional distress, fear, sadness, and pain are all discriminated. When a child's repertoire of distress signals is limited, the pain scales for normal children may no longer distinguish among behaviors.

Emerging reports provide some description of the expression of pain in the case of certain disabilities and provide scales that have face validity, some empirical validity, and perhaps clinical utility. In a case report Collignon et al. [7] described the difficulty of pain assessment in three children with CP which lead to the initial development of a 22-item scale focusing on observations made during the response to physical examination and thought to be indicative of pain [8]. Since then, a number of empiric studies have yielded important inventories of behaviors considered by observers to be pain-related among children with SNIs [9–11].

Multidimensional instruments have been designed to assess pain in children and adults with communication and cognitive impairments [12–16]. These measures have focused on the identification of a variety of possible pain cues in children with cognitive impairment [11, 14, 17, 18]. These include vocalizations (e.g., cry, scream, moan), facial expression, movement (both increased and decreased), change in muscle tone (increased and decreased), guarding/protection, and changes in everyday activity (social interaction, eating, and sleeping).

Breau and colleagues [19,20] have developed an observational assessment tool to quantify pain responses observed by parents and caregivers of cognitively and physically impaired children. Physiological changes such as changes in skin color, shivering, and sweating are included as assessment items. Their instrument provides a very helpful illustration of the vast and, at times, conflicting behaviors that are thought to be pain-related in developmentally disabled children.

An alternate approach has been offered by Hunt et al. [21] (Paediatric Pain Profile (PPP) *http://www.ppprofile.org.uk*) using individual symptom clusters to develop an individual's pain assessment. This semi-individualized measure gives predetermined categories of behaviors, which are then added to by the parent/caregiver, and provide a base and ceiling for pain behaviors, rated from 0 to 3 in severity scoring. This measure provides a highly valid, reliable, and sensitive measure for each individual child, but does not provide measures that are generalizable across children of a similar condition. In this sense, this measure gives the clinician and family a way of distinguishing an individual child's good days from bad days, and so may be well-suited for a clinical setting.

Self-report tools can be useful for some people with cognitive impairments [22]. Tools focused on establishing sensitive and specific measures of nonverbal pain displays (e.g., facial expression) [23] and biobehavioral reactivity (e.g., heart rate variability) [24] have been studied, but the clinical utility of these approaches to assessing pain in this setting remains to be determined. Irrespective of the instruments used, it is clear that systematic pain assessments should be routinely undertaken, regardless of the disability, particularly when extraordinary behavior or context dictates the possibility that pain is present.

5. Investigation of Pain in a Child with an SNI

Gena's symptoms increased in frequency, duration, and intensity, and particularly troubling was her continuous facial grimacing. Her symptoms were paroxysmal, with no antecedent behaviors, position, or event. In the rare

moments when she was not crying, her parents reported that she was irritable and typical sensory experiences that had been pleasant were now ineffective or even aversive. The night before the clinic visit Gena awoke crying. Finding that she had no fever and she was breathing rapidly, her father stopped an overnight feed and she was repositioned in bed. Her crying continued.

A work-up commenced which included CBC with differential, ESR, electrolytes, liver function tests, urinalysis, and X-rays of the chest and abdomen. A gastroenterology consult was obtained and a 24-hour pH probe followed by an upper GI series and an endoscopic examination of the esophagus and stomach were done. A neurology consultation was obtained with an EEG. A review by orthopedic surgery, along with X-rays of the spine and hip, were also done.

All of the laboratory investigations were reported to be normal or unchanged from her previous baseline. The chest X-ray was unremarkable. The abdominal film revealed stool throughout the colon, but no evidence of obstruction. The spine films showed moderate, non-progressive scoliosis. The hips were in the same dislocated position that had been reported one year earlier. There was diffuse osteopenia. The EEG revealed generalized slowing and abnormal rhythms, but no seizure activity. Gena had occasional gastric reflux, but the endoscopic examination was unrevealing. While there were findings that could have explained her pain or irritability, no unifying diagnosis appeared.

In order to identify the level of pain and to make a diagnosis in patients whose symptoms and behaviors are so far for the norm, individualized assessment strategies must be invoked, and may even need to be changed over time. The history should build upon the use of an established, symptom cluster assessment tool, such as those by Hunt [21] or Breau [12,13]. This approach might provide a profile of typical everyday behaviors, how they have changed during this period of "pain," and other associated changes in everyday function and activities. Understanding changes from an agreed baseline set of behaviors observed by experienced caregivers, compiled to reflect a longitudinal perspective, may be the most reliable measure of pain and distress available. A detailed history should include an account of known baseline behaviors or physical conditions, known stresses, and an understanding of the typical repertoire of verbal and nonverbal cues used to communicate pain and

TABLE 4-2. P-Q-R-S-T–eliciting and exploring pain symptoms.

P–palliative or provocative factors for the pain
Q–quality of pain (burning, stabbing, aching, etc.)
R–region of body affected
S–severity of pain (usually 0 to 10 scale)
T–timing of pain (after meals, in the morning, etc.)

TABLE 4-3. Differential diagnoses to consider for pain and irritability of unknown origin.

Head and Neck
• Corneal abrasion
• Otitis media/externa
• Sinusitis
• Dental infection/injury (note halitosis, bleeding, dental erosion)

Cardiorespiratory System
• Pneumonia
• Congestive heart failure (N.B. Swelling, cold extremities)

Gastrointestinal System
• Gastritis, esophagitis
• Inflammation at the stoma for a G-tube
• Subcutaneous tube migration
• Chronic constipation

Neurological System
• Dystonia [25]
• Spasticity/hypertonicity [26]
• Seizures
• Neuropathic pain

Genitourinary
• Dysuria/urinary tract infection
• Urinary stones (Immobility, bone resorption, medications and formula composition may be predisposing factors)
• Menses/premenstrual cramping or menorrhagia and other gynecological causes
• Hernia
• Testicular torsion

Skin
• Pressure sores
• Infection (under leg brace, etc.)
• Hair strangulation of digit

Musculoskeletal System
• Fractures/dislocations (i.e., risk from osteopenia/osteoporosis. Look for dislocation, angulation, erythema, bruising, and crepitus and leg length discrepancies as clues to a dislocated hip)*

a variety of affective states. One helpful technique is to ask the family to make a brief home video recording of the behavior; watching the video with the parents develops understanding and agreement about the exact nature of the complaint. The influence of the caregiver's perceptions, social setting, or the individual's tolerance to change or stress are key to understanding the child's current situation. Context of the pain behavior is crucial. Pain on changing a diaper suggests hip subluxation or sacral decubitus ulcers; pain after eating or upon lying down suggests gastroesophageal reflux, for instance. Beyond a pain history, a detailed review of all systems, medications, allergies, diet, and recent procedures remains essential. A helpful mnemonic is listed in Table 4-2.

Many key features of the physical examination require emphasis. Sufficient time and place are essential for a thoughtful and deliberate approach. Careful observation, with guidance by experienced caregivers looking for specific areas of discomfort or injury is essential. Throughout the exam, one should observe the patient's facial and vocal reactions to manipulations, as well as the reaction of the parent (as a proxy for self-report; the parent's "gut reaction" can sometimes help more than asking them for a more complex evaluation of pain behaviors). Body parts should be isolated as best as possible to avoid pain behaviors based on global reactions, which can conflict with reactions to manipulation of a specific body part. Allowing the patient to calm down and relax between examining body regions is important to avoid generalized overstimulation, which can be confounding. Ideally, the child should be moved to an examining table, completely undressed and provided with a gown or sheet for modesty and warmth. Examinations should not take place through clothing or around orthotic devices. A list of differential diagnoses can be found in Table 4-3.

*Bilateral dislocation, however, will not show such a difference. Dislocation or subluxation found on physical examination and/or X-ray does not absolutely guarantee that this is the pain source. The presence of hip dislocation or subluxation on a single exam or imaging is also not sufficient—sometimes it is the dynamic movement of the hip and lumbar area during transfers, dressing, bathing, etc, that causes pain. Examination needs to include both static- and movement-based observations. A selective nerve block with injection of a long-acting local anesthetic (bupivacaine) into the hip joint may be diagnostic as well as therapeutic. Importantly, surgical approaches to the dislocated hip can involve extensive and painful procedures, (and also not relieve all pain) so one should be certain that this is the source, and that the pain of a dislocation outweighs that of a surgical procedure.

6. Pain Management

In spite of a careful history and thoughtful approach to investigating Gena's pain, the etiology of her irritability and possible pain remained uncertain. The lack of a simple explanation was frustrating for all, leading to a feeling that "I can't diagnose, therefore I can't treat."

Pain management requires clear objectives, which are specific to the child and the developmental disability, and a comprehensive plan that includes combination pharmacologic and nonpharmacologic options. Typically, pain management needs to focus on identifying the underlying pathology, leading to a diagnosis and a treatment plan that reduces distress and facilitates a return to baseline function. However, a diagnosis may not always be possible. Careful empiric evaluation of the pain, exacerbating and mediating factors, clinical judgment, an empiric medication trial, and careful follow-up may be the only available management options. The success of pain management in this setting requires three key elements: 1) a clearly identified plan, 2) coordinated communication and decision making among the child, caregivers, and clinicians alike, and 3) a process for ongoing evaluation to keep this management plan on track, especially when the pain has not resolved.

6.1. Analgesics

Not surprisingly, typical analgesics such as acetaminophen, nonsteroidal anti-inflammatory drugs, and opioids should be considered for everyday pain. Selection of appropriate medications should ideally follow an appreciation of likely pathophysiology of the pain (e.g., acute inflammatory pain may respond to NSAIDs). In this setting, where assessment is uncertain, as needed (prn) dosing may lead to either under- or over-treatment and therefore, should be avoided. Around-the-clock dosing for a specified period of time, combined with a pain tracking tool, will be more effective in determining the efficacy of a therapy. The route of medication administration should be the least invasive and appropriate for the patient and sources of pain. Oral or G-tube route is preferable. With the added pain of injections and reduced muscle mass, intramuscular injections should be avoided. Subcutaneous delivery via indwelling catheters may be an appropriate way to administer opioids for selected, severe pain states. Topical anesthetic creams or other topical agents should be considered prior to injections, venipuncture, refills of intrathecal baclofen pumps, and other cutaneous procedures. Silver nitrate and sulcrate in zinc oxide can be very effective topical agents for controlling local irritation at gastric tube sites. It might be useful to use an "n-of-1" trial to determine therapeutic efficacy. The idea is to compare the patient's response to a medication against their own response to a placebo. This requires the use of a blinding procedure, often by a pharmacist, to use placebos and medication interventions in a randomized fashion. This can also be helpful in eliminating an expectation bias.

It is crucial to recognize that improved pain symptoms do not always mean improved function, and continued evaluation of both the symptom and functional outcomes is an essential component of pain management. For example, in using an anti-spasticity agent to improve neuromuscular tone in a child with spastic hypertonic cerebral palsy, the drug may reduce pain and reduce tone; however, reduced tone may in fact lead to diminished fine motor skills, reduced ability to stand and transfer, and apparent loss of muscle "strength." This leads to even broader effects of increased distress and decreased independence.

6.2. Drug Interactions

When multiple medications are needed to manage a patient's diverse number of conditions, drug-drug interactions can alter analgesic efficacy and drug side effects can be problematic. Careful consideration of drug interactions and new knowledge of underlying genetic metabolic differences related to hepatic metabolic isozymes help to explain how different patients can respond quite differently to the same medication combination [27]. For example, both traditional (e.g., phenobarbital, carbamazepine, phenytoin, valproic acid) and the newer (e.g., vigabatrin, lamotrigine) antiepileptic drugs are a common source of drug-drug interactions [28, 29]. Antibiotics have substantial potential to interact with commonly used analgesics. For example, erythromycin inhibits the hepatic CYP 3A4 isoenzyme that is needed for drug metabolism and reduces clearance of drugs metabolized by this pathway, such as midazolam and fentanyl [30]. Pain can be a direct side effect of some medications. For example, ranitidine can cause headaches. Therefore, reviewing the patient's medication list has several roles in pain evaluation and treatment for these complex patients.

6.3. Drug Trials

Frequently, children and infants with degenerative conditions such as a metabolic/genetic disease or HIV encephalopathy will present with pain behaviors and irritability of an unclear origin that appear to be refractory to typical analgesic or sedative medications. This is a particularly frustrating and unsatisfying situation for the children, families, and clinicians. Judicious medication trials with anticonvulsants, such as gabapentin or carbamazepine, and atypical neuroleptics (risperidone) may be helpful adjunctive treatments. If a child is hospitalized for evaluation, a trial of intravenous anticonvulsants, such as fosphenytoin, may give a more rapid answer as to the role for this class of medications in situations where generalized pain behaviors cannot be tied to an obvious nociceptive source. A similar trial of intravenous opioids can be done under inpatient conditions as well. Such acute trials can guide outpatient therapy and help the family understand the roles for the various types of medications. As noted above, inpatient drug trials require round-the-clock dosing, possibly with additional prn doses for breakthrough pain, and the use of a tracking tool to monitor analgesic effect. In this setting, even a simple bedside visual analog scale for parents, caregivers, and nurses will suffice.

6.4. Acute Pain

Acute procedural and postoperative pain management for children with developmental disabilities are also challenging, requiring the same imaginative approach used in other settings. Simple management strategies may be helpful. At the outset, keeping usual caregivers at hand may help in assessment and allow differentiation of nonspecific arousal behavior from pain behavior. Similarly, it is important to maintain ongoing communication with the inpatient treating team regarding how the patient reacts to pain and prior treatments, and improve the management of ongoing or preexisting problems. Empowering the parents or guardians to present their method of pain assessment to the treating team can facilitate pain care in a setting where the patient may not be as well known as in the physician's office. Medications used prior to surgery, such as anticonvulsants and muscle relaxants, should be continued. Nursing staff involved in managing postoperative pain require ongoing support from the pain management team, and customized assessment and management protocols should be developed for each child. As with all children, behavioral interventions can be particularly helpful options for managing acute pain. Depending on the child's ability to communicate or responsiveness to external stimulation, distraction and imagery may be a helpful adjunctive therapy. From clinical experience, physical measures such as massage, touch, heat, or cold therapy can be considered, though to date there have been no published studies evaluating these strategies for this population.

Confronting Gena's ongoing raised levels of arousal, irritability and pain, and the team's frustration, her caregivers stepped back from their focus on acute pain and the search for an underlying or unifying etiology, and reviewed her polypharmacy "cocktail." The combination of medications seemed appropriate for her various conditions.

After considering the options, an empiric trial of opioid analgesics was started. Morphine was begun with initial dosing every four hours for pain behaviors and the dose was titrated towards a reduction in the behaviors. Effects were monitored before and one hour after dosing with a validated behavioral observation pain scale by her parents. The team also discussed the use of antipsychotic medication, given the possibility that her generalized arousal was not pain-related. However, the side effect profile of these medications led the team to defer using them.

Within two weeks of starting morphine, Gena's family reported substantially reduced irritability, increased appetite, and a return to her typical activities of daily living. Close follow-up was arranged with the team and any changes to her management plan were based on a comprehensive and ongoing multidisciplinary pain management plan that included a case manager and regular communication with Gena, her family, and health care professionals.

Take-Home Points

- Keep usual caregivers at hand to assist in ongoing assessment and management of pain.
- In the absence of "gold standard" pain measures, consider each child as their own control and compare behavior and response to interventions against previous assessments.
- Maintain typical means of communications (computer, eye gaze device, etc.).
- Maintain typical means of comfort and mobility (seating system, form board, wheel chair, etc.).
- Use behavioral and nonpharmacologic interventions appropriate to child's developmental stage and pain condition.
- Attempt to match medication mechanism of action to type of pain (i.e., neuropathic, inflammatory, and nociceptive).
- Note that improved symptoms are not always associated with improved function—function should always be considered as an outcome of pain management.
- Consider novel approaches to sensory modalities in assessing effect of pain management strategies, especially where communication and cognition are limited.
- Maintain ongoing communication with usual primary care and subspecialty health care professionals for management of ongoing and preexisting conditions.
- In the case of surgical procedures, maintain all usual preoperative medications (anticonvulsant and muscle relaxants, e.g., baclofen, diazepam).
- Use a multidisciplinary approach, drawing on support from a specialized pediatric pain management team where possible.

Recommended Reading Material

Oberlander TF, Symons F. Pain in Children and Adults with Developmental Disabilities. Baltimore, MD:Paul H Brookes Publishing Co.,2006. Chapters 6, 10 and 12.

Taddio A, Oberlander TF. Pharmacological management of pain in children and youth with significant neurological impairments. In: Oberlander TF, Symons F, eds. Pain in Children and Adults with Developmental Disabilities. Baltimore, MD: Paul H. Brookes Publishing Co., 2006: 193-211.

Breau LM, Stevens B, Eckstein Grunau R. Developmental issues in acute and chronic pain in developmental dis-abilities. In Oberlander TF, Symons FJ, eds. Pain in Children and Adults with Developmental Disabilities. Baltimore: Paul Brookes Publishing Co., 2006: 89-107.

Breau LM, McGrath PJ, Zabalia M. Assessing pediatric pain and developmental disabilities. In Oberlander TF, Symons FJ, eds. Pain in Children and Adults with Developmental Disabilities. Baltimore: Paul Brookes Publishing Co., 2006: 149-172.

References

1. Merskey HE. Classification of chronic pain: Descriptions of chronic pain syndromes and definitions of pain terms. Pain 1986; suppl 3:51.
2. *http:, www.iasp-pain.org/terms-p.html. http://www. iasp-pain.org/terms-p.html. http://www.iasp-pain. org.* 2001.
3. Oberlander TF, Symon FJ. Pain in Children and Adults with Developmental Disabilities. Baltimore, MD: Paul H Brookes Publishing Co., 2006.
4. Hadden KL, Baeyer CL. Pain in children with cerebral palsy: Common triggers and expressive behaviors, Pain 2002;99:281–288.
5. Appelros P. Prevalence and predictors of pain and fatigue after stroke: A population-based study. Int J Rehabil Res 2006;29:329–333.
6. Cole LJ, Farrell MJ, Duff EP, Barber JB, Egan GF, Gibson SJ. Pain sensitivity and fMRI pain-related brain activity in Alzheimer's disease. Brain 2006;129:2957–2965.
7. Collignon P, Giusiano B, Porsmoguer E, Jimeno MT, Combe JC. Difficulties in diagnosing pain in children with multiple disabilities. Annales de Pediatrie 1995;42:123–126.
8. Giusiano B, Jimeno MT, Collignon P, Chau Y. Utilization of neural network in the elaboration of an evaluation scale for pain in cerebral palsy. Methods Inf Med 1995;34:498–502.
9. Stallard P, Williams L, Velleman R, Lenton S, McGrath PJ. Brief report: behaviors identified by caregivers to detect pain in noncommunicating children. J Pediatr Psychol 2002;27:209–214.
10. Stallard P, Williams L, Velleman R, Lenton S, McGrath PJ. Intervening factors in caregivers' assessments of pain in non-communicating children. Dev Med Child Neurol 2002; 44:213–214.
11. Stallard P, Williams L, Velleman R, Lenton S, McGrath PJ, Taylor G. The development and evaluation of the Pain Indicator for Communicatively Impaired Children (PICIC). Pain 2002;98:145–149.
12. Breau LM, McGrath PJ, Camfield CS, Finley GA. Psychometric properties of the noncommunicating children's pain checklist-revised. Pain 2002;99: 349–357.

13. Breau LM, Finley GA, McGrath PJ, Camfield CS. Validation of the noncommunicating children's pain checklist-postoperative version. Anesthesiology 2002;96:528–535.

14. Collignon P, Giusiano B. Validation of a pain evaluation scale for patients with severe cerebral palsy. Eur J Pain 2001;5:433–442.

15. Hadden KL, von Baeyer CL. Global and specific behavioral measures of pain in children with cerebral palsy. Clin J Pain 2005;21:140–146.

16. McGrath PJ, Rosmus C, Canfield C, Campbell MA, Hennigar A. Behaviours caregivers use to determine pain in nonverbal, cognitively impaired individuals. Dev Med Child Neurol 1998;40:340–343.

17. Validation of the pediatric pain profile, a behavioral rating scale to assess pain in children with severe neurological impairment. 10th World Congress on Pain; 2002; San Diego: International Association for the Study of Pain, 2002.

18. Breau LM, McGrath PJ, Camfield C, Rosmus C, Finley GA. Preliminary validation of an observational pain checklist for persons with cognitive impairments and inability to communicate verbally. Dev Med Child Neurol 2000; 42:609–616.

19. Breau LM, Camfield C, McGrath PJ, Rosmus C, Finley GA. Measuring pain accurately in children with cognitive impairments: refinement of a caregiver scale. J Pediatr 2001;138:721–727.

20. Breau LM, Stevens B, Eckstein Grunau R. Developmental Issues in Acute and Chronic Pain in Developmental Disabilities. In: Oberlander TF, Symons FJ, editors. Pain in Children and Adults with Developmental Disabilities. Baltimore: Paul Brookes Publishing Co., 2006:89–107.

21. Hunt A, Goldman A, Seers K, Crichton N, Mastroyannopoulou K, Moffat V, Oulton K, Brady M. Clinical validation of the paediatric pain profile. Dev Med Child Neurol 2004;46:9–18.

22. Fanurik D, Koh JL, Harrison RD, Conrad TM, Tomerlin C. Pain assessment in children with cognitive impairment. An exploration of self-report skills. Clin Nurs Res 1998;7:103–119.

23. Nader R, Oberlander TF, Chambers CT, Craig KD. Expression of Pain in Children With Autism. Clin J Pain 2004;20:88–97.

24. Oberlander TF, O'Donnell ME, Montgomery CJ. Pain in children with significant neurological impairment. J Dev Behav Pediatr 1999;20:235–243.

25. Kulisevsky J, Lleo A, Gironell A, Molet J, Pascual-Sedano B, Pares P. Bilateral pallidal stimulation for cervical dystonia: Dissociated pain and motor improvement. Neurology 2000;55:1754–1755.

26. Sanger TD, Delgado MR, Gaebler-Spira D, Hallett M, Mink JW. Classification and definition of disorders causing hypertonia in childhood. Pediatrics 2003;111: e89–e97.

27. Taddio A, Oberlander TF. Pharmacological management of pain in children and youth with significant neurological impairments. In: Oberlander TF, Symons F, editors. Pain in Children and Adults with Developmental Disabilities. Baltimore, MD: Paul H. Brookes Publishing Co., 2006:193–211.

28. Eriksson AS, Hoppu K, Nergardh A, Boreus L. Pharmacokinetic interactions between lamotrigine and other antiepileptic drugs in children with intractable epilepsy. Epilepsia 1996;37:769–773.

29. Sanchez-Alcaraz A, Quintana MB, Lopez E, Rodriguez I, Llopis P. Effect of vigabatrin on the pharmacokinetics of carbamazepine. J Clin Pharm Ther 2002; 27:427–430.

30. Olkkola KT, Aranko K, Luurila H, Hiller A, Saarnivaara L, Himberg JJ, et al. A potentially hazardous interaction between erythromycin and midazolam. Clin Pharmacol Ther 1993;53: 298–305.

5
Remote Management of Pediatric Pain

Paula A. Forgeron and Patrick J. McGrath

Abstract: Many children and adolescents will experience pain that is recurrent or chronic in nature, and the provision of pain care presents a challenge to many pediatricians. Pediatric pain care for patients and families who live at a distance from specialist care add another dimension to these challenges. The overall approach to pain management is the same for patients and families who live a distance from their care provider as those who live close to their care provider, but with some practical differences. This chapter reviews general approaches to pediatric pain management with attention to adapting these approaches for remote patients and families, and also highlights distance-specific approaches. Distance resources for practitioners are also reviewed.

Key words: Pediatric pain, remote treatment, chronic pain, web based pain management, adolescent pain.

Introduction

Pediatric pain is common and specialist care in this field is limited and concentrated almost exclusively in tertiary care centers. Moreover, not all tertiary pediatric centers have specialist pain clinics. Upwards of 25 percent of children and adolescents will experience recurrent and ongoing pain for 3 months or more, and up to one-third of these children (i.e., about 7 to 8 percent) will experience frequent severe pain [1]. Because access to pain specialist care is limited, most families will depend on their pediatrician or family practitioner to manage frequent, recurrent and chronic pain.

This chapter will describe the distance options available to pediatricians and family practitioners. Although children in rural and remote areas experience all forms of pain, continuous and frequent recurrent pain severe enough to interfere with activities are the most challenging to treat and, therefore, this chapter will concentrate on these pains, which we will refer to as chronic pain.

There are three major forms that remote management can take. First, there is long-distance management ("distance management") between the primary health caregiver and the patient. Secondly, there can be distance management between a specialist clinic and a patient and their family. Thirdly, there is consultation between the primary health caregiver (usually a pediatrician or family physician) and a specialist or specialty resources.

Distance methods are ubiquitous and provide a significant extension of needed care. Distance methods range from the simple and nearly universal use of telephone consultation between regular appointments, to complete treatment programs that are given at a distance. Videoconferencing consultations are starting to be offered in more areas and the early research evidence for pain management is promising [2]. Patients suffering chronic pain who live at a distance from their practitioners report significant savings in time and cost with videoconferencing consultations, compared to in-person consultations, thus increasing their satisfaction with care [3]. Strong therapeutic relationships can develop using distance treatment, even if the only contact is on the

G.A. Walco and K.R. Goldschneider (eds.), *Pain in Children: A Practical Guide for Primary Care.*
© Humana Press, a part of Springer Science + Business Media, 2008

telephone [4]. Videoconferencing can break through geographic boundaries; one of the authors of this chapter, along with a medical colleague, conducted videoconferencing with a pediatrician and nurse in Amman, Jordan to collaborate in the implementation of a pediatric pain service [5]. Our hope is that, in the near future, distance methods will mean that living far from a specialist clinician will no longer represent a decrease in treatment opportunity.

1. Pediatrician to Patient and Family

Providing care to children and families in rural and remote areas is challenging regardless of the child's condition; however, chronic pain has some unique difficulties. Chronic pain is "differentiated from acute pain in that acute pain signals a specific nociceptive event and is self-limited. Chronic pain may begin as acute pain, but it continues beyond the normal time expected for resolution of the problem or persists or recurs for other reasons" [6]. There is little understanding of pain by the general public and by many health professionals, and although chronic pain is a common experience for children and adolescents, acknowledgement and understanding within society is not. Most children with chronic pain, or their families, have not met others with similar pain experiences. The uncertainty of complex pain and the fact that, in many cases, there is no detectable injury or specific treatment add to the complexities of helping the child and family [7].

Management of all pain requires assessment, treatment, and reassessment. Assessment and management at a distance present unique challenges. The following are some suggestions.

1.1. Assessment at a Distance

The assessment of children's pain has been reviewed recently [8], but there is no one tool that is appropriate for all children in all situations. Self-report is the gold standard by which pain should be assessed in children who are old enough to use a self-report tool. The following pain assessment tools are easy to use, cost effective and have the best evidence at present to recommend their use. All of these can be used at a distance, as they do not require a health professional to be present during the assessment.

For a more in-depth review of pain assessment, see Chapter 3.

The Faces Pain Scale-Revised (see Chapter 3) can be administered by parents at home to assess the intensity of their child's pain. Children as young as four years of age have been found to reliably use this tool correctly [9]. It is available in 24 languages and free to download from *http://painsourcebook.ca/docs/pps92.html*. This website is not restricted to health professionals so parents can download this tool and have the child rate their pain prior to appointments. The instructions for use are on the website. This tool can be used regardless of the family's ethnic or language background, thereby eliminating the need to have multiple versions of the same scale.

Numeric pain scales that rely on a child being able to rate their pain on a conceptual scale ranging from 0 to 10 or 0 to 100 can be used with older children and adolescents who do not have any developmental delays. These scales require that the child be able to think and express themselves in quantitative terms [10] and therefore can be used for children as young as 9 years of age. Again, this type of scale does not require a professional background or equipment and therefore can be used at home.

Describing the location of pain can be difficult for children and adolescents. The Eland color chart [11] is a front and back body outline pain location tool. The child or adolescent picks the colors to represent their mild, moderate, and severe pain and then colors the appropriate body areas. Young children can complete this chart with the help of a parent and older children can complete the chart independently. One of the advantages of using a body outline tool with children who live at a distance is that it can easily be brought to office visits or mailed back to the clinic to help in reassessment during treatment and augment telephone assessments. When children have pain for long periods of time it is difficult for them, or their parents, to remember what the pain was like a month ago and to recognize gradual improvements over time, especially when pain is still present. The Eland color chart can provide a visual representation of the child's pain and a concrete measure of small improvements over time. This type of recording also removes the need to rely on past memory of children and families in describing pain location and intensity changes over time.

In addition to location and intensity it is essential to look for patterns and triggers of pain. A pain diary is a useful way to gather this information. A pain diary can be as simple as a calendar where the parent or child lists activities and pain intensity and duration during a given day. These can be reviewed to determine if certain situations exacerbate or decrease the child's pain. These can be mailed back to the clinic or brought to appointments, thus decreasing reliance on past memory.

Although it is essential to assess pain location and intensity to determine appropriate treatment and to reassess these parameters to evaluate treatment, it is important for children with chronic pain not to focus solely on their pain. Helping to orient the child and family towards improvements in functioning is essential. Capturing data on the activities that are limited by the pain pre- and post-treatment are important components of pain assessment. Completing a diary that captures activities can be as simple as the previously mentioned calendar to illustrate the gradual increases in function. It is helpful for all children with pain, and their parents, to know that improvements in chronic pain conditions are gradually seen over weeks, not days. This is especially important for those at a distance, as they do not have easy access to professionals to discuss concerns about the speed of their child's progress.

Assessing pain in nonverbal children is often problematic; however, research in this area has shown that nonverbal children display specific pain behaviors making it possible to differentiate pain from other causes of behavioral change. The Non-Communicating Children's Pain Checklist (NCCPC) is a valid, reliable, paper-based checklist-type pain assessment tool that is easy to use for this population [12, 13]. There are two versions, one for use in the postoperative period while in the hospital, and the other for use at home to detect chronic pain problems. The tool is designed to be completed by nonprofessional caregivers, such as parents or home care workers, and is free to download (postoperative version *http://www.aboutkidshealth.ca/PDF/AKH_Breau_post-op.pdf*; at home version *http://www.aboutkidshealth.ca/PDF/AKH_Breau_everyday.pdf*). Interpretating scores is relatively simple, as the tool includes cut-off scores, making it easier to determine clinically significant pain, and improvements in pain after treatment is initiated. This population has been found to have more pain on average then their healthy counterparts [14] and the negative impact of pain on these children is significant. Breau and colleagues found that children with cognitive impairment displayed reductions in communication, daily living skills, socialization, and motor skills on days that they experienced pain [15] (see Chapter 4 for a more in-depth discussion of pain in children with disabilities). Again, like the other assessment suggestions in this chapter, the NCCPC is a paper-based tool and parent assessments can be mailed to the clinic to help with telephone or videoconferencing reassessments. Parents find this tool useful since children with recurrent pain and/or chronic pain often may not be experiencing an exacerbation during an office visit. To supplement the NCCPC parents can videotape the child's behaviors during episodes of pain.

Despite living at a distance from their health care provider, most children can have a fairly extensive pain assessment, which is fundamental for appropriate management.

1.2. Treatment at a Distance

Most significant ongoing pain conditions require a rehabilitative, multimodal approach to treatment. This includes a combination of medications, nonpharmacological techniques, and physical therapy approaches. In most rural care settings the pediatrician or primary practitioner needs to take on the role of coordinator for the child's treatment as incorporating other modalities are widely considered to be necessary for improvement in chronic pain conditions. Chapter 8 reviews the medications that are most helpful in various types of pain conditions. Most chronic pain medications are administered orally and therefore do not require patients to be in the hospital or live close to their pediatrician. Seldom are interventional techniques, such as epidural analgesia, used in pediatric chronic pain treatment.

Psychological techniques such as relaxation, thought stopping, guided imagery, and distraction can be taught by a local child psychologist who is well versed in a rehabilitation approach. In addition to teaching these techniques, the pediatric psychologist can diagnosis comorbid conditions such as anxiety disorders or depression, which are known to exacerbate an existing pain condition.

Although they may not have pain-specific expertise, they will have knowledge and skills to teach more general cognitive-behavioral techniques that can help reduce pain. However, it is important for psychologists who are working with pain patients to understand the basics of chronic pain and the specific applications of evidence-based psychological treatments to this population [16].

Physical therapists can work with children experiencing chronic pain at a distance to help increase activity. The physical therapist can be viewed as a coach, to prompt gradual return to activity. This is especially helpful as some children and adolescents fear activities that increase pain and, as a result, general physical deconditioning occurs. Although a physical therapist with pain-specific expertise would be preferable, this is not always available. It is necessary that the physical therapist, like all health professionals involved in the child's pain care, understand the rudiments of pediatric pain treatment [17] so that activity is paced for the individual child. Pushing beyond a state of readiness usually does not help and may decrease the child and family's commitment to remain engaged in a conditioning program. On the other hand, holding back on progressing through the exercises until the pain subsides may not be productive either. It may be helpful to review the status of the patient with the physical therapist. The therapist can better help the child work through a certain level of pain if the they know that no harm will come of it (e.g., for foot pain in the absence of fracture, infection or tumor, weight-bearing exercises can be safe and appropriate).

Education on chronic pain conditions is important for both parents and children. At times children with chronic pain and their parents may appear defensive during an office visit. Research has illustrated that children and parents have encountered disbelief on the part of clinicians when repeated investigations find no cause for the child's pain. Although this is a necessary step, normal results may contribute to children and their parents feeling as though no one believes them or are unable to help with their child's pain problem [7]. Parents and children viewed medical encounters as positive if the physician believed that the child was having pain, even if there was no diagnosis for the pain [7]. Providing assurance that they are believed and you are willing to work with

them to improve the child's pain and functioning is one of the first important therapeutic actions. This may be even more important for families living at a distance from care, as they undoubtedly will encounter individuals for whom the concept of chronic pain in children is new. Being a distance from their pediatrician or family practitioner may separate them from the support they need when they encounter disbelief in their communities. Education for both parents and children can help them restructure their responses to pain exacerbations and strategize ways to cope with the chronic pain the child experiences.

The World Wide Web has made an abundance of health information available to parents. A study by Provost et al. [18] used an online survey to capture data from over 2,600 patients and health professionals in Europe and the United States. These authors concluded that the use of the Internet for health purposes is growing in importance to the patient–physician relationship. Parents with a child suffering chronic pain are no different in their pursuit for answers and tend to actively search the Internet for information, as many times there is no one definitive cure for these types of pain conditions. The amount of information available can be daunting to pediatricians and general practitioners who are trying to keep apace with many childhood conditions. As with any other health-related topic, not all pain websites are accurate sources of information—a concern for both patients and health care providers [18].

A recent article by Oermann et al. [19] evaluated 40 public information websites obtained from Google and MSN searches using key phrases for pain management in children. They used the Health Information Technology Institute (HITI) criteria for assessing the quality of the health information found on the sites. The HITI criteria consist of seven main categories to assess, with subcategories in each. The main categories are credibility, content, disclosure, links, design, interactivity, and caveats. Only nine of the 40 websites evaluated met all the HITI criteria. Readability was the most likely category not to meet criteria. This means that many parents and children may need help with understanding the information on the websites. Over 18 million sites were retrieved from a Google search using the phrase "pain management for children." Therefore, it is important that health care providers be able to direct families towards the best websites available. The top three from the Oermann study are Pain Management for Children (*http://www.health-first.org/health_info/your_health_first/kids/pain.cfm*), Making Cancer Less Painful (*http://pediatric-pain.ca/mclp/mclp.html*) and Reducing Pain from Surgery: What a Parent Should Know (*http://www.ynhh.com/choice/reducingpain.html*). Another credible public website with a section on pain is About Kids Health, hosted by the Toronto Hospital for Sick Kids (*http://www.aboutkidshealth.ca/PNHome.asp*). This site has information on both acute and chronic pain, medications, physiology, and cognitive behavioral techniques with child- and adult-friendly graphics.

Few lay books exist that discuss chronic pain in children. However, two that parents have found useful are *Conquering Your Child's Chronic Pain: A Pediatrician's Guide for Reclaiming a Normal Childhood*, written by Dr. Lonnie Zeltzer [20], and *Relieve Your Child's Chronic Pain* written by Dr. Elliot J. Krane [21]. These books cover important information on parenting a child with chronic pain and include chapters on medication, nonpharmacological techniques, and school-related issues. The book by Zeltzer also lists pain specialty clinics in North America with contact information. Other books on pain that are helpful and include information on managing acute pain episodes are *Pain Pain Go Away* by McGrath, Finley, Ritchie, and Dowden [22] and *Making Cancer Less Painful* by McGrath, Finley, and Turner [23].

1.3. Schools at a Distance

School can be a major source of stress for children with ongoing pain. Not only do children miss school due to pain, but pain also impacts the child's ability to comprehend information when they are in school. Walker et al. found that life stress may play a significant role in sustaining pain symptoms [24], and that in addition to stressors associated with their disease, children with recurrent abdominal pain identified difficulty with comprehending homework assignments as a source of stress [25]. Many teachers are not aware of the impact recurrent and chronic pain can have on a child's academic abilities. As noted by Brown [26], a decrease in work assignments may be necessary if a child is unable to keep up.

Although school visits by health professionals are effective in collaborating with teachers and improving understanding of the child's condition and needs, this is not possible for many physicians, especially if the child lives at a distance. Parents alone may not be as effective in negotiating school adaptations as a combination of parents and health professionals. Many children and parents find it is anxiety-producing to try to explain school absence to teachers and peers, especially when there is no specific etiology known [26]. Telephone conferences are one way that school meetings can be accomplished; however, these can be time consuming for a busy practitioner. Alternatively, direct contact by telephone with a school official, in addition to a letter outlining some of the common features of chronic pain and patient-specific recommendations, can be very helpful. Some of the specific issues for children can include the state of school bathrooms for children with gastrointestinal-related pain (with respect to cleanliness, accessibility, and safety), the management of a pain episode at school and test or performance anxiety [26].

A sample letter used by our pediatric pain clinic (reprinted with permission) is provided as an example (see Appendix A). This letter is usually sent after the first or second clinic appointment, as prevention of school issues is more effective than crisis intervention and helps decrease school stress. The section on specific adaptations for the student needs to be modified to fit each individual patient; however, the information on chronic pain is general in nature.

There is usually a need to follow-up with phone calls to principals and/or teaching staff, especially at the beginning of each new school year. There is little knowledge of chronic pain conditions in the general public and, since many children with pain conditions do not have visible physical abnormalities, periodic reminders that the pain is ongoing are necessary.

1.4. When to Refer to a Pain Service

- Child missing school despite interventions or out of school for more than a month
- Initial interventions did not impact pain intensity or function
- Unable to determine cause of pain or pain that is disproportionate to believed causation

- Child showing signs and symptoms of depression
- Child's pain condition could benefit from interventional techniques
- Suspected Complex Regional Pain Syndrome Type 1 (reflex sympathetic dystrophy) or Type 2 (causalgia)

2. Pediatric Pain Specialist Care to Patient and Family

Despite the need to travel it is important that children be referred for expert advice and treatment if they meet any of the criteria listed above. When children live at a distance the need to involve a physician that is geographically closer is usually an important component of care. There are several different formats by which children's pain clinics offer support and treatment to distance patients. Some clinics assess and recommend treatments that are provided by the pediatrician or family physician, similar to many other specialist referrals. However, most pediatric pain clinics are interdisciplinary in nature with a psychologist, physical therapist, clinical nurse specialist or nurse practitioner, as well as the pain physician, all collaborating to administer treatment (see Chapter 14 for a more in-depth discussion). Therefore, in many cases the pediatric pain service remains the principal provider of the child's pain care. To facilitate treatment with distance patients, professionals in these clinics generally remain in contact and monitor patient progress via e-mail, telephone, mail, and videoconferencing, which supplement face-to-face contact. Liaison between the pediatric pain team and the primary practitioner is essential, as many of these children will have exacerbations that need more aggressive treatment locally and/or other health conditions that may impact their chronic pain condition.

2.1. Pediatric Pain Clinic Assessment at a Distance

Due to the interdisciplinary nature of most pediatric pain clinics and the global impact of chronic pain on a child and the family, a holistic pain assessment is completed. This type of pain assessment includes elements that target the affective, functional and family impact components of the child's pain, as well as physical components. It is the integration of an interdisciplinary approach that makes it possible to encompass strategies that target the various components of pain and improve disabling chronic pain conditions.

New innovative approaches are on the horizon to assist in capturing data on a child's pain. Electronic pain assessment tools are being developed. Personal Digital Assistants (PDAs) equipped with pain diary software are being studied. One recent study involving 60 children—30 children randomized to the electronic diary group and 30 children to the paper diary group—found a significantly higher completion in the data requested in the electronic diary group (83 percent), compared to the paper diary group (47 percent) [27]. All the children in the study were between the ages of 8 and 16 years and asked to complete the diaries for a 7-day period. Both diaries asked for 19 different items to be documented, ranging from pain intensity to functional impairment due to pain. Children in this study found both diaries easy to use. The PDAs are portable and can be equipped with alarm reminders to cue children and adolescents to complete data entry. Another study showed that children and adolescents found electronic devices fun and easy to use [28] and therefore were more likely to complete the diaries, thus improving assessment. The importance of a complete assessment cannot be understated as treatment is based on assessment and reassessment. Therefore, increased use of electronic versions of pain diaries may enhance the accuracy of data that clinicians use to decide on treatments.

2.2. Pediatric Pain Clinic Treatment at a Distance

Integrated treatment by the health professionals of the pediatric pain specialty clinic include approaches such as medication, pain education, cognitive behavioral techniques, specific physical therapy techniques aimed at desensitization and improving conditioning, and strategies to facilitate self-care by parents and children. Other treatment strategies to decrease the impact of the child's pain condition on the entire family, treatment for child anxiety and depression, and steps for reintegration into school may need to be included. After the initial assessment, some of the treatments can be delivered by collaborating with colleagues in the respective disciplines who are geographically closer to the patient, but who may not have pediatric pain expertise.

Most pain physicians have expertise in medications and medical interventions. Due to their expertise, pediatric pain physicians are comfortable with treating patients at a distance and monitoring the escalations in doses of medications as required. Most pediatric pain clinics are associated with a specific hospital and, therefore, pediatric pain physicians have admitting privileges. There are times when admission to the hospital for a chronic pain condition may be necessary for more aggressive pain treatment, such as epidural analgesia or intravenous infusions to control pain until other long-term rehabilitative techniques such as cognitive behavioral therapy can be taught.

2.3. Pediatric Pain Clinic and Schools at a Distance

Pediatric pain clinics are able to work with schools in similar ways as mentioned above including telephone, video or telephone conferences, and letters. In addition, the physical therapist or occupational therapist can address issues related to seating, mobility, and graded participation in gym class. Psychologists are qualified in assessing learning disabilities, anxiety, and cognitive impairments of pain and therefore can contribute significantly by suggesting specific strategies for helping the child reach academic outcomes. The clinical nurse specialist (CNS) or nurse practitioner (NP) have expertise in most aspects of pain including physiology, pharmacology, nonpharmacological approaches to pain relief, as well as expertise on strategies to work with parents and community partners. Therefore, the CNS or NP can help educate and support both the family and teaching staff to improve outcomes.

2.4. Pediatric Pain Clinic and Distance Specific Treatments

Research is emerging on the use of Internet and CD-ROM-based distance programs for children and youth with chronic pain conditions. A recent clinical trial by Hicks et al. [29] illustrated the effectiveness of a web-based program on the pain ratings of youths (9 to 16 years old) experiencing either recurrent abdominal pain, recurrent headache, or both. They found a significant improvement in summed pain ratings at one and three months post-web-based treatments with weekly telephone follow-up, compared to the control group (wait listed). This study used a web-based approach of information sharing for the youths and their parents. Seven chapters were included in the manual and delivered one week at a time. Information in the chapters included cognitive-behavioral approaches such as deep breathing, relaxation, and thought stopping. Other chapters covered basic information on headaches and abdominal pain, and physical pain management strategies such as cold and heat. Topics such as managing pain episodes at school and pacing were also covered. In addition to the web-based manual, participants in the treatment arm received a package by mail that included personalized relaxation and imagery techniques, and a thought journal that was to be used in combination with the cognitive restructuring strategies discussed in the web-based manual. Subjects were contacted each week by a psychologist, either by phone or e-mail. Parents were contacted twice during the seven weeks by phone. The results indicate that the 71 percent and 72 percent of youths in the treatment group had 50 percent or more reduction in pain at one month and three months post-program, respectively. By comparison the youths in the control group only had a 19 percent and 17 percent improvement in their pain. Both youth and parents found the web-based program helpful, effective, and flexible, and enjoyed the ability to do the program from home as they lived at a distance from tertiary care. The number needed to treat in this study was two, indicating a high rate of effectiveness with this approach. Certainly as more studies become available, distance treatments such as the one described will be offered by pediatric pain clinics. "Help Yourself Online" is available for order on CD-ROM(CAD \$30, including shipping). For information about ordering, please see the following web page: *http://www.usask.ca/childpain/research/hicks/hyo-available.htm*. Clinicians or researchers wishing to implement the program must have access to their own web space and must meet other conditions for non-profit use listed on the above page.

A study by Connelly et al. [30] showed a decrease in headache severity in children 7 to 12 years when they followed a 4-week CD-ROM educational/activity package that was mailed to their home, in comparison to a control wait list group. Similar studies that used a minimal contact method to teach children cognitive-behavioral techniques to manage headaches illustrate that efficacious treatment options are available for distance patients. Not all effective distance programs need to be computer-based. Written materials such as workbooks and relaxation audiotapes are approaches that have been found to be effective at improving headache pain. In a study by McGrath et al. improvements in headache pain were found with a single visit session in combination with a workbook for home and a telephone coach [31]. These studies all illustrate that psychological techniques provided in a minimal contact method are effective at decreasing pain in children and adolescents, which is key when working with patients who live at a distance from treatment facilities. Pediatric psychologists working on a referral pediatric pain team can provide this type of treatment for children with ongoing pain problems, ranging from CD-ROM interventions to individualized paper-based instruction.

3. Professional-to-Professional Consultation

The traditional forms of professional-to-professional consultation are by e-mail, telephone, or videoconferencing. In addition, there are other options to seek expert advice on children's pain care. The Pediatric Pain List is an e-mail discussion list that was established in 1993 and includes over 750 multidisciplinary health professionals from over 40 countries. Members of the list ask each other difficult assessment and management questions. They also share experiences, policies, and resources to improve pain management for children. The following is an example of a discussion on the list.

A family nurse practitioner from Tennessee posted the following complex case, requesting help:

We presently have a 17-year-old female with ulcerative colitis and colostomy. She has been admitted to the hospital several times since having her colostomy surgery last year. She has been placed on hydromorphone IV/PO, amitriptyline and sumatriptan for headaches. She is in the hospital today for constant abdominal pain that she describes as sharp and getting progressively worse. She has not had complete relief of abdominal pain since surgery. Rates pain 10/10 and reports pain is only controlled with meperidine 75 mg that she is able to get q 4 hrs prn, but she reports that the medication decreases pain to 0/10, but only lasts two hours. She was placed on meperidine prior to me seeing her today. She is allergic to morphine. I would like input as to what pain medications that you all have found to provide relief with ulcerative colitis pts with persistent abdominal pain. She presents as having neuropathic pain due to the sharp pain that is getting progressively worse and is mildly controlled with opioids. However, her GI physician seems to think it is more a stomach virus.

A pediatric anesthesiologist and medical director of a pediatric chronic pain service in Canada posted this reply:

We have seen a number of patients like this. I regard it as usually being a manifestation of central sensitization secondary to repeated episodes of pain, inflammation and surgical intervention—"visceral hyperalgesia," for want of a better term. A "stomach virus" that lasts a year doesn't seem likely, although this type of pain can certainly flare up with a transient viral gastroenteritis. She needs management by a multidisciplinary chronic pain team, providing medication, physical interventions, and cognitive-behavioral therapy.

In terms of medications, gabapentin and amitriptyline are most often helpful because this really is a neuropathic pain. Opioids may have a place, but should be on a regular schedule. Meperidine is almost always a poor choice. Are you sure that she is really "allergic" to morphine?

Lonnie Zeltzer's book is excellent for families suffering from chronic pain, and has a particular emphasis on abdominal pain.

The Pediatric Pain List is free and can be subscribed to at *http://pediatric-pain.ca/ppml/*.

Many professional associations have open access to resources on pain issues through their websites. The International Association for the Study of Pain (*http://www.iasp-pain.org/*) offers open access to PAIN: Clinical Updates, a short synopsis of the present state of the research and practice on a wide range of clinical issues written by international experts. For example Psychological Interventions for Acute and Chronic Pain in Children is available at *http://www.iasp-pain.org/AM/Template.cfm ?Section=Home&Template=/CM/ContentDisplay. cfm&ContentID=2271*, and Why Children's Pain

Matters is available at *http://www.iasp-pain.org/ AM/Template.cfm?Section=Home&Template=/ CM/ContentDisplay.cfm&ContentID=2265.*

The American Pain Society (APS) found at *http://www.ampainsoc.org/* has open access links to various position statements that are pediatric-specific, including acute pain assessment and management (*http://www.ampainsoc.org/advocacy/ pediatric2.htm*) and pediatric chronic pain (*http:// www.ampainsoc.org/advocacy/pediatric.htm*). Other more general policy statements on such topics as the unethical use of placebos and use of opioids in ongoing pain conditions are also available through the APS website.

The Pediatric Pain Letter (*http://pediatric-pain. ca/ppl/*) provides open access to peer-reviewed commentaries on pain in infants, children, and adolescents. In publication since 1996, it is currently published three times per year and includes book reviews and announcements of events related to pediatric pain, in addition to clinical issues. Current and past issues are available online. Topics covered range from issues pertaining to recurrent and chronic pain, such as school functioning, to acute pain issues like post-operative pain management.

Other professional sites that contain useful information include the Pediatric Pain Source book (*http://painsourcebook.ca/*) where assessment tools and policies are available. Unfortunately, most professional journals are not open access and require subscriptions. Most university libraries have electronic subscriptions to a large number of journals, but these are usually available only to those in the university community. PubMed, the web-based service of the United States National Library and National Institutes of Health, is open access (*http://www.ncbi.nlm.nih.gov/entrez/*) and leads to many open access articles. Some provincial or state medical societies also have online journal and textbook subscriptions available to their members.

In addition to already established Internet-based supports, networks can be established locally to provide a more personal form of support, education, and sharing of resources. Networks are relatively simple and cost-effective to establish and can consist of a group of organizations or individuals that work together on common goals [32]. In comparison to larger Internet e-mail discussion lists, networks provide a means to deal with complex issues locally and to pool resources and expertise. An example of a children's pain network is the Maritime Pediatric Pain Network in Atlantic Canada. An anesthesiologist and clinical nurse specialist with pediatric pain expertise established this network. A physician and a nurse representative from each of 13 regional hospitals, covering a large geographic area, were invited to attend a weekend workshop to determine the needs of health professionals in the representatives' hospitals. The purpose of this initial weekend was to establish the goals of the network and create the mechanisms to meet those goals. These individuals now act as pain champions within their hospital. Due to the relatively small group in attendance there was ample opportunity to meet one another and build collaborative relationships. All of the represented hospitals provide care to both adults and children. All of the nurses in attendance had expertise in pediatrics. The physicians included mostly pediatricians as well as several anesthesiologists and family physicians. None of the represented hospitals had health professionals with pediatric pain expertise, except for the one tertiary children's hospital which runs both an inpatient and outpatient pain service. The network has been running for almost three years. Activities of the network to date include the establishment of an e-mail list, five site visits by the founding anesthesiologist and clinical nurse specialist, one site visit by a pediatrician to the tertiary center, telephone consultations for complex acute and chronic pain, chronic pain referrals, and the sharing of hospital policies and resources such as pain assessment tools and opioid infusion policies. The five site visits not only included traditional presentations on children's pain but, more importantly, informal discussions about specific hospital barriers to improving pain practice. Collaborative relationships have been built between all the participants and there is bidirectional sharing of resources amongst all hospitals, not simply a one-way dissemination from the tertiary care health center to others. Networks like this are not difficult to organize; however, they do require a champion to initiate them and keep them active until the benefits of membership become apparent. Membership can consist of individuals from a variety of professions that have an interest in improving children's pain management.

4. Ethical/Legal Issues

The ethical and legal issues with distance methods are very similar to those with face-to-face methods of assessment and treatment [33]. For example, it is important to ensure patient confidentiality is not breached in all clinical situations. In typical clinical situations, this would involve training of staff, physical security for records and design of the clinic to allow for private conversations. The issues with distance methods are the same, but the implementation may involve a secure server instead of a solid wall.

Similarly, the assessment and treatment approach should be appropriate for the patient. Just as one would not question a patient in a language that they do understand, one should not expect a patient to use a computer if they are computer illiterate.

In some situations professional liability coverage may be different for e-health than it is for more typical treatments. Telemedicine licensure requirements vary by state and may pose limitations on practice, especially related to reimbursement [34]. Professionals should be aware of any specific guidelines their professional body has determined for e-health treatment.

Finally, although there may be advantages to distance treatment, if an intervention is only available by high-speed internet and a computer, then it will not be available to families who do not have high-speed internet in their homes, especially those at lower income levels. Additionally, many health plans may not cover distance treatment and this may be a major impediment to delivering services at a distance.

5. Conclusion

The prevalence of pediatric recurrent and chronic pain is now being recognized. Access to pain care is needed to improve the lives of the children who suffer; however, the availability of specialty clinics is less than the demand and most are located in large centers. Most families will need to rely on their pediatrician or general practitioner for help with easing their child's suffering. Several forms of distance treatment are available to assist pediatricians and patients with chronic pain conditions. Professional-to-professional assistance can

range from pediatric pain e-mail discussion lists to locally developed networks. Pediatricians can help distance patients by monitoring improvements with paper-based assessment tools and telephone and Internet contact, as well as by referring parents and children to helpful websites for education. Interdisciplinary specialty clinics can help patients at a distance by collaborating with local professionals, creating home treatment plans including web or CD-ROM-based cognitive-behavior interventions and education. Innovations in distance care are providing patients with effective care close to home.

Take-Home Points

- Acknowledge belief in the patient's report of pain
- Assessment
  - Diary for pain triggers
  - Intensity rating (FPS-R, numeric, Eland, NCCPC)
  - Function
- Treatment
  - Access and coordinate with local professionals (psychologist, physical therapist, acupuncturist)
  - Education for parents
  - Education for child
  - Nonpharmacologic
  - Pharmacologic
  - Technology
- Schools
  - Proactive approach
  - General letter
  - Specifics for patient
- Professional distance supports
  - Trustworthy websites
  - Discussion forums/E-mail lists
  - Pain service referral

References

1. Perquin CW, Hazebroek-Kampschreur A, Hunfeld J, Bohnen AM, van Suijlekom-Smit LW, Passchier J, van der Wouden JC. Pain in children and adolescents: a common experience. Pain 2000;87:51–58.

2. King C, Workman B. Using videoconferencing technologies to deliver clinical pain management services to nursing home residents. J Telemed Telecare 2004; 10(suppl1): 100-101.

3. Peng, PWH, Stafford MA, Wong DT, Salenieks ME. Use of telemedicine in chronic pain consultation: A pilot study. Clin J Pain 2006; 22: 350-352.

4. Lingely-Pottie P, McGrath PJ. A therapeutic alliance can exist without face-to-face contact. J Telemed Telecare 2006;12: 396-9.

5. Finley GA, Forgeron PA. Developing Pain Services Around the World. In: Finley GA, McGrath PJ & Chambers CT (Eds.) Bringing Pain Relief to Children. New Jersey: Humana Press Inc. 2006: 177-198.

6. American Pain Society. Principles of analgesic use in the treatment of acute pain and cancer pain (4th ed.). 1999. Glenview, IL: American Pain Society.

7. Carter B. Chronic pain in childhood and medical encounter: Professional ventriloquism and hidden voices. Qual Health Res 2002; 12: 28-41.

8. Stinson JN, Kavanagh T, Yamada J, Gill N, Stevens B. Systematic review of the psychometric properties, interpretability and feasibility of self-report pain intensity measure for use in clinical trial in children and adolescents. Pain. 2006; 125:143–157.

9. Hicks CL, von Baeyer CL, Spafford P, van Korlaar, Goodenough B. The Faces Pain Scale - Revised: Toward a common metric in pediatric pain measurement. Pain 2001;93:173-183.

10. Von Baeyer C. Children's self-reports of pain intensity: Scale selection, limitations and interpretations. Pain Res Manag 2006; 11: 157- 162.

11. Eland JM, Anderson JE. The experience of pain in children. In: Jacox AK, ed. Pain: A Sourcebook for Nurses and Other Health Professionals. Boston: Little, Brown and Company, 1977: 453-473.

12. Breau L, McGrath PJ, Camfield CS, Finley GA. Psychometric properties of the Non-Communicating Children's Pain Checklist-revised. Pain 2002; 99: 349-357.

13. Breau L, Finley GA, McGrath PJ, Camfield C. Validation of the non-communicating children's pain checklist-postoperative version. Anesthesiology 2002; 96: 528-535.

14. Breau LM, Camfield CS, McGrath PJ, Finley GA. The incidence of pain in children with severe cognitive impairments. Arch Pediatr Adolesc Med 2003; 157: 1219-1226.

15. Breau LM, Camfield CS, McGrath PJ, Finley GA. Pain's impact on adaptive functioning. J Intellect Disabil Res 2007; 51: 125-134.

16. McGrath PJ, Goodman JE. Pain in childhood. In: P.J. Graham (Ed.), Cognitive Behaviour Therapy for Children and Families, 2nd ed., Cambridge: Cambridge University Press. 2004. 426-442.

17. Moseley L. Unraveling the barriers to reconceptualization of the problem in chronic pain: The actual and perceived ability of the patients and health professionals to understand the neurophysiology. J Pain 2003; 4: 184-189.

18. Provost M, Perri M, Baujard V, Boyer C. Opinions and e-health behaviours of patients and health professionals in the U.S.A. and Europe. Stud Health Technol Inform 2003; 95: 695-700.

19. Oermann M, Lowery NF, Thornley J. Evaluation of web sites on management of pain in children. Pain Manag Nurs 2003; 4: 99-105.

20. Zeltzer L, Blackett-Schlank C. Conquering Your Child's Chronic Pain: A Pediatrician's Guide for Reclaiming a Normal Childhood. New York: Harper Collins Publishers, Inc. 2005.

21. Krane, EJ, Mitchell D. (2005). Relieve Your Child's Chronic Pain. California: Fireside Books.

22. McGrath PJ, Finley GA, Ritchie J, Dowden SJ. Pain, Pain, Go Away: Helping Children with Pain. 2nd ed. Halifax: Dalhousie University. 2003.

23. McGrath PJ, Finley GA, Turner C. Making Cancer Less Painful: A Handbook for Parents. Halifax: IWK Health Centre. 1992.

24. Walker LS. Helping the child with recurrent abdominal pain return to school. Pediatr Ann 2004; 33: 128-136.

25. Walker LS, Smith CA, Garber J, Van Slyke DA, Claar RL. The relation of daily stressors to somatic and emotional symptoms in children with and without recurrent abdominal pain. J Consult Clin Psychol 2001; 69:85-91.

26. Brown RT. Managing Pediatric Pain at School. In: Finley GA, McGrath PJ, Chambers CT, eds. Bringing Pain Relief to Children: Treatment Approaches. New Jersey: Humana Press Inc; 2006: 113-129.

27. Palmero TM, Valenzuela D, Stork PP. A randomized trial of electronic versus paper pain diaries in children: impact on compliance, accuracy, and acceptability. Pain 2004; 107: 213-219.

28. Stinson JN, Petroz GC, Tait G, Feldman, BM, Steiner D, McGrath PJ, Stevens, BJ. e-Ouch: Usability testing of an electronic chronic pain diary for adolescents with arthritis. Clin J Pain 2006; 22: 295-305.

29. Hicks CL, von Baeyer C, McGrath PJ. Online psychological treatment for pediatric recurrent pain: a randomized evaluation. J Pediatr Psychol 2006; 31: 724-736.

30. Connelly M, Rapoff MA, Thompson N, Connelly W. Headstrong: a pilot study of a CD-ROM intervention for recurrent pediatric headache. J Pediatr Psychol 2006; 31: 737-747.

31. McGrath PJ, Humphreys P, Keene D, Goodman JT, Lascelles MA, Cunningham SJ, The efficacy and efficiency of a self-administered treatment for adolescent migraine. Pain 1992; 49: 321-324.
32. Chisholm RF. On the meaning of networks. Group and Organization Management. 1996; 21: 216-235.
33. Canadian Council on Health Services Accreditation. Telehealth Supplementary Criteria. Canada: Canadian Council on Health Services Accreditation. 2006.
34. Sable C. Telecardiology: Potential impact on acute care. Crit Care Med. 2001; 29: N159-N165.

Appendix A

Dear (Principal)

(Patient name) has just recently started to work with (physician name). He/she suffers from a chronic pain condition that impacts his/her everyday life.

Chronic pain is due to maladaptive nerve processing within the central nervous system. Unlike acute pain, chronic pain does not serve a benefit and limiting one's actions may not necessarily prevent further damage. Conversely, acute pain is what we experience when we are hurt and is a useful alert system for the body. Acute pain usually involves damage to muscles, tendons and/or other tissue, and it usually limits our movements to prevent further damage to the body's injured area.

Although (patient's name) has started on medication for his/her condition it may take several months before there is any improvement in his/her pain. He/she still experiences moderate to severe pain on a daily basis and the pain is present most of the time in varying degrees. There are times when he/she is able to participate fully in school, like most adolescents, but then there are times when his/her ability to cope with such ongoing pain limits his/her activities.

Adolescents who live with complex chronic pain face many challenges. Pain makes it difficult to concentrate at times and, therefore, even when (patient's name) is in class he/she may not fully comprehend the content and may need extra help on occasion. Pain can also make it difficult to complete work at home and can disrupt sleep, which leads to further problems with concentration and attention. Most people with chronic pain can complete tasks, but may need more time and effort because of these effects.

One of the most difficult aspects of such a complex pain condition is that many teens (children) meet adults and peers who don't believe their pain. Most people have experienced pain at some point in their lives and try and relate someone else's pain to their experiences. However, most of us have never experienced chronic pain that is unrelenting and therefore our experiences are not helpful. It is a result of the unrelenting nature of pain, and the fluctuating increases in the pain intensity, that impact one's ability to cope which explains why some days an adolescent (child) with complex pain is able to do more than on other days.

Although stress and anxiety do not cause pain, they do contribute to exacerbations of pain conditions. The increase in an individual's pain as a result of stress and anxiety is physiologically mediated. The release of excitatory neurotransmitters and hormones during stress and anxiety increases the number and strength of pain signals reaching the brain due to the chemical interference in the pain dampening system in the spinal cord and an increase in receptor sensitivity to pain.

School attendance and social interaction have been recognized as important components of a chronic pain rehabilitation program for adolescents (children). Although adolescents (children) with chronic pain may miss school more than some other students, the benefits they derive from school attendance are essential for their physical and social recovery. In fact, social activity, such as participation in extracurricular groups, is a key to reducing the risk of depressive symptoms in teens (children) with chronic pain. Those who are not allowed to take part in these activities can become isolated and suffer from depressive symptoms which, in turn, have negative effects on academic performance. Thus, it is very important that (patient name) be allowed to participate in school social activities regardless of his/her academic performance.

There are times when (patient's name) pain becomes severe and occurs for no apparent reason; this is the nature of complex chronic pain. (Patient's name) has indicated that in these situations he/she may have to stay home or go home as he/she is no longer able to concentrate and finds resting helpful. However, if a quiet room is available where (patient name) could rest or work independently, even if this means missing a class, he/she may be able to attend the rest of his/her classes that day.

In discussions (patient's name) has identified the following strategies that may be helpful to him/her so that he/she can meet the necessary academic outcomes. Many of these are the same accommodations that other schools have been able to offer to students we work with. First, (patient name) has identified that he/she can find it difficult to focus and take notes in most of his/her classes. We recommend that another student be provided with a carbon book so that copies of notes would be available for (patient name) daily, or that the teachers could provide him/her with notes. Although he/she may not need these everyday it is difficult at the outset of class for (patient name) to know if his/her pain level will rise and therefore interfere with his/her ability to both concentrate on the lecture and take notes. Second, due to the amount of time missed for tests it would be helpful if (patient name) could write the tests, but only have them count if they do not negatively impact his/her grades as the stress and anxiety associated with writing tests under these conditions can exacerbate his/her pain for the reasons mentioned above.

On occasion (patient name) may miss classes due to his/her pain or to attend appointments. We are aware that the School Board has a policy on the number of days missed in a term with respect to a student's successful completion of a course. We are hopeful that (patient's name) health condition will be kept in mind when reviewing his/her absence and that he/she will not be penalized for his/her health condition.

I am very hopeful that, with continued support by the faculty at (school name) and the treatment plan, (patient name) will have a successful school year both academically and socially.

We appreciate your help in this matter and if I can be of any further assistance or if more information on chronic pain would be helpful, please do not hesitate to contact me.

Part II
Acute Pain Management

6

Pain Management in the Primary Care Office

General Considerations and Specific Approaches

Neil L. Schechter

Abstract: Many things seen in everyday practice are uncomfortable or painful. Although research for common causes of pain have lagged behind some of the more attention-commanding etiologies (e.g., cancer), primary caregivers face a steady stream of less intense causes of pain. Most of the time, simple interventions can significantly reduce the burden of these pains. Educating parents about expectations for entities such as teething, ear infection, colic, and pharyngitis, coupled with straightforward interventions, can bring good results. Creating a "pain-friendly" office can relieve anxiety in the children and their parents, and lower the stress level for all involved. Office staff can learn simple techniques to help children cope with potentially painful aspects of their visit.

Key words: Teething pain, colic, primary care, pediatric, office management, minor pain, pediatric pain.

Introduction

During the past 20 years there has been an outpouring of research on pain management in children. Most of the new information that has emerged, however, is focused on the tertiary setting. As a result, postoperative pain, pain in newborns, procedure pain, and cancer pain are usually well addressed, and hospitals are much friendlier places for children than they were.

Unfortunately, children seen in ambulatory facilities have not benefited equally from this new information. Many of the strategies that are so effective in inpatient settings are not applicable to outpatient facilities due to the short length of most outpatient visits and the typically less severe and ephemeral nature of the pain that is encountered during these visits. Despite the inadequacy of hospital-based approaches, research interest to develop new strategies for office pain problems has been limited for a number of reasons. Pain in ambulatory settings, as previously mentioned, is often self-limited and lacks the sense of urgency and poignancy that accompanies pain problems in the hospital. Thus, the level of sympathy generated for the child who is terrorized by injections or is crying due to otitis media pain is often far less than that for the child who has just undergone scoliosis surgery or chemotherapy for a CNS tumor. As a result, researchers have not been drawn to investigate common pain problems, which are often trivialized by the more extreme nature of inpatient pain.

Such attitudes are unfortunate, but do not mitigate the fact that office-based pain problems impose a significant burden on children. The sheer volume of these relatively minor pains is staggering. There are hundreds of millions of injections given in offices and relatively simple techniques, if applied routinely, can reduce the pain they engender. Such interventions may also reduce the 10 percent of children [1] who become needle phobic, a frustrating problem for parents and providers which can dominate outpatient encounters and reduce their efficiency. The pains of acute infections and minor sprains and strains, although inevitable, can be reduced somewhat by available treatments if used appropriately.

Common acute pain problems may be attributed to normative processes such as teething, "growing

G.A. Walco and K.R. Goldschneider (eds.), *Pain in Children: A Practical Guide for Primary Care.*
© Humana Press, a part of Springer Science + Business Media, 2008

pains," or colic, from infections such as otitis media or pharyngitis, from minor injuries, or from the routine procedures to maintain health or evaluate illness such as immunizations, urinary catheterizations, or phlebotomy. In this chapter, a smorgasbord of common acute pain problems typically seen in the pediatric office will be reviewed. Other frequently encountered pain problems such as pain induced by necessary office procedures and chronic pains are discussed elsewhere throughout this volume. Finally, some suggestions about the creation of a "pain-friendly" office will be offered.

1. Pains in Normal Growth and Development

Normal developmental processes are sometimes accompanied by pain. Teething, colic, and growing pains are classic examples which require discussion.

1.1. Teething

It is conventional wisdom that tooth eruption is associated with many different symptoms including pain, irritability, drooling, biting, sleeping, and eating problems. In a cross-sectional survey of Australian child health professionals, the average number of symptoms ascribed to teething varied from 2.8 in pediatricians, to 4.4 in dentists, and 9.8 in nurses [2]. Parents expressed even stronger beliefs that teething was associated with a host of symptoms. Specific studies of teething, however, have called these assumptions into question. One study meticulously compared parents' reports of the child's mood, wellness/illness, drooling, eating, and stooling with simultaneous examination by a dental hygienist of the child's tooth eruption. This study did not confirm that tooth eruption in infants was reliably associated with other symptoms. An evidence-based review [3] of the area suggests that attributing symptoms to teething should be done only when other possible causes of those symptoms have been ruled out.

It does appear, however, that teething is associated with discomfort and there has been very little research on the management of teething pain. As with most pain problems, strategies to ameliorate teething pain include both nonpharmacological

and pharmacological, but none of these have been subjected to rigorous study.

Nonpharmacologic strategies include some old standby remedies: chilled teething rings (solid rings are superior to liquid-filled ones because they avoid the possibility of leakage); hard biscuits, breadsticks or frozen breads (a bagel is a good choice); pacifiers, and pressure on the gums (for example, rubbing them with gauze).

Pharmacologic strategies are a bit more controversial. There are topical anesthetic preparations which contain benzocaine, lidocaine, and choline salicylate available for teething. Anecdotal reports of their efficacy exist, but adverse events such as overdosage and methhemoglobinemia have been associated with their use as well. Some of these preparations also contain alcohol, which should be avoided in infants. Systemic analgesics such as acetaminophen, if dosed appropriately, are safe and may provide some relief for teething pain. Homeopathic remedies such as preparations containing chamomile are also frequently used by parents, although their efficacy is unknown.

In summary, teething, which typically occurs between 6 months and 2 years of age, has been associated with pain and irritability, as well as a number of other symptoms. Physicians should be certain that the reported symptoms are not secondary to other illnesses and, if attributed to teething, nonpharmacologic strategies and oral analgesics are probably first line treatment.

1.2. Colic

Based on a thorough review by Barr and Geertsma [4], the term "colic" describes a behavioral syndrome of recurrent crying that occurs during the first 3 months of life. They suggest that it is characterized by three typical behavioral patterns: 1) increased crying clustering in the late afternoon beginning in the second month and decreasing in the fourth month, 2) crying associated with distress behaviors (clenched fists, arched back, legs drawn into abdomen, facial grimacing) and are difficult to soothe and 3) paroxysmal crying bouts which are unpredictable and seemingly unrelated to meals or to the events in the infant's environment. As a result of these features, colic has often been thought of as a pain syndrome although this remains only a supposition. The etiology of colic remains unknown, but is most likely multifactorial.

The diagnosis of colic is made by history and by a normal physical examination. Typically, the crying pattern has been described as occurring more than three hours per day, for at least three days per week, occurring for more than three weeks (and usually lasting about three months). Babies with colic are often described as "gassy," implying a gastrointestinal origin, but the excessive crying itself may lead to aerophagia—which may be responsible for the gassiness—so this is not a reliable marker. GERD and formula intolerance (lactase deficiency, cow milk allergy) should be ruled out as an explanation for the colicky behavior.

A host of interventions for colic have been attempted with mixed results. Pharmacologically, two agents have been advocated. Simethicone is often suggested, but carefully controlled studies do not show it to be more effective than placebo. Dicyclomine has shown some efficacy in randomized trials, but it is associated with a number of side effects including sedation, apnea, and seizures and, as a result, it is not indicated for children under 6 months of age. "Gripe water," which contains alcohol and sodium bicarbonate, is a popular over-the-counter preparation for colic, but there are no formal studies of its efficacy.

Nonpharmacologic strategies are the mainstay of treatment in colic. Parental carrying of the infant using slings or backpacks is often helpful. Studies have been contradictory about the impact of carrying babies for prolonged periods of time (four to five hours per day) on preventing subsequent crying, but such a strategy may be effective for a given child. Rocking the child, using a swing, going for a car ride, tight swaddling, non-nutritive sucking, as well as the use of devices which soothe the child through vibration or white noise have all been promoted and may be helpful. Finally, dietary changes in the breast-feeding mother and formula changes in the infant may be helpful for a subset of children with colic.

In the end, the treatment of colic involves ruling out organic explanations for the fussy behavior, validating parental frustration while reassuring them that this behavior is time-limited, suggesting the importance of respite, and offering a series of noninvasive interventions so parents can feel they are at least doing something while this process comes to a natural conclusion.

1.3. Growing Pains

Growing pains are intermittent, bilateral, muscular, nonarticular pains that occur at night and are not associated with systemic symptoms. They occur in children between the ages of 3 and 12 years, most typically between 4 and 8. This phenomenon is quite common, with a prevalence estimate in one large study being 37 percent in children between ages 4 and 6.

The etiology of growing pains remains unknown, but it does not appear to be related to periods of pronounced growth. Poor posture, overuse, hypermobility, restless leg syndrome, as well as a host of psychological factors have been implicated, but most studies are small and the data are inconclusive. It may well be that its origin is multifactorial. Because of its lack of association with growth, Goodyear-Smith [5] has suggested that the condition be renamed "recurrent limb pain in childhood."

The diagnosis of growing pains is one of exclusion. The pain is not localized and not at one specific point. It typically occurs at night and is gone by the morning. There is no residual limping or evidence of other systemic illness. Growing pains typically occur in the anterior thigh, calf, and posterior knee and not in the joints. It usually occurs in both legs, although not necessarily at the same time. The pain is intermittent and there are pain-free nights. The physical examination is completely normal with no erythema, swelling, or limitation of movement. Laboratory and imaging data are usually not helpful, but controversy remains as to whether accumulation of such information is sufficiently reassuring to families (as well as to practitioners) to warrant the additional expense.

The typical treatments for growing pains are nonspecific and include stretching and strengthening exercises during the day, use of a heating pad, and systemic analgesics such as ibuprofen and acetaminophen. Practitioners should reassure parents that they know what the entity is (not only what it is not) and that these symptoms do not represent a serious disorder. Like teething and colic, these symptoms are self-limited and symptomatic treatment is all that is necessary.

2. Pain Associated with Acute Infections

Many common infections in childhood are associated with pain, and it is often the pain which brings the child to the medical office. Historically, the emphasis on treating these pains has been the elimination of the underlying infection which is presumed to be causing it. Unfortunately, such an approach does not immediately address the symptoms that brought the child to the doctor in the first place. In this section, we will discuss two of the many common infections in children that are associated with pain—otitis media and pharyngitis. The general principles outlined in this discussion are applicable to other common infections which are also associated with pain.

2.1. Otitis Media

Otitis media is the most common infection seen in pediatric offices. In some surveys, 80 percent of children will have had at least one episode of otitis by the age of 3 years. Otalgia is a frequent presenting symptom associated with otitis. In a study in the early 1980s, the pain associated with acute otitis was considered severe in 42 percent, moderate in 40 percent and absent in 18 percent [6]. In a more recent study of almost 3,000 French children [7] the average pain in children 5 years of age or younger presenting with otitis was 5.75/10, and, in children older than 5, was 6.15. On the second day, even with analgesia, the pain was about half (2.82 and 3.23, respectively) and essentially gone on the third day. These studies suggest that otitis is associated with at least moderate pain in most children and that pain might last for at least 48 hours.

Treatment for most painful infections typically involves treating the underlying disease itself, usually with antibiotics as well as systemic analgesia and local treatment. For otitis, the impact of antibiotic treatment on both the disease and the associated pain is controversial. In randomized clinical trials, 60 percent of children were essentially pain-free within 48 hours, whether or not they were receiving antibiotics. Between 2 and 7 days after presentation, 14 percent of the nonantibiotic group and 6 percent of the antibiotic group had pain.

Most authorities, therefore, suggest that antibiotics have a minor role in pain reduction.

Systemic analgesics remain the mainstay of treatment. In the one study that compared analgesics head to head, Bertin [8] reported that with three-times-daily dosing, ibuprofen provided slightly better pain relief than acetaminophen. Fixed preparations of acetaminophen and opioids (such as codeine) are typically recommended for more severe pain.

A few key points should be emphasized regarding outpatient analgesic usage. It is essential that parents be given detailed instructions on dosing over-the-counter medication to their children. In one study over 50 percent of children receiving acetaminophen or ibuprofen were administered the wrong amount [9]. Most errors resulted primarily in underdosing. Given the number of formulations available and the complexity of measurement, physicians should be certain that parents are aware of the exact dose they should administer and are capable of measuring it. Dosing guidelines for the use of fixed acetaminophen/ibuprofen-opioid preparations, typically used for more severe pain, should also be given in detail, and physicians should be certain that parents understand them. Because of the configuration of presently available formulations, overuse will more likely result in acetaminophen poisoning, not opioid overdosage as might be surmised by parents. An alternative is to separate the opioid (typically codeine or oxycodone) from the acetaminophen or ibuprofen, although this may introduce more confusion for parents. Finally, recent work on pharmacogenomics has identified the fact that a significant number of individuals have reduced capacity to metabolize codeine and therefore receive limited analgesic efficacy from it [10]. Persistent pain, despite seemingly adequate doses of codeine, might warrant changing to an alternative opioid such as oxycodone which does not depend on the missing enzyme.

Local treatment of ear pain has long had anecdotal support, but only recently have specific treatments been investigated. Hoberman and colleagues [11] examined the impact of Auralgan® (a mixture of antipyrine, benzocaine, oxyquinolone and glycerin) on ear pain and found that it significantly reduced ear pain within 30 minutes after instillation. In fact, McWilliams and colleagues [12] incorporated anticipatory guidance about ear pain, as well as a prescription for antipryine/benzocaine drops, to parents at the 15-month well child visit. They found a dramatic reduction (80 percent) in emergency department visits and urgent care visits for ear pain in this group. Naturopathic herbal extracts have also been shown to reduce ear pain [13]. Warm compresses and warmed oil placed in the ear have been used for many years, although never studied formally.

2.2. Pharyngitis

Acute pharyngitis is another frequent source of pain in children and a common cause of physician visits. The intensity of pharyngitis pain is quite variable and it is clear that streptococcal pharyngitis is associated with severe pain (4/5), while non-streptococcal pharyngitis is associated with significantly less pain. In the same data set used to assess otitis pain, Narcy and colleagues [14] also examined pharyngitis pain. They found that, on average, children both over and under five years reported similar pain intensity (5.4/10) on presentation with pharyngitis. This group did not classify the etiology of the pharyngitis. Despite the associated level of discomfort and its impact on functioning such as swallowing, the pain of pharyngitis has been poorly studied and is infrequently addressed. Sagarin and Roberts [15] expressed concern about a review of acute pharyngitis in the *New England Journal of Medicine* which did not address the pain of pharyngitis. They stated that patients with throat pain come to the physician for relief of the pain associated with swallowing and are typically given only antibiotics which will be of little immediate help, and of no help if the pharyngitis is of non-bacterial origin.

As with otitis media, the treatment of the pain associated with pharyngitis has three components —antibiotic treatment if there is a bacterial etiology, systemic analgesics, and local treatment. For the most part, pharyngitis is a self-limited disease. Ninety percent of children and adults will be well after 1 week, regardless of the origin of the pharyngitis and prescription of antibiotics. Antibiotic treatment does reduce the period of pain in individuals whose pharyngitis is associated with group A streptococcal infection, but as previously mentioned, has no effect on other causes of pharyngitis.

The limited research on analgesic treatment of pharyngitis also parallels otitis media. In one of the only available studies, Bertin [16] and colleagues performed a randomized double-blind multicenter trial of ibuprofen versus acetaminophen versus placebo for treatment of symptoms of pharyngitis in children. At 48 hours, pain had resolved in 80 percent of the patients on around-the-clock ibuprofen, 70 percent on around-the-clock acetaminophen, and 55 percent of children on placebo. Unlike otitis, another systemic agent has demonstrated efficacy in pharyngitis. Steroids (parenteral betamethosone or oral dexamethasone) coupled with antibiotics have been shown to reduce the pain of exudative pharyngitis in adolescents. Local treatment with anesthetic sprays, lozenges, and gargles are often used, although none have received formal investigation.

2.3. Summary

In summary, the treatment of pain associated with acute infection involves antibiotic treatment where appropriate (which often has limited impact), systemic analgesics (nonsteroidal anti-inflammatory agents seem to be slightly more effective than acetaminophen), and local treatments. A similar model applies to the pain of other infections such as urinary tract and viral mouth infections.

3. Pain Associated with Minor Injuries

Musculoskeletal injuries account for 6 percent of visits to pediatric primary care offices. Most stem from acute trauma or overuse syndromes and their numbers have dramatically increased due to the skyrocketing interest and participation of children and adolescents in athletics. In a study of high school athletes over a 2-year time span, 81 percent of football players, 75 percent of wrestlers, and 35 percent of track athletes reported injuries [17].

Typically these injuries are strains or sprains. Sprains are wrenching or twisting injuries to ligaments. They most often involve the ankles, knees, or wrists. Sprains can be graded as 1 (slight stretching and some damage to ligament), 2 (partial tear of the ligament), or 3 (complete tear of the ligament). Strains are injuries to a muscle or tendon caused by stretching or overuse. Common sites for strains are the back and hamstrings, but the hands and elbows can also be strained. Strains and sprains are relatively uncommon in younger children because their growth plates are weaker than their muscles and tendons and, as a result, young children are more prone to fractures

The acute inflammation associated with strains and sprains is characterized by pain, swelling, erythema, and increased warmth. The child may guard the involved area and refuse to move or bear weight on it. The diagnosis is made by history and physical examination with the assistance of imaging studies as indicated.

The typical treatment of minor musculoskeletal trauma is reflected in the acronym PRICE which stands for Protection, Rest, Ice, Compression and Elevation. Protection implies splinting, bracing, or immobilization to prevent further injury. Because the pain associated with acute injury, unlike chronic pain, does have a warning function, it is therefore best to avoid activities which cause pain for the first few days following an injury. Icing (cryotherapy) is preferred in the first 48 to 72 hours following strains or sprains. Cold offers multiple benefits—it provides analgesia and reduces both edema and muscle spasm. In studies where cryotherapy was used immediately following injury, as compared to later (after 36 hours) or to heat, there was a dramatic difference in the time to full recovery between the groups. Compression, typically via a compressive wrap, also reduces swelling. Wrapping should begin at the distal end of the injury and move proximally. Elevation of extremities above the level of the heart reduces edema and should be attempted if possible.

Recent data suggest that prolonged immobilization is probably detrimental and may contribute to the development of complex regional pain syndrome (formerly reflex sympathetic dystrophy). As a result, it is important that once the initial swelling/inflammation has decreased, the limb should be mobilized. This may require supportive physical therapy. Physical therapists also have a number of other modalities that may facilitate healing at their disposal, and a referral should be made if there is any concern about prolonged healing or dysfunction following an injury.

Analgesia is an important part of the equation. Typically, nonsteroidal anti-inflammatory agents such as ibuprofen are more effective than acetaminophen for musculoskeletal pain [18]. They not only provide direct pain relief, but reduce inflammation which acetaminophen does not. They should be considered around-the-clock initially and then subsequently as needed. If the child will be attending physical therapy, it is sometimes beneficial to preemptively provide analgesia prior to the session to reduce the pain associated with movement. There have been recent reviews of the use of topical nonsteroidal anti-inflammatory agents which uniformly endorse their efficacy for the relief of localized musculoskeletal pain. These preparations may be hard to access, but seem appropriate for use in the adolescent athlete.

Finally, if children experience recurrent sprains, they should be evaluated for hypermobility, which may be associated with recurrent injury and lead to chronic pain if not adequately addressed [19].

4. Creating a Pain-Friendly Office

In this chapter, and others throughout this volume, pain problems that may present at the pediatric office are described. Obviously, this list is not exhaustive and anyone who works in such a setting can suggest dozens of other pain problems that they have confronted. Unfortunately, very few of these have been formally studied in ways that would satisfy even the broadest demands of evidence-based medicine. Despite this lack of information about the evaluation and treatment of specific pains, there are enough commonalities between them that allow for the generation of principles as well as specific strategies that have been generally associated with pain reduction. Awareness of these principles and their integration into the fabric of the practice will help create an office that is truly "pain-friendly" [20].

4.1. Setting the Stage

It is important to inform parents from the outset that the office is committed to minimizing the pain associated with illness and procedures. This can be accomplished either through face-to-face discussion at the initial visit or through signage or brochures. It should not be implied that pain will be entirely eliminated in all situations as some pain is, unfortunately, inevitable in medical care. Instead the emphasis should be that, in this office, the staff considers provision of comfort to be a guiding principle of their care and will be considered in all decisions. Parents, therefore, should have expectations that pain relief will be offered whenever possible, but their expectations should be appropriate to the situation. At this initial meeting, the important role that parents have in pain reduction and amplification should be discussed.

4.2. Education

Education of children, their parents and the medical staff is the cornerstone of a uniform approach to pain management in the office.

4.2.1. Parents and Children

Education of parents and children around pain-related topics is beneficial both in advance of a pain problem and in the middle of one. This education has two purposes: 1) giving the child and parents a realistic sense of the pain that can be expected (preparation) and 2) teaching strategies that they can use to ameliorate pain.

We know that the anticipation of a feared event is often worse than the event itself. There is an extensive literature in both children and adults that demonstrates that adequate preparation clearly reduces the pain an individual experiences from an anticipated noxious stimulus. It might be beneficial, therefore, for pediatric offices to have fact sheets available that offer information about what to expect regarding the pain from common procedures and illnesses.

Similarly, brochures or discussion can review strategies that might help. Many of these strategies are discussed throughout this book, but they include developmentally appropriate preparation, parental demeanor during the procedure, and a host of distraction and calming techniques that parents can use, depending on the unique personality characteristics of their child. Parents who seek additional information can be referred to books for parents that specifically address this topic (L. Zeltzer, *Conquering Your Child's Chronic Pain* [21], L. Kuttner, *A Child in Pain* [22] and E. Krane, *Relieve Your Child's Chronic Pain* [23]).

4.2.2. Staff Education

Ongoing staff education is necessary to initiate and maintain a "pain-friendly" office. This is most easily accomplished by designation or self-selection of an office "champion" who will be responsible for keeping up with new information and helping to integrate it into the practice. Research in postgraduate medical education suggests that training in small groups at the site of care is most effective. Therefore, ongoing discussions in the office would seem to be far preferable to attending conferences out of the area. For example, if new local anesthetics, needles, analgesic combinations, and soothing strategies become available, the office champion can arrange for educational programs to introduce them. It is often helpful to survey patients or do chart audits around comfort issues. These procedures can either reassure the staff that they are doing a good job, or point out that additional changes are necessary.

Although many medical practitioners have developed their own distraction and relaxation techniques and strategies, it may be helpful to have a formal training session in the office to emphasize the importance of these approaches and reinforce the need for their uniform application. A pediatric psychologist from the community or another practitioner who is particularly interested in this area can conduct a workshop in the office if additional expertise is thought to be necessary. If any provider is interested in an in-depth experience in hypnosis, the Society for Developmental and Behavioral Pediatrics conducts yearly seminars on this topic. Knowing how to talk to and soothe a child is invaluable for essentially all aspects of pediatric care.

Finally, it is important for health care providers to have easy access to protocols that offer algorithms to help with pain management. For example, because there are a number of analgesics available and the average pediatrician uses them infrequently, he or she is far more likely to prescribe them if there is a protocol that outlines the choices, doses and side effects.

4.3. Cultivating Relationships with Outside Providers

Many chronic pain problems require a multidisciplinary approach which is not possible to offer in the typical office. A simulation of a multidisciplinary team can be generated through the identification of practitioners in other disciplines in the community who are comfortable caring for children in pain.

Physical therapy has much to offer individuals with both acute and chronic pain. It is critical that the therapist encourage the child toward steady growth, but does not overwhelm him or her. Unfortunately, many physical therapists are not trained in pediatrics or particularly interested in children. Cultivating a relationship with a physical therapy practice which has pediatric expertise and equipment is therefore highly beneficial. Additionally, we have found that many pain problems respond well to aquatherapy, where a warm pool reduces some of the impact of the techniques; therefore, a program with access to a pool is an added benefit.

In addition to a physical therapist, identifying a pediatric psychologist who is comfortable with the problems surrounding chronic pain is also very helpful. Many pain problems are exacerbated by or cause stress. Psychologists have many approaches that may benefit children with pain problems. Cognitive behavioral techniques can help provide relaxation and distraction, and coping skills. Psychologists can address sleep hygiene and school reintegration if those are problems, and can serve as a liaison between the family and the school. They can teach the family to help the child return to full functioning and reinforce non-pain behaviors. If depression or anxiety are playing a significant role in promoting pain and are not responsive to the psychologist's intervention, he or she may have a relationship with a psychiatrist who may offer psychotropic medications to address these issues.

4.4. Office Environment

The final piece in the creation of a pain-friendly office is the physical environment itself. Although most pediatric offices are bright and cheery, they should offer materials that can provide or promote distraction both in the waiting room and the examining room. DVD players, pinwheels, party blowers, fish tanks, and interesting books for parents to read should be part of the landscape. Sucrose solution should be available for young infants during painful procedures. Furniture should be comfortable so that both the child and parents feel relaxed and unhurried.

5. Summary

Pain is often a fellow traveler with medical illness and often inevitable while performing office procedures. Chronic pain is also a common complaint in primary care. Recognizing that pain is a problem worthy of consideration is the first step towards addressing it. It is important to alert parents to the fact that pain reduction or prevention is one of the office's primary concerns. A number of simple physical, pharmacological, and psychological strategies can reduce pain in most situations. The efficacy of those techniques is greatly enhanced by having literature available, involving parents in the process and fostering connections with other practitioners in the community. Although fear of pain can clearly interfere with the child's and family's relationship with the pediatric health care provider, addressing pain proactively can help build and strengthen that relationship.

Take-Home Points

- Given the large percentage of office visits that result from pain, primary care physicians can have a large impact on children's pain.
- Colic is common, distressing, and increasingly thought not to be a pain syndrome.
- Care of common distressing phenomena of childhood (e.g., colic, growing pains, teething) rely more on good rapport with families and simple interventions, as research has lagged in this area.
- The pain of infections and minor trauma has not been well-studied, but consistent application of basic interventions and parent education can improve.
- A "pain-friendly office" can be created with a small investment of resources, yet effectively reduce anxiety and pain in patients and families.
- Multidisciplinary care for chronic pain conditions can be initiated directly from the primary care office by establishing links with local physical therapists and psychologists. Such liaisons can reduce the burden on the primary care physician that would result from trying to treat a complex pain problem alone.

References

1. Hamilton JG. Needle phobia: a neglected diagnosis. J Fam Pract 1995;41:169–175.
2. Wake M, Hesketh K, Lucas J. Teething and tooth eruption in children: A cohort study. Pediatrics 2000;106:1374–1379.
3. Tighe M, Roe MFE. Does a teething child need serious illness excluding? Arch Dis Child 2007;92:266–268.
4. Barr RG, Geertsema MG. Colic: The pain perplex. In: Schechter NL, Berde CB, Yaster M. Pain in Infants, Children, and Adolescents. Philadelphia: Lippincott, Williams, and Wilkins, 2003:751–761.
5. Goodyear-Smith F, Arroll B. Growing pains. BMJ 2006;333:456–457.
6. Hayden GF, Schwartz RH. Characteristics of earache among children with acute otitis media. Am J Dis Child 1985;139:721–723.
7. Narcy P, Reinert R, Olive G, et al. Therapeutic management and objective evaluation of pain in children consulting for acute otitis media (abstract). 7th International Symposium on Pediatric Pain. Vancouver, Canada: June, 2006.
8. Bertin L, Pons G, D'Athis P, et al. A randomized, double-blind, multicentre controlled trial of ibuprofen versus acetaminophen and placebo for symptoms of acute otitis media in children. Fundam Clin Pharmacol 1996;10:378–392.
9. Li SF, Lacher B, Crain EF. Acetaminophen and ibuprofen dosing by parents. Pediatr Emerg Care 2000;16:394–397.
10. Fagerlund TH, Braaten O. No pain relief from codeine…?: An introduction to pharmacogenomics. Acta Anaesth Scand 2001;45:140–149.
11. Hoberman A, Paradise JL, Reynolds EA and Urkin,J. Efficacy of Auralgan for treating ear pain in children with acute otitis media. Arch Pediatr Adolesc Med 1997;151:675–678.
12. McWilliams D, Jacobson R, Van Houten H, Naessens J. Can anticipatory guidance and a preemptive prescription prevent ER visits for ear pain (abstract). Pediatric Academic Society Annual Meeting, April 30, 2006.
13. Sarrell EM, Mandelberg A, Cohen HA. Efficacy of naturopathic extracts in the management of ear pain associated with acute otitis media. Arch Pediatr Adolesc Med 2001;155:796–799
14. Narcy P, Reinert R, Olive G, et al. Therapeutic management and objective evaluation of pain in children consulting for acute pharyngeal pain (abstract). 7th International Symposium on Pediatric Pain. Vancouver, Canada: June, 2006.
15. Sagarin MJ, Roberts J. Acute Pharyngitis (correspondence). N Engl J Med 2001;344:1479–1480.
16. Bertin L, Pons G, d'Athis, et al. Randomized double-blind multicenter, controlled trial of ibuprofen versus acetaminophen for symptoms of tonsillitis and pharyngitis in children. J Pediatr 1991;119:811–814.
17. Garrick JG, Requa RK. Injuries in high school sports. Pediatrics 1978;61:465–467.
18. Clark E, Plint AC, Correll R, et al. A randomized controlled trial of acetaminophen, ibuprofen, and codeine for acute pain relief in children with musculoskeletal trauma. Pediatrics 2007;119:460–467
19. Engelbert RH, Bank RA, Sakkers RJ, et al. Pediatric generalized joint hypermobility with and without musculoskeletal complaints: A localized or systemic disorder? Pediatrics 2003;111:e248–254.
20. Schechter NL, Blankson V, Pachter LM, et al. The Ouchless Place: No pain, children's gain. Pediatrics 1997;99:890–894.
21. Zeltzer LK, Schlank CB. Conquering Your Child's Chronic Pain. New York: Harper Collins, 2005.
22. Kuttner L. A Child in Pain: How to Help, What to Do. Point Roberts, WA: Hartley and Marks, 1996.
23. Krane E, Mitchell D. Relieve Your Child's Chronic Pain: A Doctor's Program for Easing Headaches, Abdominal Pain, Fibromyalgia, Juvenile Rheumatoid Arthritis, and More. New York: Fireside, 2005.

7
Topical Anesthetics and Office-Based Procedures

William T. Zempsky and Neil L. Schechter

Abstract: Minor procedures performed by the primary care practitioner are a source of pain and anxiety for children and their families. This includes procedures such as injections, venipuncture, and bladder catheterizations. A paradigm which includes developmentally appropriate preparation, distraction, topical and local anesthesia, and complementary techniques will make the child more comfortable, calm the parent, and allow the procedure to be completed successfully.

Key words: Procedural pain, immunization, needle pain, children, topical analgesics.

Introduction

The primary care office is often the site of minor procedures which are a source of discomfort and worry for children and their families. Injections, phlebotomy, urinary catheterizations, nasal and throat swabs—all are annoyances at least, and for some children a major preoccupation, which dominates the medical encounter and limits the opportunity for relationship building and for calm health supervision. Research regarding strategies for improving the child's experience with these procedures has expanded during recent years. The clinician can use a variety of strategies including preparation, distraction, and the application of topical anesthesia to make these procedures go more smoothly.

1. Needle Procedures: Immunizations, Venous Access, and Heel Lance

While immunizations are certainly the predominant procedure performed in the outpatient office, clinicians who care for children may be called upon to perform venipuncture or venous access as well as heel lance procedures. At a minimum, they should understand and be able to counsel their patients on the approach to pain in these scenarios. Many strategies for reducing pain during these procedures are similar so they will be addressed together in this chapter.

All health care providers who work with children have encountered this scenario—a child eyeing them warily as they enter the room looking for evidence of the bulging pocket that hides the inevitable needle. Most children are afraid of needles and, by some estimates, 10 percent of children meet criteria for needle phobia [1, 2]. In fact, hospitalized children fear needles more than they do major surgeries [3]. Although injections have long been a part of pediatric practice, there has been a dramatic increase in the number of immunizations over the past 10 years. Now the average child may receive 20 immunizations in the first 2 years, and close to 30 throughout childhood. Therefore, it is likely that at least one injection will accompany every visit to the doctor in the early years. For children who are temperamentally predisposed, this creates the opportunity for significant anticipatory anxiety about the visit, inefficiency during it, and,

G.A. Walco and K.R. Goldschneider (eds.), *Pain in Children: A Practical Guide for Primary Care.*
© Humana Press, a part of Springer Science + Business Media, 2008

in general, a tension between the child and provider that inhibits good medical care.

There are strategies available from multiple sources that can reduce some of the pain associated with needle procedures. In general, techniques that are associated with pain reduction can be categorized based on when they are used (*prior to* or *during* the needle procedure).

1.1. Prior to the Needle Procedure

1.1.1. Preparation

Adequate preparation prior to procedures has been shown to decrease distress in the child and parent. There is an extensive literature supporting its efficacy for dental procedures, venipuncture and surgery [4–6], but there are few studies examining the impact of preparation for pediatric immunizations in the office. Extrapolating from those literatures, a number of recommendations regarding preparation can be made.

Parents should be fully informed about the reason for the procedure and given a realistic appraisal of the side effects and the pain associated with it. Parents should be queried about their perception of the child's coping style as well as what strategies might complement it. Finally, they should be taught techniques that they can use to "coach" their child through the pain of this and subsequent procedures. These strategies might include reading a favorite book to the child or telling favorite stories, breathing, blowing bubbles, or involving the child in a fantasy.

For children, preparation should be guided by the child's age, developmental level, and temperamental style. In general, specific content (what will happen and how it will feel) is far more relevant for children over the age of 2 years. For younger children (toddlers and preschoolers), preparation should occur as close to the time of the procedure as possible to prevent escalating anxiety. If possible, children should be given a choice for the type of distraction technique to use. For more detail on preparation for painful procedures, please see Chapter 10.

1.1.2. Site

For intramuscular injections, there is general agreement among most major professional organizations regarding the site of administration. In published consensus statements [7-10] most groups endorse the use of the anterior-lateral thigh in children under 18 months and the deltoid in children over 3 years of age. For children between 18 months and 2 years of age, there remains some debate among authorities.

These sites were chosen for theoretical reasons and not necessarily based on strong medical evidence. The anterolateral thigh was selected for infants because of its relatively large muscle mass and its lack of vital structures. The deltoid was chosen for older children because by age 3 its muscle mass is usually sufficient to allow for injection, and because some data suggest that injection in the thigh in older children is associated with more pain and incapacitation than the arm [11]. In practical terms injection pain in the thigh may prevent walking, which becomes problematic for parents as children grow in size.

There is a body of information, primarily sourced in the nursing literature, that suggests that a more appropriate site for immunizations in children of all ages is the ventrogluteal, or "hip," site [12, 13]. This site is identified by "placing the palm of your hand over the greater trochanter, index finger over the anterior-superior iliac tubercle, and middle finger along the posterior iliac crest." The needle should be injected perpendicularly into the center of the V formed by the fingers. A series of papers have supported its safety and lack of systemic reactions, but this site is not now endorsed by many major medical organizations [12, 13].

The best site for venipuncture and intravenous placement depends on many factors, one of the least of which is pain. Most practitioners would consider the antecubital fossa as a less painful area. However, this area is problematic for intravenous line placement because it is more difficult to restrict movement. It is likely that pain related to venous access procedures will be minimized by selecting an area where the vein can be accessed most easily and where stabilization of the site (if necessary) is assured. When there is a choice, venipuncture is preferable to heel lance for blood sampling in neonates, as it is clearly less painful.

1.1.3. Needle Type

For injections, although it may appear intuitive that a shorter needle will cause less pain, the available data suggest that the opposite is, in fact, true. Shorter needles seem to be associated with increased swelling, redness, and pain while longer needles are more likely to penetrate muscle and have fewer adverse effects. There has been some debate, however, about the exact length of needle necessary to penetrate muscle. Different research paradigms confounded further by different injection techniques have yielded differing conclusions. As a result, the Royal College of Paediatrics and Child Health felt there was insufficient evidence to make firm statements regarding needle length. The Red Book, however, suggests a needle length of 5/8″ for newborns to 2 months, and 1″ for infants. For toddlers and young children, it recommends 5/8″ to 1″ if the deltoid is used and 1¼″ if the anterolateral thigh is used. For adolescents, 1″ to 2″ needles are felt to be appropriate.

A few studies that suggest that the higher gauge (thinner) needle will cause the least amount of pain upon insertion for venous access procedures [14, 15]. Needle bevel design also seems to play a role, with bevels that provide easier penetration being less painful. Anecdotally, the technical skill of the clinician also plays a role in the pain of the procedure, but teasing out the factors associated with this skill is difficult.

For heel lance, several studies have demonstrated that automatic lancets reduce the pain and distress associated with this procedure [15–17]. In a comparison of automated devices, the BD QuikHeel® lancet (Becton Dickinson, New Jersey) was superior in reducing pain and ensuring procedure success. Again, heel lancing is a procedure where the skill of the clinician is key to minimizing distress; if blood flows smoothly, the procedure is completed quickly.

1.1.4. Injectate Properties

Different properties of the immunization itself may impact the pain associated with it. There has been very limited research in this area, although a few general principles can be garnered from the available work.

It appears that the higher the pH of the injectate, the less pain. This has been studied in the MMR where dramatic differences were identified between the commonly used MMR immunization and two different preparations, both of which had higher pHs. More research is necessary to see if

this principle can be applied to other immunizations.

There is ample evidence to show that injecting a colder substance appears to hurt more than injecting a warmer substance [18]. It would make sense to extrapolate this to immunizations, as many preparations are kept refrigerated until immediately before injection. Unfortunately, in the one study that examined this concept for immunizations, Maiden and colleagues [19] evaluated the pain in adults of a diphtheria-tetanus injection under three different conditions—cold, rubbed (between the palms for one minute) and warmed to body temperature. They found no difference in associated pain. Again, this is an area that requires additional research.

Finally, the type of diluent used may impact the discomfort associated with the injection. The MMR, varicella, and HIB vaccines are not premixed and require dilution. In research examining the impact of the diluent on other injections (ceftriaxone and benzathine penicillin), it is quite clear that using lidocaine instead of sterile water dramatically reduces pain associated with injection. Research on the impact of changing the diluent for immunizations is necessary before consideration of this practice can be entertained.

1.2. During the Procedure

1.2.1. Parental Demeanor

There is now strong evidence that one of the most critical factors in the child's response to an injection is the demeanor and attitude of his or her parent during the procedure [20–24]. Excessive reassurance, apologies, begging, pleading, and negotiating all seem to promote distress rather than alleviate it. Although the reasons for this phenomenon are not completely understood, children may interpret those responses as representing, at least, parental ambivalence toward the procedure and assume that intensification of their response may move the parent toward aborting the injection. The available literature supports maintaining a matter-of-fact attitude emphasizing humor, talk not related to the procedure, and "coaching" the child to use coping strategies [20–24]. Coping strategies should be discussed with the child and parent before the procedure, practiced at home, and put in place during the immunization. Such techniques promote mastery, compared to repeated expressions of sympathy which do not promote active coping.

1.2.2. Distraction

A number of distraction techniques for pain reduction are available with documented efficacy. For children, age and temperamental style will dictate the specific strategy employed. For infants, distraction consists primarily of stroking and softly talking to the child. For children over 3 years of age, a number of techniques utilizing breathing are available such as bubble blowing, different types of deep breathing, and the use of party blowers and pinwheels. Other distraction techniques for older children include reading a favorite book, telling familiar stories, and the active use of fantasy and reframing. Key to the success of these strategies is the appropriate match of the technique to the child's personality and coping style. The techniques work best when the child and parent collaborate, under non-stressful conditions to practice them, and to apply them when needed.

1.2.3. Topical Anesthetics

The choice of topical anesthetics has expanded in recent years (Table 7-1). These agents have been most well studied for venipuncture and venous access procedures, though some have been shown to be effective for injections as well. Unfortunately, none of these agents has been demonstrated to be successful for heel lance. Topical anesthetics use should be encouraged for all venous access procedures and, due to time and expense, topical anesthetic use for immunizations should be considered on a patient by patient basis.

The most commonly used topical anesthetics include EMLA® Cream (Eutectic Mixture of Local Anesthetics) and LMX4® (4% liposomal lidocaine). EMLA® has been extensively studied and is effective for a variety of procedures including venous cannulation, venipuncture, immunization, subcutaneous port access, and lumbar puncture. Though EMLA® has been associated with methemoglobinemia [25, 26], it has been shown to be safe when used appropriately, even in premature infants. EMLA® requires at least a 60 minute application time to provide adequate topical anesthesia. EMLA® does not affect immunogenicity when used prior to immunization.

LMX4® is a cream-based formulation and, when applied for 30 minutes, it has similar anesthetic efficacy for venous access and venipuncture to EMLA® applied for 60 minutes. Though the absence of prilocaine may make LMX4® inherently safer, there are limited data on the risk of systemic effects of this product especially, in infants and prematures. LMX4® has not been well studied for procedures outside of venous access.

Vapocoolant sprays such as ethyl chloride and flourimethane work in about 30 seconds and are inexpensive. There is contradictory evidence regarding their efficacy for injection pain and they have not been shown to be efficacious for venous access procedures [27–29]. Some children find their administration unpleasant.

The use of topical anesthetics in the primary care setting has been limited by speed of onset and cost. While cost still remains an issue, several new topical anesthetics provide more rapid anesthesia than currently available creams. These systems utilize different mechanisms that penetrate the stratum corneum and speed the onset of topical anesthesia.

Lidocaine iontophoresis (Numby Stuff® IOMED, Inc. and LidoSite™ Topical System, B. Braun Medical Inc.) provides anesthesia in about 10

TABLE 7-1. Topical anesthetics.

Drug	Brand name	Onset of action
Lidocaine/Prilocaine Cream	EMLA®	60 minutes
4% Liposomal Lidocaine	LMX4®	30 minutes
Lidocaine/Tetracaine Patch	Synera®	20–30 minutes
Lidocaine Iontophoresis	Lidosite®	10 minutes
Lidocaine Hydrochloride Monohydrate Product	Zingo®	1–3 minutes
Vapocoolant Spray	Pain Ease®	30 seconds

Note: Trade names are used for example only, and do not imply brand preference.

minutes. Iontophoresis is the transfer of charged molecules into the skin under the influence of electric current. Lidocaine, which is positively charged, can be delivered rapidly into the skin using iontophoresis. Lidocaine iontophoresis has been demonstrated to be superior to EMLA® as a topical anesthetic for venous access. Lidocaine iontophoresis also decreases the pain of injection, but has not been specifically evaluated for immunization pain. Lidocaine iontophoresis does not produce systemic lidocaine levels during routine use. However, some patients experience tingling, itching, or burning with this technology, which has limited its acceptance for lidocaine delivery.

Lidocaine Hydrochloride Monohydrate Product (Zingo™, Anesiva, Inc., South San Francisco) utilizes a prefilled, needleless system to deliver lidocaine for topical anesthesia. When the system is activated, compressed helium gas is released, which accelerates powdered lidocaine into the skin. Anesthesia is achieved painlessly in about one minute. Studies have not been done for injections, but some show efficacy for both venipuncture and venous access procedures [30, 31].

Lidocaine/tetracaine patch (Synera™, Endo Pharmaceuticals) includes a controlled heating system, which accelerates transcutaneous delivery and analgesic effect of local anesthetics. Anesthesia is achieved in 20 minutes for venous access. Tetracaine and the heat supplied by the patch both have vasodilatory effects which may facilitate venous access. This product has not been studied for immunization although the surface area of the patch is relatively large, making it potentially useful for this application.

1.2.4. Complementary Analgesia for Infants

Although sweetened liquids have been used empirically for pain reduction in infants for generations, recent studies have provided evidence for this phenomenon [32–36]. Administering a sucrose solution has been shown to reduce the pain of heel lance, venipuncture, and immunization for babies. Sucrose analgesia is effective in newborns and is present until babies are about 6 months old, at which time it is no longer measurable. Sucrose of various concentrations and glucose have all been shown to provide some pain relief for babies, but most studies use a 24 percent sucrose solution.

Sucrose can be instilled into the mouth using a syringe or via a sucrose-sweetened pacifier. This should be done one to two minutes prior to the procedure for optimal effect.

Non-nutritive sucking (sucking on a pacifier) has also been shown to provide analgesia in neonates undergoing procedures such as heel lance. In addition skin to skin contact and breastfeeding during the procedure have also been demonstrated to be analgesic. Given the safety of these methods, logistical barriers to their implementation should be eliminated.

For heel lance, in particular, swaddling of the infant has been shown to decrease the distress associated with the procedure. In addition, massaging the ipsilateral leg for 2 minutes prior to heel lance can decrease exhibited pain behaviors.

1.2.5. Physical Methods

Direct pressure at the injection site is another technique that reduces needle pain. It probably floods the painful area with non-noxious stimuli that effectively dilute the painful stimulus. Pressure can be applied either with a finger or with a device such as the Shot Blocker™—a horseshoe-shaped tufted plastic device through which the injection can be given. Both of these techniques have been studied and appear to offer modest pain reduction [37–39].

1.2.6. Simultaneous Injection

Some practitioners with adequate staff elect to give multiple injections simultaneously, as opposed to sequentially, when several immunizations are scheduled. Such an approach makes intuitive sense as it reduces anticipatory anxiety in the child. Studies examining the impact of this technique in young children and in older children both reached the same conclusion—obvious pain reduction could not be identified in the child, but parents clearly preferred simultaneous injections [40, 41].

2. Urinary Catheterization

Urinary catheterization, whether to collect a urine sample or as part of a diagnostic procedure, can be painful and anxiety provoking.

It is clear that preparation for both the parent and the child can markedly improve the success and outcome of the procedure. Preparation includes a complete explanation of the procedure, a definition of the parental role and some coaching for the child on relaxation techniques. For centers that have the capability, an experienced child life worker can support both the patient and the parent prior to and during the procedure. Distraction techniques as discussed in the previous section should be utilized.

Instillation of lidocaine *prior* to catheterization clearly reduces the pain associated with this procedure [42]. However, if lidocaine is used as a lubricant at the time of catheterization, this is less effective. To provide optimal anesthesia, a cotton ball soaked in lidocaine lubricant should be held at the urethral meatus for one to two minutes. Then, depending on the child's size, 0.5 to 2 cc of lubricant should be instilled into the urethra three times with two minutes of waiting time between each instillation. The bladder catheter is then passed through the urethra.

For infants undergoing catheterization, sucrose, non-nutritive sucking, and the opportunity for maternal contact should all be considered as part of the analgesic regimen. Urethral catheterization is less painful than suprapubic aspiration in this age group [43] and should be the procedure of choice for diagnostic urine collection.

In some children undergoing bladder catheterization for diagnostic imaging, sedation may be necessary. Common agents utilized in this setting include midazolam and nitrous oxide. These procedures should be completed according to published guidelines and with appropriate monitoring and expertise in place.

3. Summary and Other Procedures

There are a range of other procedures that are performed in the primary care setting, from wart and foreign body removal to throat swabs and nasal aspirates. Regardless of the procedure, the clinician should pay attention to the framework described in this chapter of developmentally appropriate preparation, distraction, topical and local anesthesia, and complementary techniques to make the procedure to be less painful and more comfortable for the child, thus leading to a successful result.

Take-Home Points

- Preparation of patient and family can reduce anxiety and pain of procedures
- Several topical anesthetics are available and can be used to good effect for needle procedures. Choosing among them is based on cost and timing considerations
- Distraction, swaddling, positive parental statements and a number of other simple interventions can help during painful procedures
- Physical considerations include needle length and gauge, type of diluent for injection, temperature of the injectate, and speed of injection

References

1. Agras S, Sylvester D, Oliveau D. The epidemiology of common fears and phobias. Compr Psychiatry 1969;10:151–156.
2. Fassler D. The fear of needles in children. Am J Orthopsychiatry 1985;55:371–377.
3. Menke E. School-aged children's perception of stress in the hospital. Child Health Care 1981;9:80–86.
4. Kolk AM, van Hoof R, Fiedeldij Dop MJ. Preparing children for venepuncture: The effect of an integrated intervention on distress before and during venepuncture. Child Care Health Dev 2000 26:251–260.
5. Melamed BG, Yurcheson R, Fleece EL, Hutcherson S, Hawes R. Effects of film modeling on the reduction of anxiety-related behaviors in individuals varying in levels of previous experience in the stress situation. J Consult Clin Psychol 1978;46: 1357–1367.
6. Kain ZN, Caldwell-Andrews AA. Preoperative psychological preparation of the child for surgery: An update. Anesth Clin N Am 2005;23:597–614.
7. Committee on Infectious Diseases, American Academy of Pediatrics. Red Book: 2003 Report of the Committee on Infectious Diseases, 26th ed. Elk Grove Village, IL: American Academy of Pediatrics, 2003.
8. Royal College of Paediatrics and Child Health. Position Statement on Injection Technique, 2002.
9. World Health Organization. Expanded Programme on Immunization. Geneva: World Health Organization, 1998.
10. County of Los Angeles Department of Public Health. Immunizations: Minimizing pain and maximizing comfort. The Public's Health 2001;1:1–2.
11. Ipp MM, Gold R, Goldbach MC, Maresky DC, Saunders N, Greenberg S, Davy T. Adverse reactions to diphtheria, tetanus, pertussis-polio vaccination at

18 months of age: Effect of injection site and needle length. Pediatrics 1989;83:679–682.

12. Cook IF, Murtagh J. Comparative reactogenicity and parental acceptability of pertussis vaccines administered into the ventrogluteal area and anterolateral thigh in children aged 2, 4, 6, and 18 months. Vaccine 2003;21:3330–3334.

13. Cook IF, Murtagh J. Ventrogluteal area: A suitable site for intramuscular vaccination in infants and toddlers. Vaccine 2006;24:2403–2408.

14. Arendt-Nielsen L, Egekvist H, Bjerring P. Pain following controlled cutaneous insertion of needles with different diameters. Somatosensory and Motor Research 2006;23:37–43.

15. Hefler L, Grimm C, Leodolter S, Tempfer C. To butterfly or to needle: The pilot phase. Ann Intern Med 2004;140:935–936.

16. Shah V, Taddio A, Kulasekaran K, O'Brien L, Perkins E, Kelly E. Evaluation of a new lancet device (BD QuikHeel) on pain response and success of procedure in term neonates. Arch Pediatr Adolesc Med 2003;157:1075–1078.

17. Vertanen H, Fellman V, Brommels M, Viinikka L. An automatic incision device for obtaining blood samples from the heels of preterm infants causes less damage than a conventional manual lancet. Arch Dis Child Fetal Neonatal Ed 2001;84:F53–55.

18. Bartfield JM, Crisafulli KM, Raccio-Robak N, Salluzzo RF. The effects of warming and buffering on pain of infiltration of lidocaine. Acad Emerg Med 1995;2:254–257.

19. Maiden MJ, Benton GN, Bourne RA. Effect of warming adult diphtheria-tetanus vaccine on discomfort after injection: a randomized controlled trial. Med J Aust 2003;178:433–436.

20. Schechter NL, Zempsky WT, Cohen LL, McGrath PJ, McMurtry CM, Bright N. Pain reduction and pediatric immunizations: Evidence-based review and recommendations. Pediatrics 2007;119:e1184–1198.

21. Manimala M, Blount RL, Cohen LL. The influence of parental reassurance and distraction on children's reactions to an aversive medical procedure. Child Health Care 2000;29:161–177.

22. Megel ME, Hesner R, Matthews K. Parents' assistance to children having immunizations. Issues Comp Pediatr Nurs 2002;25:151–165.

23. Duff AJA. Incorporating psychological approaches into routine paediatric venepuncture. Arch Dis Child 2003;88:931–937.

24. Eland JM. Minimizing pain associated with prekindergarten intramuscular injections. Issues Compr Pediatr Nurs 1981;5:361–372.

25. Gunter JB. Benefit and risks of local anesthetics in infants and children. Paediatric Drugs 2002;4:649–672.

26. Frayling IM, Addison GM, Chattergee K, Meakin G. Methaemoglobinaemia in children treated with prilocaine-lignocaine cream. BMJ 1990;301:153–154.

27. Reis EC, Holubkov R. Vapocoolant spray is equally effective as EMLA Cream in reducing immunization pain in school aged children. Pediatrics 1997;100:e5.

28. Abbott K, Fowler-Kerry S. The use of refrigerant anesthetic to reduce injection pain in children. J Pain Symptom Manage 1995;10:584–590.

29. Maikler VE. Effects of a skin refrigerant/anesthetic and age on the pain responses of infants receiving immunizations. Res Nurs Health 1991;14:397–403.

30. Zempsky WT, Bean-Lejewski J, Kauffman RE, Koh JL, Malviya SV, Rose JB, Richards PT, Gennevois DJ. Needle-free powder lidocaine delivery system provides rapid and effective analgesia for venipuncture or cannulation pain in children: The randomized double-blind COMFORT-003 trial. Pediatrics 2008;121:979–987.

31. Zempsky WT, Robbins B, Richards PT, Leong MS, Schechter NL. A study evaluating venipuncture pain in children receiving a novel needlefree powder lidocaine delivery system for rapid local analgesia. J Pediatr 2008;152:405–411.

32. Lewindon PJ, Harkness L, Lewindon N. Randomized controlled trial of sucrose by mouth for the relief of infant crying after immunization [comment]. Arch Dis Child. 1998;78:453–456.

33. Barr RG, Young SN, Wright JH, Cassidy KL, Hendricks L, Bedard Y, Yaremko J, Leduc D, Treherne S. Sucrose analgesia and Diptheria-Tetanus-Pertussis immunizations at 2 and 4 months. J Dev Behav Pediatr 1995;16:220–225.

34. Kracke GR, Uthoff KA, Tobias JD. Sugar solution analgesia: the effects of glucose on expressed mu opioid receptors. Anesth Analg 2005;101:64–68.

35. Anseloni VC, Ren K, Dubner R, Ennis M. A brainstem substrate for analgesia elicited by intraoral sucrose. Neuroscience 2005;133:231–243.

36. Gibbins S, Stevens B. Mechanisms of sucrose and non-nutritive sucking in procedural pain management in infants. Pain Res Manag 2001;6:21–28.

37. Barnhill BJ, Holbert MD, Jackson NM, Erickson RS. Using pressure to decrease the pain of intramuscular injections. J Pain Sympt Manage 1996;12:52–58.

38. Chung JW, Ng WM, Wong TK. An experimental study on the use of manual pressure to reduce pain in intramuscular injections. J Clin Nurs 2002;11:457–461.

39. Bernstein BA, Schechter NL, Bogin FJ, O'Donnell HD. Efficacy of a skin surface pressure device in reducing pain during immunization. Abstract:E:PAS2007:61:8402.5. Poster Presentation at the Annual

Meeting of the Pediatric Academic Societies, Toronto: May 8, 2007.

40. Bogin FJ, Bernstein BA, Payton JS, Schechter NL, Ristau B. A comparison of the pain associated with simultaneous (SIM) vs. sequential (SEQ) immunization injection given at the 9 and 12 month well child visits. Pediatr Res 2004;55:210A.

41. Horn MI, McCarthy AM. Children's responses to sequential versus simultaneous immunization injections. J Pediatr Health Care 1999;13:18–23.

42. Gerard LL, Cooper CS, Duethman KS, Gordley BM, Kleiber CM. Effectiveness of lidocaine lubricant for discomfort during pediatric urethral catheterization. J Urol 2003;170:564–567.

43. Kozer E, Rosenbloom E, Goldman D, Lavy G, Rosenfeld N, Goldman M. Pain in infants who are younger than 2 months during suprapubic aspiration and transurethral bladder catheterization: A randomized, controlled study. Pediatrics 2006;118: e51–56.

8

Analgesic Medications for Acute Pain Management in Children

John Barns Rose

Abstract: Pain is one of the most common complaints leading a parent or guardian to seek medical attention for their child. In addition to evaluating the child to determine the source for the pain, it is important for the pediatrician to be well versed in medications to manage acute pediatric pain to ensure that the child is comfortable. In this chapter the author presents an overview of oral analgesic medications useful in managing mild to moderate acute pediatric pain, as well as a discussion of intravenous analgesic therapy, including patient-controlled analgesia and continuous opioid infusions, for managing moderate to severe acute pain in children.

Key words: Analgesic, opioids, pharmacotherapy, acute pain, pediatric.

Introduction

Advances in developmental neurobiology and pediatric pharmacology, coupled with an expanding clinical experience in pediatric pain management, has resulted in a dramatic increase in methods to effectively treat acute pain in children of all ages [1].

Pain is termed "acute" or nociceptive when it results from tissue injury, inflammation, or infection. Usually acute pain is most severe initially and gradually resolves as the injured or inflamed tissue heals over the course of days to weeks. Nociception generally consists of four basic steps: transformation of a noxious inflammatory, mechanical, or thermal stimulus into a neural impulse in the periphery; transmission of the neural impulse from the periphery to the central nervous system; modulation (amplification or diminution) of the impulse in the central nervous system; and perception of the stimulus. Pharmacologic therapy can be targeted at one or more of these processes.

Pharmacogenetic differences among individuals also contribute to variability in the response to analgesic medications. This, in turn, can account for the clinical observation that some individuals appear to experience more or less pain than other individuals with a similar illness, surgery, or injury.

A good example of this is provided by codeine, one of the most commonly utilized oral analgesics in children. Codeine is a derivative of morphine that must undergo O-demethylation in the liver by a P-450 enzyme, CYP2D6, to form morphine as a metabolite. This conversion must occur for analgesia to result from codeine administration [2]. The parent molecule of codeine has no analgesic effects (see below). Between 4 to 10 percent of the population lacks the CYP2D6 enzyme required for this transformation and thus these individuals derive no analgesic benefit from codeine. Other genetic variations of CYP2D6 increase the conversion of codeine to morphine, resulting in increased analgesic effects as well as an increase in the incidence of adverse events. Data presently are coming forth regarding the pharmacogenetics of μ receptors, revealing differences in receptor number and response to morphine among individuals with various mutations [3].

Nociceptive or acute pain is usually responsive to antipyretic, analgesic, nonsteroidal anti-inflammatory agents (NSAIDs), opioids, regional anesthesia, and several nonpharmacological interventions (see

G.A. Walco and K.R. Goldschneider (eds.), *Pain in Children: A Practical Guide for Primary Care.*
© Humana Press, a part of Springer Science + Business Media, 2008

Chapters 2, 15, 16). Mild to moderate acute pain is often managed successfully with NSAIDs administered orally. For example, a recent study of acute musculoskeletal pain in children 6 to 17 years old found that while ibuprofen 10 mg/kg orally, acetaminophen 15 mg/kg orally, and codeine 1 mg/kg orally all resulted in analgesia, ibuprofen was the most effective analgesic in terms of the absolute reduction in pain score from baseline [4]. Moderate pain may require the addition of an oral opioid to the analgesic regimen. Moderate to severe pain may require the use of intravenous opioids to rapidly titrate medication to the desired effect (see below), followed by analgesic administration at regularly scheduled intervals, continuous infusion and/or programmable, computerized patient-controlled analgesia (PCA) pump.

The aim of this chapter is to provide a brief overview of the analgesic medications available for acute pain management in children, PCA, and continuous opioid infusions.

1. Nonsteroidal Anti-Inflammatory Drugs

NSAIDs are used for mild to moderate pain. They are used alone or in combination with opioids. Although they are often categorized as weak analgesics, for pain associated with tissue inflammation they may be superior to opioids. Their use is not associated with the common adverse reactions associated with opioid therapy: respiratory depression, sedation, physical dependence, nausea, vomiting, constipation, or pruritis. All NSAIDs work by inhibition of cyclooxygenase (COX), the enzyme responsible for metabolizing arachidonic acid. A number of factors can initiate an inflammatory reaction, including thermal or mechanical trauma, infectious agents, antigen–antibody complexes, or ischemia. Once released by traumatized or damaged cell membranes, arachidonic acid is metabolized by COX to form prostaglandins and thromboxanes. Prostaglandins and thromboxanes then sensitize peripheral nerve endings and vasodilate vessels causing pain, erythema, and inflammation. A number of COX isoenzymes have been identified. The constitutive form of COX (COX-1) is present throughout the body. Prostaglandins produced by

COX-1 are necessary for a variety of essential functions including: regulation of kidney blood flow, protection of gastric mucosa from damage secondary to gastric acid secretion, and platelet aggregation. Therefore, complications from the use of nonselective COX inhibitors such as ibuprofen, ketorolac, and naproxen include gastric ulceration, bleeding, and impaired renal function. The biggest risk factor for NSAID-induced renal failure is preexisting renal disease, so NSAID use in that situation should be pursued carefully, if at all. COX-2 is an inducible isoform of cyclooxygenase. It is induced by inflammatory mediators in traumatized cells. COX-2 is also a constitutive isoform since it is present in the brain and kidney in the absence of inflammation. Most NSAIDs are nonselective COX inhibitors. The theoretical advantages of using the COX-2 inhibitors relate to a reduction in the incidence of adverse drug reactions. Unfortunately, the initial enthusiasm for COX-2 inhibitors has been tempered by the observation of increased cardiovascular morbidity, myocardial infarction, and stroke due to thrombotic events in adults treated for prolonged periods with these drugs. As a result, two COX-2 inhibitors, rofecoxib and valdecoxib, were withdrawn from the market. At present, the future of COX-2 inhibitors in children is uncertain. There is little difference in analgesic efficacy between the many drugs that are now available. Choice of an agent depends upon other factors such as cost, the desired dosing interval, underlying medical conditions, and the patient's fasting status. Table 8-1 displays dosing and common dosage forms for a variety of NSAIDs.

1.1. Nonspecific Cyclooxegenase Inhibitors

1.1.1. Acetylsalicylic Acid (Aspirin)

Acetylsalicylic acid (aspirin) is the oldest NSAID. However, its use as an analgesic in pediatric patients has nearly stopped due to its association with Reye's syndrome. Aspirin is still used for some pediatric patients suffering from rheumatologic conditions [5].

1.1.2. Acetaminophen

Acetaminophen, the most widely used NSAID for the treatment of fever and pain, is different from

TABLE 8-1. Nonsteroidal anti-inflammatory drugs (NSAIDs).

Drug	Preparation	Dose	Interval	Maximum daily dose	Comments
Aspirin	Tabs: 81 mg, 325 mg Chewable tabs: 81 mg	PO: 10–15 mg/kg	PO: 4–6 hr	90 mg/kg/day	Not recommended for acute pediatric pain management
Acetaminophen	Tabs: 325 mg, 500 mg Chewable tabs: 80 mg, 160 mg Elixir: 160 mg/5 ml Drops: 80 mg/0.8 ml Suppositories: 80 mg, 120 mg, 325 mg, 650 mg	PO: 10–15 mg/kg Rectal (single dose): 35 – 45 mg/kg Rectal (repeated dose): 20 mg/kg	PO: 4 hr Rectal: 6 hr Rectal (premature newborns): 12 hr	Children: lesser of 90 mg/kg/day or 4 gm Infants: 75 mg/kg/day Newborns: (> 32 wks PCA): 60 mg/kg/day (28-32 PCA: 40 mg/kg/day	
Ibuprofen	Tabs: 200 mg, 400 mg, 600 mg, 800 mg Chewable tabs: 50 mg, 100 mg Elixir: 100 mg/5 ml Drops: 50 mg/1.25 ml	PO: 6–10 mg/kg	PO: 6–8 hr	Lesser of 40 mg/kg/day or 2.4 gm	
Naproxen	Tabs: 220 mg, 250 mg, 375 mg, 500 mg Elixir: 25 mg/ml	PO: 5–10 mg/kg	PO: 8–12 hr	20 mg/kg/day	
Etodolac	Tabs: 400 mg, 500 mg; Capsules: 200 mg, 300 mg; Extended release: 400 mg, 600 mg	PO: 5–10 mg/kg Extended release: 10-20 mg/kg	PO: 8–12 hours Extended release: 24 hours	PO and extended Release: 20 mg/kg/day	Approved for children 6–16 years old with JRA
Ketorolac	Injectable: 15 mg/ml, 30 mg/ml Tabs: 10 mg	IV: 0.5 mg/kg PO: 10 mg	IV: 6 hr PO: 6 hr	IV: Lesser of 2 mg/kg/day or 120 mg/day PO: 40 mg/day	Combined IV and PO maximum: 5 days of therapy or 20 doses

the other NSAIDs. High levels of peroxides in inflammatory tissue appear to inhibit the ability of acetaminophen to block COX. Peroxide concentrations are low in the brain, thus acetaminophen is an effective COX inhibitor centrally, a potent antipyretic, and a mild analgesic. Because it is a weak COX inhibitor in the periphery, it lacks the troublesome side effects of other NSAIDs, but it is a weak anti-inflammatory agent. In the United States, acetaminophen is available for oral or rectal administration. An intravenous preparation is available elsewhere. Of concern is the fact that acetaminophen is frequently misused, and acetaminophen overdose can lead to hepatic necrosis and failure [6]. Under normal circumstances, acetaminophen is metabolized in the liver primarily by glucuronidation and sulfation. However, in acetaminophen overdose, an oxidation pathway predominates via cytochrome P450. This oxidation pathway results in the production of a highly hepatotoxic metabolite.

1.1.3. Ibuprofen

Ibuprofen is another widely used drug in this class and is available in several formulations for pediatric administration. Adverse events are rare when used for a short time in treating acute pain and inflammation due to injury, infection, or illness. For analgesia, ibuprofen can be given as a single dose of 15 mg/kg orally. However, for repeated doses in children aged 6 months to 12 years, ibuprofen should be given orally as 10 mg/kg every 6 hours (maximum daily dose 40 mg/kg).

1.1.4. Naproxen

Naproxen has a longer half-life than ibuprofen, allowing it to be given every 8 to 12 hours. Its safety in newborns and infants has not been established. The usual dose is 5 to 10 mg/kg orally, administered every 8 to 12 hours (maximum daily dose 20 mg/kg).

1.1.5. Etodolac

Although etodolac is classified as a nonspecific COX inhibitor, it has been shown to be relatively selective for COX-2 in animals. It has also been approved for use in children 6 to 16 years old with juvenile rheumatoid arthritis. It is available in tablet form (etodolac 400 mg and 500 mg), capsules (etodolac

200 mg and 300 mg) and an extended release preparation (etodolac extended release 400 mg and 600 mg) allowing once per day dosing. The maximum daily dose is 20 mg/kg/day, which can be divided in doses every 8 to 12 hours, or it can be taken once per day with the extended release preparation.

1.1.6. Ketorolac

Ketorolac is the only NSAID available for intravenous and oral administration in the United States, making it useful in the treatment of postoperative pain in patients who are not able to take medications orally. However, caution is warranted in using ketorolac as acute renal failure, gastrointestinal bleeding, and hypersensitivity reactions have been reported in pediatric patients. Some conclude that short-term use (less than five days) of ketorolac 0.5 mg/kg intravenously every six hours (maximum dose = 30 mg) in children 1 to 16 years old who do not have any known contraindication to NSAID use is safe [7].

1.2. COX-2 Inhibitors

Selective COX-2 inhibitors, including celecoxib, have not been approved for use in pediatric patients, except for juvenile rheumatoid arthritis (see Chapter 23) in patients over 2 years of age.

2. Opioids

Opioids are the mainstays of treatment for moderate to severe nociceptive pain. Unlike NSAIDs, which act peripherally by enzyme inhibition, opioids exert their pharmacologic effects by binding to specific opiate receptors on pre- and postsynaptic cell membranes in the central nervous system, resulting in the inhibition of excitatory neurotransmitter release from presynaptic terminals and hyperpolarization of the postsynaptic neuronal membrane. Opiate receptors are linked to regulatory G proteins when bound to an opioid analgesic. By regulating ion channels, G proteins cause hyperpolarization of the neuron, rendering it less excitable. Several types and subtypes of opiate receptors have been identified. The μ receptor (so named because of its affinity for morphine) is found in the cortex, thalamus, and periaqueductal gray regions of the brain, as well as in the substantia gelatinosa of the spinal cord. The μ receptor has been further subtyped to include μ_1 (mediating supraspinal analgesia and dependence) and μ_2 (mediating respiratory depression, intestinal dysmotility, sedation, and bradycardia). Most opioids in clinical use today exert their analgesic effects when administered systemically at supraspinal μ receptors. However, with spinally administered opioids, effects are predominantly mediated by μ receptors in the substantia gelatinosa of the spinal cord. The κ receptor is found primarily in the substantia gelatinosa of the spinal cord, but is also found in the brain. It is associated with spinal analgesia, sedation, miosis, inhibition of antidiuretic hormone, and mild respiratory depression. The δ receptor mediates analgesia and euphoria and has been located in the pontine nucleus, amygdala, and deep cortex. Sigma (σ) receptor activation by some opioids, especially the mixed agonist–antagonist drugs like butorphanol and nalbuphine, is thought to mediate unpleasant psychomimetic effects, including dysphoria and hallucinations.

2.1. Agonists and Antagonists

An agonist binds and occupies a receptor site, initiating a change in cell function that produces a pharmacologic effect. Morphine, meperidine, fentanyl, oxycodone, and hydromorphone are all examples of opioid agonists. A partial agonist, e.g., buprenorphine, binds the opiate receptor (μ-receptor), but produces a reduced response compared to a pure agonist (e.g., morphine). Mixed agonist-antagonists, such as nalbuphine, are agonist at certain receptors (analgesia mediated via κ- and σ- receptors) and antagonists at others (μ receptor). The antagonists bind to a receptor (usually μ receptors), but do not result in a change in cell function. They do prevent access to the receptor by an agonist, thus "antagonizing" the action of the agonist. Examples of opioid antagonists include naloxone, naltrexone, and nalmefene.

2.2. Adverse Drug Reaction

The adverse drug reaction (ADR) profiles for all opioids in a study population look similar. So, in

answer to one of the more common questions parents ask: the risk of side effects or addictive potential between one opioid and another are similar. The most common opioid-related ADRs include nausea, vomiting, sedation, pruritis, urinary retention, respiratory depression, ileus, and constipation. Less common effects include myoclonic movement, dysphoria, hallucinations, and seizures. However, there is a great deal of variability in the incidence of these undesirable effects for specific opioids among individuals within a study population. "Opioid switching" is a term used for transitioning a patient who is experiencing an intolerable side effect or lack of efficacy due to one opioid analgesic, to another opioid in an attempt to improve tolerability and/or efficacy of opioid therapy for pain. Although this is a common practice and many believe it to be an effective strategy, there are no randomized, controlled trials to prove the efficacy of opioid switching. Thus, if a child who is receiving morphine experiences an intolerable side effect such as vomiting, it may be worthwhile to try a different opioid such as hydromorphone.

2.3. Recommended Doses

The recommended doses of several commonly used opioids are provided in Table 8-2. There is wide individual variability in analgesic response to opioids, so the doses recommended are intended to guide initial dosing. Careful and repeated assessment of patients receiving analgesics is required to determine analgesic efficacy and to look for analgesic complications. Commonly, the initial dose selected will need to be modified upward or downward based on clinical circumstances.

2.4. Morphine

Isolated from opium in the early 19th century and named for the Greek god of dreams (Morpheus), morphine is the standard opioid analgesic used for treating moderate to severe pain in children. It is conveniently administered by a number of routes for acute pain management: oral, subcutaneous, intramuscular, intravenous, epidural, intrathecal, and intra-articular. Morphine is primarily metabolized in the liver by glucoronidation to form an inactive (morphine-3-glucoronide, M3G) and an active metabolite (morphine-6-glucuronide, M6G).

TABLE 8-2. Opioid dosing regimens.

Opioid	Route/age group	Dose/interval
Morphine	Oral, immediate release: Infants and Children	0.3 mg/kg every 3–4 hr
	Oral, sustained release: Older Children and Adolescents	0.25–0.5 mg//kg every 8–12 hr
	IV Bolus:	
	Preterm neonate	10–25 mcg/kg every 2–4 hr
	Full-term neonate	25–50 mcg/kg/hr every 3–4 hr
	Infants and children	50–100 mcg /kg every 3 hr
	IV Infusion:	
	Preterm neonate	2–10 mcg/kg/hr
	Full-term neonate	5–20 mcg/kg hr
	Infants and children	15–30 mcg/kg/hr
Hydromorphone	Oral: Infants and children	40–80 mcg/kg every 4 hr
	IV bolus: Infants and children	10–20 mcg/kg every 3 – 4 hr
	IV infusion: Infants and children	3–5 mcg/kg/hr
Fentanyl	Oral transmucosal*	10–15 mcg/kg (oralet)
	Intranasal*	1–2 mcg/kg
	Transdermal*	12.5, 25, 50, 75, 100 mcg/hr patches
	IV bolus	0.5–1 mcg/kg every 1–2 hr
	IV infusion	0.5 mcg/kg/hr
Meperidine	IV bolus: Infants and children	0.5–1 mg/kg every 3–4 hr
Nalbuphine	IV bolus:	
	Preterm neonate	10–25 mcg/kg every 2–4 hr
	Full-term neonate	25–50 mcg/kg every 2–4 hr
	Infants and children	50–100 mcg/kg every 2–4 hr
Codeine	Oral	0.5–1 mg/kg every 4 hr
Oxycodone	Oral	0.1–0.15 mg/kg every 4 hr
Hydrocodone	Oral	0.1–0.2 mg/kg every 4 hr
Tramadol	Oral	1–2 mg/kg every 6 hr (Maximum dose: lesser of 100 mg or 2 mg/kg; Maximum daily dose: lesser of 400 mg or 8 mg/kg/day)

*Not recommended for acute pediatric pain management in outpatient, unmonitored settings, or in patients not already tolerant to opioids.

Both M3G and M6G are excreted by the kidneys. Although M6G is about 100 times more potent than the parent morphine compound in laboratory animals, it penetrates the blood-brain barrier less effectively, and in clinical practice it is only twice as potent as morphine. This fact can become significant in the face of renal insufficiency when M6G can accumulate, leading to central nervous system and respiratory depression. Several factors can predispose the preterm and even term neonate to an increased risk for respiratory and CNS depression with morphine therapy. First, clearance and elimination half-life are prolonged in the newborn. Though these functions mature quickly, reaching adult values by two months of age, a single dose of morphine can last longer and repeated doses can result in a dangerous accumulation of morphine and M6G. Second, the morphine is less protein bound, leading to an increased fraction of unbound, pharmacologically active drug to penetrate the blood-brain barrier. Therefore, it is important to monitor the degree of analgesia and the types and severity of side effects produced by any dose of morphine, and to adjust the dose and dosing interval accordingly [8–11].

2.4.1. Fentanyl

The highly lipophilic, phenylpiperidine-related, synthetic opioid, fentanyl readily penetrates the blood-brain barrier, and is 50 and 100 times more potent than morphine. After intravenous administration it has a relatively rapid onset and short offset due to rapid redistribution to pharmacologically inactive sites, making it a preferred analgesic for short, painful procedures when close monitoring of the patient's vital signs and mental status is possible, and when personnel with expertise in airway support and management are immediately available.

It is not useful for routine acute pediatric pain management outside of direct medical supervision. Fentanyl actually has a relatively long total body elimination half-life: 233 ± 137 minutes in three- to 12-month-old infants, 244 ± 79 minutes in infants aged over one year and 129 ± 42 minutes in adults [12]. This means that with high doses, repeated doses, or continuous infusions, fentanyl can saturate pharmacologically inactive sites and accumulate in the plasma. Duration of effects such as analgesia and respiratory depression then become dependent upon fentanyl's metabolism and excretion, and not redistribution. In practice, this phenomenon may present as persistent sedation in a patient who had received an infusion of fentanyl after the infusion is discontinued. The term "context-sensitive halftime" is used to describe this change in pharmacokinetics. Like morphine, fentanyl undergoes glucoronidation in the liver, but all metabolites are pharmacologically inactive making it safe for administration to patients with renal insufficiency and failure. The inactive metabolites are primarily excreted by the kidney. Also like morphine, fentanyl is highly bound to α_1-acid glycoprotein in the plasma. Thus, newborns who have reduced α_1-acid glycoprotein have a higher percentage of free unbound fentanyl, increasing its potential for CNS and respiratory depression.

In addition to intravenous and epidural administration, fentanyl can be administered by intranasal, transmucosal, and transdermal routes. Fentanyl is also available in a candy matrix (fentanyl oralet) for transmucosal absorption and is administered as a premedication for children undergoing painful procedures. Transmucosal absorption is approximately 25 to 33 percent, bypasses the hepatic first-pass effect, and is therefore more efficient than oral administration. Analgesic effects begin within 20 minutes of transmucosal administration and last for approximately 2 hours. If somnolence is observed the oralet should be taken away from the child.

Fentanyl can be administered transcutaneously by a patch that consists of a semipermeable membrane and a drug reservoir. The fentanyl patch is applied to the skin with a contact adhesive. The patches come in a variety of strengths to deliver fentanyl at a rate of 12.5, 25, 50, 75 or 100 µg/h for three days. There is a relatively long time to onset, but after the patch is removed a small depot of fentanyl remains in the skin. The fentanyl patch and the fentanyl oralet are not appropriate for opioid-naive patients with acute pain at home or any medically unsupervised setting since the analgesic effects cannot be safely titrated or, in the case of the fentanyl patch, rapidly achieved.

2.4.2. Hydromorphone

Hydromorphone is one of many semisynthetic derivatives of morphine made by a simple modification of the parent compound. This modification makes hydromorphone 10 times more lipophilic and five times more potent than morphine. It has a similar duration of action (four to five hours) and plasma half-life (two to three hours) as morphine [13]. Preparations exist for oral, subcutaneous, intramuscular, intravenous, and epidural administration (see Table 8-2). Many clinicians familiar with this drug believe that it is associated with less nausea, vomiting, and pruritis than morphine when administered in equianalgesic doses. Others believe there is no significant difference in adverse drug reactions between the two drugs.

2.4.3. Meperidine

Meperidine, like fentanyl, is a synthetic opioid related to phenylpiperidine. Unlike fentanyl, however, meperidine is only one-tenth as potent as morphine. Meperidine undergoes hepatic metabolism by hydrolysis and N-demethylation producing an active metabolite—normeperidine—which is one-half as potent as an analgesic, but has the potential to cause seizures. It is rarely used for acute pediatric pain management since repeated administration may result in normeperidine accumulation and produce tremors or seizures. A potentially fatal syndrome of excitation, delirium, hyperpyrexia, and convulsions has been seen in patients who received meperidine concomitantly with monoamine oxidase inhibitors and in patients with hyperthyroidism. It is still used to treat postoperative shivering, as well as shivering associated with amphotericin or blood product administration.

2.4.4. Methadone

Methadone is better known for its treatment of opioid abstinence syndromes in adults than it is for acute pediatric pain management. It is a synthetic opioid that has a single-dose potency similar to morphine. Even though it has the longest and most unpredictable elimination half-life (15 to 40+ hours), there is some interest in using methadone for acute postoperative pain management in children because it can produce stable blood levels for prolonged periods of time, can be administered every 6 to 12 hours, and has an excellent bioavailability (around 80 percent) after oral administration. The usual starting dose is 0.1 mg/kg orally and 0.05 to 0.1 mg/kg intravenously. Analgesia can be seen within 10 to 20 minutes following intravenous administration, and in 30 to 60 minutes after oral administration. Thus, titrating methadone with incremental doses of 0.05 mg/kg IV every 15 to 20 minutes is possible. Once satisfactory analgesia is achieved, additional methadone at 0.05 to 0.1 mg/kg IV can be administered every 6 to 12 hours as needed. Due to accumulation (leading to delayed sedation) and the potential for prolonging the cardiac QT interval, methadone is recommended for use by persons with expertise in its use and monitoring.

2.4.5. Codeine

Codeine is a synthetic derivative of morphine and one of the most commonly prescribed oral analgesics in pediatric patients. Although it has an oral bioavailability of 60 percent, codeine has a very low affinity for opiate receptors and the parent compound is not responsible for the observed analgesia. As noted in the introduction, about 5 to 10 percent of administered codeine is converted into morphine after O-demethylation in the liver by a P-450 oxidase pathway. Up to 10 percent of patients in some populations lack the enzyme that converts codeine to morphine, and these individuals get no analgesic benefit from codeine. Analgesic effects are seen within 20 minutes with peak effects at between one and two hours in individuals capable of the codeine-to-morphine conversion. Its elimination half-life is 2.5 to 3 hours.

Codeine is usually administered with acetaminophen for conditions that are moderately painful. Careful attention should be paid to the acetaminophen dose when administering formulations of codeine combined with acetaminophen to avoid acetaminophen toxicity. Because a significant number of people do not experience analgesic benefits from codeine, and because codeine is associated with severe nausea and vomiting in some patients, we prefer to use oxycodone as a first-line oral opioid analgesic in children. Only when a child has been on codeine in the past, and the family requests codeine because it worked well, do we continue to prescribe this drug.

2.4.6. Oxycodone and Hydrocodone

Oxycodone and hydrocodone are semisynthetic thebaine derivatives structurally related to morphine. They are available in liquid and tablet form alone or in combination with acetaminophen. Oxycodone is also now available in combination with ibuprofen. Oxycodone is roughly 1.5 times *more* potent than oral morphine (or 15 times more than codeine), and hydrocodone is about 1.5 times *less* potent (or 7 times more than codeine). After oral administration, they have a bioavailability of 60 percent. Analgesia begins within 20 to 30 minutes and peaks at between 1 and 2 hours. They have an elimination half-time of 2.5 to 4 hours and duration of effect of 4 to 5 hours. Oxycodone and its active metabolite oxymorphone may accumulate in patients with renal insufficiency, leading to respiratory depression if the dose and interval are not adjusted. A sustained-release form of oxycodone is available, but many families resist this drug because of the negative press it has received related to its abuse. The sustained action forms of oxycodone and morphine are not generally for use in opioid naïve patients, and the tablet forms must be swallowed whole.

2.4.7. Tramadol

An atypical opioid, tramadol is an effective and safe analgesic for acute pain in children [14, 15]. The primary mechanism for producing analgesia is tramadol's central inhibition of norepinephrine and serotonin reuptake. Weak μ-receptor agonism is thought to be a secondary mechanism resulting in analgesia. Tramadol is estimated to be 10 to 15 times less potent than morphine and has a favorable side effect profile compared to other opioid analgesics, making it an attractive alternative for analgesic therapy in children. It does not cause respiratory depression, sedation, or constipation. Nausea, vomiting, and dizziness may occur as frequently as with other opioid analgesics. Seizures are a rare complication of tramadol therapy. Exceeding dosing guidelines, prescribing tramadol in patients taking psychoactive medications (tricyclic antidepressants, selective serotonin reuptake inhibitors, monoamine oxidase inhibitors and neuroleptics, and other drugs known to reduce seizure thresholds), and administering tramadol to patients with a known seizure disorder or head injury, all appear to increase the risk for seizures. Tramadol is available as a 50 mg scored tablet. It is also available in combination with acetaminophen (37.5 mg tramadol/325 mg acetaminophen). The recommended dose of tramadol is 1 to 2 mg/kg (maximum dose 100 mg) every 6 hours (maximum daily dose the lesser of 8 mg/kg/day or 400 mg/day).

2.4.8. Nalbuphine

The mixed μ-receptor antagonist and κ-receptor agonist, nalbuphine is often used to antagonize opioid-related, μ-receptor mediated adverse drug reactions such as pruritus, nausea, vomiting, and urinary retention. Nalbuphine is also occasionally used to treat pain because it produces analgesic effects through κ-receptor agonism and, thus, theoretically may have an advantage over the μ-receptor agonists in treating patients with pain secondary to biliary tract pathology, or pain due to intestinal dysmotility. Nalbuphine doses up to 200 mcg/kg IV are roughly equivalent to morphine with respect to analgesia. However, increasing the nalbuphine dose beyond this point does not result in greater analgesia (the "ceiling effect"). κ-mediated effects (e.g., sedation, dysphoria and euphoria) may occur with increasing doses or with repetitive lower doses. Other primarily μ-mediated effects such as physical dependence are reported much less frequently with chronic nalbuphine administration. Patients receiving μ agonists for long periods may experience withdrawal symptoms if they are treated with nalbuphine. Nalbuphine is primarily administered intravenously, but has been administered orally. Oral bioavailability is only 20 to 25 percent. It undergoes hepatic metabolism and has an elimination half-life of 5 hours.

2.4.9. Naloxone

Naloxone is a potent μ, δ, and κ antagonist. It is used to antagonize respiratory depression and coma due to opioid overdose (naloxone 10 μg/kg SC or IV) and in lower doses (naloxone 0.25 to 2 μg/kg/h IV) it is useful in treating sedation, nausea and vomiting, urinary retention, or, most commonly, intractable pruritus associated with opioid administration [16]. A syndrome of hypertension, tachycardia, dyspnea, tachypnea, pulmonary edema, nausea, vomiting, and ventricular fibrillation has been reported in opioid-dependent patients, or in patients who are receiving high doses of opioids for severe pain and who receive excessive doses of naloxone rapidly for the treatment of respiratory depression and coma. It is preferable in these circumstances to provide ventilatory assistance while titrating smaller amounts of naloxone (0.5 to 1 μg/kg IV, repeated at one minute intervals) to the desired effect. Naloxone is rapidly metabolized in the liver and has a plasma elimination half-life of 60 minutes. Therefore, its duration of action is less than that of the μ agonists it is intended to antagonize. Continued close observation is required in all patients who have received naloxone to reverse respiratory depression to prevent a catastrophic return of respiratory depression when the effects of naloxone are gone.

3. Approaches to Opioid Use

Intravenous analgesic therapy is often the safest and quickest way to effectively manage severe acute pain in children. A key, practical concept is *titration*. As discussed, each child may respond differently to an opioid; cause and the intensity of pain may also differ, and the margin of respiratory reserve may be slim in some circumstances. By giving smaller doses of opioid than typically listed in textbook tables (e.g., 0.05 mg of morphine every 10 minutes IV, rather than a single dose of 0.1 mg/kg), and reassessing the patient before repeating the dose, comfort can be achieved without excessive sedation or respiratory compromise. Just as one can titrate an acid against a base to neutralize it, opioids can be used to titrate against pain without compromising safety. Oral analgesics have a delayed onset of action and it is difficult to titrate oral opioids quickly to the desired level of analgesia for children experiencing severe pain, particularly if they are at home or in the office setting. Because their peak effects may not be seen for 1 to 2 hours after dosing, repeating oral opioid doses over short periods of time can result in delayed respiratory and CNS depression as these drugs accumulate. Thus, hospitalization for intravenous analgesic therapy is sometimes warranted. In this section patient-controlled analgesia (PCA) and continuous intravenous opioid infusions will be discussed briefly. It should be mentioned that strict adherence to institutional policies regarding monitoring patients receiving intravenous opioids continuously or by PCA is mandatory.

3.1. Patient-Controlled Analgesia

Patient-controlled analgesia is suitable for use in hospitalized children with acute pain over 6 years old in moderate to severe pain. Computerized PCA infusion pumps allow the patient to self-administer opioids by using a button, which when pressed or activated delivers a prescribed dose of an opioid "on demand."

PCA requires that several parameters for the individual patient be established including a demand dose, lockout interval, continuous or basal infusion (if any), and a 1-hour limit (see Table 8-3). The demand dose is the dose of analgesic programmed for the patient to receive during a given time period or lockout interval, as long as the patient has not exceeded the programmed 1-hour limit of opioid. A typical lockout interval for most opioids is 7 to 10 minutes and, during this time, the patient may only receive one demand dose regardless of the number of attempts to activate the demand button. At our institution we typically program a maximum of five demand doses per hour when a standard demand dose is ordered. It is also possible to program a continuous (basal) infusion of opioid which the patient will receive in addition to any demand doses administered. The pump records the patient's history of attempts and

actual opioid injections, allowing caregivers to adjust analgesic delivery based on patient need.

Over the course of time patients are able to maintain a more stable plasma opioid level, resulting in lower peaks and higher troughs in plasma opioid levels when compared to regimens where opioids are administered intermittently on an every 3- to 6-hour basis. Obviously, avoiding the peak opioid levels in these circumstances may reduce the incidence of ADRs such as respiratory and CNS depression. Avoiding the troughs in plasma opioid levels associated with intermittent opioid administration can result in fewer episodes of severe "breakthrough pain." PCA is effective because it allows patients (or proxies, see below) to titrate the amount of analgesic they desire based on the amount of pain they are experiencing.

PCA is considered safe since the individual demand doses are relatively small and, if the patient begins to get sleepy due to frequent PCA demand dose administration, the patient will drop the button and stop activating the PCA pump until he or she is more awake and experiencing more pain. PCA is highly satisfactory to patients, families, and nursing staff because it is safe, effective and it gives patients some control over managing their pain [17]. If another individual (family member or hospital staff) pushes the demand button for a sleeping patient, CNS and respiratory depression can ensue. Thus, only the patient is allowed to use the PCA button unless the institution in question has a PCA by proxy (parent or nursing PCA) policy. Only after nurses and parents have completed a formal, structured orientation about PCA by proxy should this intervention be instituted. PCA by proxy has been shown to provide effective and safe analgesia to patients younger than 6 years old, as well as children with cognitive and physical disabilities who would otherwise not be able to use PCA [18].

TABLE 8-3. Guidelines for computerized PCA infusion pumps in children.

Drug	Demand dose (mcg/kg)	Lockout interval (min)	Basal infusion (mcg/kg/hr)	1 hour limit (mcg/kg)
Fentanyl	0.25	7–8	0–0.15	4
Morphine	20	7–8	0–20	100
Hydromorphone	4	7–8	0–4	20

3.2. Continuous Opioid Infusions

Continuous intravenous opioid infusions are frequently used to control moderate to severe pain in hospitalized children who are unable to use a PCA pump effectively due to physical or cognitive impairments or those who are less than 6 years old [19]. As with PCA infusions, continuous opioid infusions provide a more stable plasma opioid level than opioids administered intermittently and thus may result in fewer ADRs and more effective analgesia. The recommended starting doses for morphine and hydromorphone are the same as the basal infusion rates for those drugs listed in Table 8-3.

4. Nontraditional Analgesics

Other classes of medications are thought by many to possess analgesic properties, or at least to be beneficial in a variety of conditions resulting in chronic pediatric pain. However, there is little to guide the clinician in the pharmacologic management of chronic pain in children because there are no large, randomized, controlled trials. Most of the evidence to support the use of these medications in children is extrapolated from experience in adults suffering from chronic pain.

4.1. Antidepressants

The analgesic effect of antidepressants in adults with chronic pain has been appreciated for some time and is the subject of many systematic reviews. Antidepressants have been used for a variety of conditions including: diabetic neuropathy, postherpetic neuralgia, trigeminal neuralgia, atypical facial pain, headaches, back pain, complex regional pain syndrome I & II, fibromyalgia, and other neuropathic pain conditions. Use of tricyclic antidepressants (TCA) is still common, as the initial enthusiasm for the newer agents (i.e., selective serotonin reuptake inhibitors [SSRI] and selective serotonin and norepinephrine reuptake inhibitors [SSRNI]) has waned, though newer antidepressants are generally better tolerated than TCAs, because they may be less effective in alleviating pain.

One report that supports the use of antidepressants in children with chronic pain involves the use of amitriptyline 0.25 to 1 mg/kg orally at bedtime for headache prophylaxis [20]. This study involved 192 children 12 ± 3 years old with migraine, migraine with aura or tension headache. Follow-up was available in 146 children a mean of 67 ± 32 days after initiating therapy. The frequency decreased from roughly 17 to 9 headaches per month. The severity and duration of headache were also reduced. The authors reported that amitriptyline was well tolerated with few side effects reported by the patients studied.

It should be remembered that the analgesic efficacy of amitriptyline and other antidepressants has not been established in children. However, many experienced clinicians believe that antidepressants may reduce pain and help with insomnia, reactive depression, and anxiety which often accompany chronic pain conditions. A few general precautions should be emphasized for consideration prior to initiating TCA therapy. In menstruating adolescents, a pregnancy test should be considered prior to initiating antidepressant therapy since antidepressants should not be used during the first trimester of pregnancy.

When antidepressant therapy is initiated in children and adolescents, regular face-to-face assessments are required to monitor for suicidal ideation since there is an increased risk for suicide in this population after antidepressant therapy is started. It is recommended that these evaluations occur weekly for 4 weeks, then monthly for 3 months, and as needed thereafter. Serious consideration should be given to obtaining a consultation with a child psychiatrist prior to initiating antidepressant therapy in children and adolescents. A complete history and physical exam should be performed, and 12 lead EKG should be considered to rule but conduction disturbances such as prolonged QT syndrome, since concomitant use of TCAs in this population increases the risk for tacchyarrhythmias, and sudden death has been reported. Common adverse drug reactions associated with TCA use include daytime sedation, dry mouth, tachycardia, and dizziness. These typically occur at relatively low doses early in treatment. Many patients adapt to these effects without a dose adjustment. Less common adverse effects which are associated with long-term therapy at higher doses and require a reduction in dose, include urinary hesitancy, blurred vision, and constipation. Abrupt cessation of TCA therapy after prolonged use can result in a withdrawal syndrome. Symptoms including insomnia, dysphoria, agitation, diaphoresis, abdominal cramps, and diarrhea may occur. Therefore, if the patient has been on relatively high doses for a many months, TCAs should be tapered gradually before discontinuation.

The best guide to therapy is the patient's clinical response. There are no data that correlate dose with desired effects. In general a low dose is started and increased every three to four days until the desired effect is achieved or an intolerable side effect is experienced. Patients who experience a beneficial effect often do so within a week of initiating therapy. The most commonly employed TCA and initial dosing in our practice is amitriptyline 0.25 mg/kg (maximum amitriptyline dose 1 mg/kg) orally at bedtime. However, if sedative effects are to be minimized, nortriptyline, desipramine, or imipramine can be used.

4.2. Anticonvulsants

Anticonvulsants, like antidepressants, have been the subject of many systematic reviews in adult patients which suggest modest analgesic efficacy for a variety of chronic and neuropathic pain conditions [21]. There are no RCTs of anticonvulsant therapy for chronic pediatric pain conditions. However, anticonvulsants are frequently used alone or in combination with a TCA for chronic pediatric pain. The major limitations to anticonvulsant use are the potential for disturbing side effects such as dizziness, unsteady gait, drowsiness, and exacerbation of behavioral disorders. Infrequently more serious adverse events occur with some anticonvulsants, including bone marrow suppression and hepatic dysfunction. Because gabapentin has the most favorable adverse event profile, it has become the preferred anticonvulsant for chronic pediatric pain.

Analgesic efficacy of gabapentin has been reported in a variety of chronic pediatric pain conditions including complex regional pain syndrome, cancer pain, phantom limb pain, and other neuropathic conditions. It is available as an elixir (250 mg/ 5 mL), capsules (100 mg, 300 mg, and 400 mg) and tablets (600 mg and 800 mg). The dosing is ramped up over three days to avoid unpleasant side effects including dizziness, unsteady gait, and drowsiness. On day one the initial dose is gabapentin 5 mg/kg orally at bedtime; on day two, gabapentin 5 mg/kg

orally every 12 hours is administered, and on day three and thereafter, gabapentin is administered in a dose of 5 mg/kg orally every 8 hours. The dose can be increased incrementally on a weekly basis until the desired effect is achieved or to a maximum dose of gabapentin 15 mg/kg orally every 8 hours. Monitoring CBC and hepatic function tests is not necessary. Gabapentin should be weaned off when the course of therapy is completed, as cases of withdrawal phenomena have been seen [22]. Other anticonvulsants such as oxcarbazepine and pregabalin have anecdotal support for use in children and young adults. The use of topiramate for headaches is outlined in Chapter 18.

Take-Home Points

- A wide range of opioid, NSAID and nontraditional medications are available to treat a variety of pain types.
- Titration is an optimal way to approach opioid dosing, to maximize comfort and safety, while minimizing side effects.
- Many adverse effects of opioids are idiosyncratic, so changing from one to another can resolve many problems such as itching, dysphoria, and nausea.
- Patient-controlled analgesia is a safe and effective mode of treatment for children 7 years and older, with PCA by proxy appropriate under limited circumstances.
- Nontraditional analgesics such as anticonvulsants and antidepressants have a role in certain pain conditions, and can be effective and safe when used with care.

References

1. Berde CB, Sethna NF. Analgesics for the treatment of pain in children. N Engl J Med 2002;347:1094–1103.
2. Caraco Y, Sheller J, Wood AJ. Pharmacogenetic determination of the effects of codeine and prediction of drug interactions. J Pharmacol Exp Ther 1996;278:1165–1174.
3. Chou WY, Wang CH, Liu PH, Liu CC, Tseng CC, Jawan B. Human opioid receptor A118G polymorphism affects intravenous patient-controlled analgesia morphine consumption after total abdominal hysterectomy. Anesthesiology 2006; 105:334–337.

4. Clark E, Plint AC, Correll R, et al. A randomized, controlled trial of acetaminophen, ibuprofen and codeine for acute pain relief in children with musculoskeletal trauma. Pediatrics 2007;119:460–467.

5. Cron RQ, Sharma S, Sherry DD. Current treatment by United States and Canadian Pediatric Rheumatologists. J Rheumatol 1999;26:2036–2038.

6. Dlugosz CK, Chater RW, Engle JP. Appropriate use of nonprescription analgesics in pediatric patients. J Pediatr Health Care 2006;20:316–325.

7. Houck CS, Wilder RT, McDermott JS, Sethna NF, Berde CB. Safety of intravenous ketorolac therapy in children and cost savings with a unit dosing system. J Ped 1996;129:292–296.

8. Kart T, Christrup LL, Rasmussen M. Recommended use of morphine in neonates, infants, and children based on the literature: Part 1 - pharmacokinetics. Paediatr Anaesth 1997;7:5–11.

9. Kart T, Christrup LL, Rasmussen M. Recommended use of morphine in neonates, infants, and children based on the literature: Part 2 - clinical use. Paediatr Anaesth 1997;7:93–101.

10. Hunt A, Joel S, Dick G, et al. Population pharmacokinetics of oral morphine and its glucoronides in children receiving morphine as immediate-release liquid or sustained-release tablets for cancer pain. J Pediatr 1999;135:47–55.

11. Bouwmeester NJ, Anderson BJ, Tibboel D, et al. Developmental pharmacokinetics of morphine and its metabolites in neonates, infants, and young children. Br J Anaesth 2004;92:208–212.

12. Singleton MA, Rosen JI, Fisher DM. Plasma concentrations of fentanyl in infants, children, and adolescents. Can J Anaesth 1987;34:152–155.

13. Quigley C, Wiffen P. A systematic review of hydromorphone for acute and chronic pain. J Pain Symptom Manage 2003;25:169–178.

14. Finkel JC, Rose JB, Schmitz ML, Birmingham PK, Ulma GA, Gunter JB, Cote CJ, Cnaan A, Medve RA, Schreiner MS. Evaluation of the efficacy and tolerability of oral tramadol hydrochloride tablets for the treatment of post surgical pain in children. Anesth Analg 2002;94:1469–1473.

15. Rose JB, Finkel JF, Arguedas-Mohs A, Himelstein BP, Schreiner MS, Medve RA. Oral tramadol for the treatment of pain of 7-30 days duration in children. Anesth Analg 2003;96:78–81.

16. Kendrick WD, Woods AM, Daly MY, et al. Naloxone versus nalbuphine infusion for prophylaxis of epidural morphine-induced pruritus. Anesth Analg 1996;82:641–647.

17. Berde CB, Lehn BM, Yee JD, et al. Patient-controlled analgesia in children and adolescents: a randomized, prospective comparison with intramuscular administration of morphine for post-operative pain in children. J Pediatr 1991;118:460–466.

18. Monitto CL, Greenberg RS, Kost-Byerly S, et al. The safety and efficacy of parent-nurse-controlled analgesia in patients less than 6 years of age. Anesth Analg 2000;91:573–579.

19. Esmail Z, Montgomery C, Courtrn C, et al. Efficacy and complications of morphine infusions in postoperative paediatric patients. Paediatr Anaesth 1999;9:321–327.

20. Hershey AD, Powers SW, Bentii AL, et al. Effectiveness of amitriptyline in the prophylactic management of childhood headaches. Headache 2000;40:539–549.

21. Chong MS, Hester J. Diabetic painful neuropathy: current and future treatment options. Drugs 2007;67:569–585.

22. Norton JW. Gabapentin withdrawal syndrome. Clin Neuropharmacol 2001;24:245–246.

9
Pain Management in the Emergency Department
A Primer for Primary Care Providers

Michael K. Kim

Abstract: Pediatric emergency departments (ED) have become much more focused on the evaluation and treatment of painful conditions in children. Evidence-based pain management with nonpharmacologic and pharmacologic interventions are provided routinely for children in pain and in need of painful procedures. Implementing the multidisciplinary team approach in the ED will ensure decreased anxiety and pain during the evaluation in the ED. Approaches to procedural sedation and analgesia, simple painful procedures and abdominal pain in EDs have gained significant advances and will be a great resource for primary care providers. This chapter reviews significant advances in pain management in the ED and offers recommendations that will assist primary care physicians to provide the best and expeditious care for acutely ill or injured children with pain.

Key words: Emergency department, acute pain, trauma, acute abdomen.

Introduction

With the explosion of clinical advances over last 25 years, pain management in pediatric practices and pediatric emergency medicine has also flourished. The most significant study findings of importance are the long-term negative impacts such as alteration of pain response and perception after unrelieved acute pain, as well as increased pain score during subsequent procedures after inadequate pain management during the initial painful procedure [1–4]. The prevalence of pain complaints in children visiting primary care facilities, outpatient care centers or EDs is significant. Most children with mild pain may be cared for at the primary health care facility. However, children with moderate to severe pain usually require urgent and comprehensive assessment and intervention, including aggressive pain management. The limitations of primary care facilities for these patients include lack of: monitoring equipment and personnel, diagnostic and intervention equipment, effective pain medications, time for observation, and direct access to consultants. Guided by the advances in pain research, pediatric emergency departments have incorporated a variety of interventions to provide immediate and comprehensive pain assessment and interventions for many painful conditions. In this chapter we will review some of the significant advances in pain management in the ED and offer recommendations to assist primary care physicians with providing the best and expeditious care for acutely ill or injured children with pain.

1. Advances in ED Pain Management

There are several areas of advancement in pain management in the ED setting that may be of importance to primary care physicians, including procedural sedation and analgesia, simple procedural pain management, and abdominal pain management.

1.1. Procedural Sedation and Analgesia

The preferred term of "procedural sedation and analgesia" (PSA) refers to administration of sedative, analgesic, or dissociative drugs to relieve

G.A. Walco and K.R. Goldschneider (eds.), *Pain in Children: A Practical Guide for Primary Care.*
© Humana Press, a part of Springer Science + Business Media, 2008

anxiety and pain associated with diagnostic and therapeutic procedures. Most common indications for procedural sedation and analgesia are painful procedures (e.g., fracture reductions, complicated laceration repairs, I & D of abscess), and diagnostic imaging that are frequently performed in emergency departments. PSA administered during a child's initial encounter with a painful procedure may help reduce distress in subsequent procedures [4].

The use of DPT (Demerol®, Phenergan®, Thorazine®) or chloral hydrate in the past for major orthopedic interventions and imaging studies was associated with significant complications and has been replaced by pharmacologic agents such as fentanyl, midazolam, ketamine, profopol, short acting barbiturates, and etomidate, that have proven track records in safety and efficacy in the ED setting [5]. Many of the procedures formerly used in the operating room may now be performed in ED by emergency physicians or subspecialists trained in administering PSA. Another popular and efficacious method of the fracture reduction method is regional block or Bier block which does not require deep sedation for those with potential physiological risks such as moderate to severe medical problems or inadequate NPO time [6]. In general, the NPO (nil per os, or fasting state) guidelines published by the American Society of Anesthesiologists (ASA) are followed for most PSA performed in the ED. Therefore, patients referred for PSA should be kept NPO in accordance with these guidelines (Table 9-1).

1.2. Simple Procedural Pain Management

Children undergoing simple yet painful procedures, such as laceration repairs, have long endured them without the benefit of topical anesthesia and

TABLE 9-1. American Society of Anesthesiologists NPO guidelines.

Clear liquids	2 hours
Breast milk	4 hours
Infant formula	6 hours
Non-human milk	6 hours
Light meal	6 hours

Note: These are guidelines for general anesthesia and sedation. There is some individual discretion in the application of NPO guidelines so it is extremely useful to directly contact the ED physician before referral.

sedation or behavioral interventions to decrease procedural distress. There are two separate, yet interrelated, distress factors in procedures—pain and anxiety.

To reduce pain, various topical anesthetics, as discussed Chapter 7, can markedly reduce procedural pain. Most commonly used agents to date in the ED are sucrose, lidocaine-adrenaline-tetracaine (LAT), EMLA® or LMX4®, Pain Ease®, and buffered lidocaine. Using pacifiers with sucrose has become a standard treatment for neonates undergoing common ED procedures such as blood draws, IV placements, and lumbar punctures [7, 8].

LAT is commonly used in the pediatric ED as an anesthetic agent to repair small to medium-sized lacerations in the face or scalp [9]. The use of LAT eliminates the pain from local anesthetic injection and anesthesia is achieved in just 30 minutes after application. For intact skin, research has also suggested placement of topical anesthetics such as LMX4®, which is effective in 30 minutes.

Intravenous access is a common painful procedure in the ED, and current protocol includes applying a topical anesthetic cream in triage prior to intravenous access [10, 11]. Pain Ease®, a vapocoolant spray, has proven to be effective in simple needle associated procedures such as blood draws, IV placements, and IM vaccinations, providing anesthesia in mere seconds after spraying [12]. Injectable lidocaine still has a significant role, and there are several methods to decrease the stinging sensation from its injection. They include buffering with sodium bicarbonate (1:9 sodium bicarbonate: lidocaine), warming it to body temperature, using the smallest needle possible, and slow injection [13–16].

Most of these agents can be used in the primary care setting; however, the anxiety component during simple procedures can be difficult to manage. Studies indicate that having a child life specialist prepare the child for the procedure, provide distraction, and teach coping techniques is extremely beneficial for children undergoing painful procedures, and is helpful to the providers as well [17–19]. Pharmacologic methods of anxiolysis include nitrous oxide (titrated to 50:50 nitrous oxide:oxygen) and oral midazolam (~0.5 mg/kg) to reduce procedural distress [20–23]. Although the ED may have more resources than the average primary care practice, the principles can be applied. For example, nurses and physician's assistants can learn and apply the same skills as child life workers and topical analgesics are readily available. When referring a patient to the ED, it is helpful to advise the family about some of these interventions and encourage them to ask about them as the situation indicates.

1.3. Acute Abdominal Pain

Abdominal pain is a common presenting complaint to any health care facility. Most patients have mild pain that can be diagnosed and treated at the primary care facility, but some require immediate referral to an ED for comprehensive evaluation and intervention. Appendicitis is high on the differential diagnosis list for acute abdominal pain. The ED can provide both immediate evaluation and, according to the severity of pain, analgesia prior to any imaging or tests. The traditional or old surgical dogma of "no pain meds for acute abdominal pain until a diagnosis is made" has been challenged by pediatric studies, resulting in provision of comfort without decrease in safety or diagnostic accuracy [24–26]. Many agencies, including AHRQ, advocate early administration of analgesia [27]. The goal in evaluating abdominal pain in children is to provide definitive intervention with early pain relief.

2. Nonpharmacologic Interventions

As attention has shifted onto comfort care in the ED, more pediatric EDs offer a range of non-medication therapies. The most commonly used and effective nonpharmacologic interventions for painful conditions in the ED setting are provided by child life specialists, pediatric nurses, and care providers who are well-versed in the emotional needs based on developmental stages of the patients [17–19]. In addition, many pediatric EDs have multimedia equipment including videos, movies, games, and other technical gadgets to distract frightened children. Simple distractions such as soap bubbles and picture books are not overlooked, though.

3. Pharmacologic Interventions

The limited availability of advanced pain medications in the primary care setting is an important reason for referring a child with pain. If first level analgesics, such as NSAIDs and oral opioids, are either unavailable or ineffective, the ED can provide more intensive treatments, such as parenteral administration of opioids for moderate to severe pain. As with any situation where the response to the medication may be unpredictable, or when a patient is or may be unstable, *titration* is the optimal approach to dosing opioids (see Chapter 8 for full discussion). Another important pharmacologic intervention that can be started in the ED is patient-controlled analgesia (PCA). Sickle cell disease patients routinely benefit from initiation of PCA in the ED as the pain is inadequately managed by intermittent dosing.

4. Preparing the Patient for an ED Visit

Prior to referral, explaining what to expect in the ED, including wait time, likely evaluation and interventions, may significantly reduce anxiety of the patient and family. Administering pain medications such as acetaminophen or ibuprofen in the office is recommended and if patient will most likely need an IV, blood draw or LP, placement of topical anesthetic such as LMX4® or EMLA® prior to transfer may help expedite care and reduce pain and distress.

Before any decision is made to refer, discuss the case regarding assessment, goals of treatment and types of intervention in the ED with the ED physician and to agree on transport arrangement to ensure a smooth transition of the care (Table 9-2). There are several options to transport the patient to the ED. The quickest method for the sickest patients is to call the local EMS (911). If available, a transport team can be utilized. When a patient is deemed stable, parent transport by car is an option. However, the severity of pain, need for relief, urgency of the condition, distance to ED, cost, primary care provider's comfort, and parental comfort should be weighed in the joint decision for method of transport.

TABLE 9-2. Checklist prior to ED referral.

- Determine the need for and goals of the referral
- Contact ED physician to discuss the case; determine preliminary course of evaluation in ED
- Determine interventions needed in the office prior to transfer (NSAIDs, topical analgesia, NPO)
- Arrange transportation
- Prepare patient and family
- Send copies of documents, test results, X-rays or reports

5. Pre-Hospital Pain Management

Most EMS systems have pre-hospital pain management protocols. Despite the existence of these protocols, the pain management in the field by EMS providers has been inadequate. In a report by Hennes et al. only 3.0 percent of children with fractures received pain medications, compared to 10.5 percent of adults with fractures [28]. Several barriers have been identified for this inadequacy and discrepancy, including lack of education, assessment difficulties, and many negative incentives. Systems barriers include inconsistent medical control and complexity of the multiple tiered EMS system [29]. Educational attempts to overcome these barriers have shown significant improvements in the rate of pain assessment documentation, from 14.5 to 53.3 percent, and an increase in the rate administration of pain medication from 7.2 percent to 33.3 percent for children with painful conditions in the field prior to arrival in the ED [30].

Take-Home Points

- Significant advances in pain management have been made in the pre-hospital and ED setting.
- Many painful conditions are evaluated and treated promptly with comprehensive pain management (e.g., trained personnel, proper equipment, child life workers, parenteral analgesics).
- Many painful procedures can be performed in the ED with minimal distress.
- Pain management can begin in the primary care physician's office with simple analgesics and application of topical anesthetics.
- The ED can be a resource for pain management information and referral for specific diagnostic studies or consultants.

- Consultation with the ED physician may be the most important step in caring for and referring a patient in pain.

References

1. Johnston C, Stevens BJ. Experience in a neonatal intensive care unit affects pain response. Pediatrics 1996;98:925–930.
2. Taddio A, Goldbach M, Ipp M, Stevens B, Koren G. Effects of neonatal circumcision on pain response during vaccination in boys. Lancet 1995;345:291–292.
3. Taddio A, Katz J, Ilersich AL, Koren G. Effects of neonatal circumcision on pain response during subsequent routine vaccination. Lancet 1997;349:599–603.
4. Weisman SJ, Bernstein B, Schechter NL. Consequences of inadequate analgesia During painful procedures in children. Arch Pediatr Adolesc Med 1998;152:147–149.
5. Krauss B, Green SM. Procedural sedation and analgesia in children. Lancet 2006;367:766–780.
6. Constantine E, Steele D, Eberson C, Boutis K, Amanullah S, Linakis J. The use of local anesthetic techniques for closed forearm fracture reduction in children: a survey of academic pediatric emergency departments. Pediatr Emerg Care 2007; 23:209–211.
7. Stevens B, Taddio A, Ohlsson A, Einarson T. The efficacy of sucrose for relieving procedural pain in neonates—a systematic review and meta-analysis. Acta Paediatr 1997;86:837–842.
8. Carbajal R, Chauvet X, Couderc S, Olivier-Martin M. Randomised trial of analgesic effects of sucrose, glucose, and pacifiers in term neonates. BMJ 1999;319: 1393–1397.
9. Ernst AA, Marvez-Valls E, Nick TG, Mills T, Minvielle L, Houry D. Topical lidocaine adrenaline tetracaine (LAT gel) versus injectable buffered lidocaine for local anesthesia in laceration repair. Western J Med 1997;167:79–81.
10. Eichenfield LF, Funk A, Fallon-Friedlander S, Cunningham BB. A clinical study to evaluate the efficacy of ELA-Max (4% liposomal lidocaine) as compared with eutectic mixture of local anesthetics cream for pain reduction of venipuncture in children. Pediatrics 2002;109:1093–1099.
11. Fein JA, Callahan JM, Boardman CR, Gorelick MH. Predicting the need for topical anesthetic in the pediatric emergency department. Pediatrics 1999;104:e19.
12. Cohen Reis E, Holobukov R. Vapocoolant spray is equally effective as EMLA cream in reducing immunization pain in school-aged children. Pediatrics 1997;100:e5.
13. Klein EJ, Shugerman RP, Leigh-Taylor K, Schneider C, Portscheller D, Koepsell T. Buffered

lidocaine: analgesia for intravenous line placement in children. Pediatrics 1995;95:709–712.

14. Davidson JA, Boom SJ. Warming lignocaine to reduce pain associated with injection. BMJ 1992;305: 617–618.

15. Krause RS, Moscati R, Filice M, Lerner EB, Hughes D. The effect of injection speed on the pain of lidocaine infiltration. Acad Emerg Med 1997;4:1032–1035.

16. Bartfield JM, Gennis P, Barbera J, Breuer B, Gallagher EJ. Buffered versus plain lidocaine as a local anesthetic for simple laceration repair. Ann Emerg Med 1990:19:1387–1389.

17. Stevenson MD, Bivins CM, O'Brien K, Gonzalez del Rey JA. Child life intervention during angiocatheter insertion in the pediatric emergency department. Pediatr Emerg Care 2005;21:712–718.

18. Christian B, Thomas DO. A child life program in one pediatric emergency department. J Emerg Nursing 1998;24:359–61.

19. Krebel MS, Clayton C, Graham C. Child life programs in the pediatric emergency department. Pediatr Emerg Care 1996;12:13–15.

20. Luhmann JD, Schootman M, Luhmann SJ, Kennedy RM. A randomized comparison of nitrous oxide plus hematoma block versus ketamine plus midazolam for emergency department forearm fracture reduction in children. Pediatrics 2006;118:e1078–1086.

21. Krauss B. Continuous-flow nitrous oxide: searching for the ideal procedural anxiolytic for toddlers. Ann Emerg Med 2001;37:61–62.

22. Luhmann JD, Kennedy RM, Porter FL, Miller JP, Jaffe DM. A randomized clinical trial of continuous-flow nitrous oxide and midazolam for sedation of young children during laceration repair. Ann Emerg Med 2001;37:20–27.

23. Cote CJ, Cohen IT, Suresh S, Rabb M, Rose JB, Weldon BC, Davis PJ, Bikhazi GB, Karl HW, Hummer KA, Hannallah RS, Khoo KC, Collins P. A comparison of three doses of a commercially prepared oral midazolam syrup in children. Anesth Analg 2002;94:37–43.

24. Kim MK, Strait RT, Sato TT, Hennes HM. A randomized clinical trial of analgesia in children with acute abdominal pain. Acad Emerg Med 2002;9: 281–287.

25. Goldman RD, Crum D, Bromberg R, Rogovik A, Langer JC. Analgesia administration for acute abdominal pain in the pediatric emergency department. Pediatr Emerg Care 2006;22:18–21.

26. Green R, Bulloch B, Kabani A, Hancock BJ, Tenenbein M. Early analgesia for children with acute abdominal pain. Pediatrics 2005;116:978–983.

27. Making health care safer: a critical analysis of patient safety practices. Evidence Report/Technology Assessment, Number 43. AHRQ Publication No. 01-E058, July 2001. Agency for Healthcare Research and Quality, Rockville, MD. Subchapter 37.2. Acute Pain Services, *http://www.ahrq.gov/clinic/ptsafety/chap37a.htm#37.2*

28. Hennes H, Kim M, Pirrallo R. Prehospital pain management: A comparison of providers' perception and practice. Prehosp Emerg Care 2005;9:32–39.

29. Hennes H, Kim M. Prehospital pain management: Current status and future direction. Clin Pediatr Emerg Med 2006;7:25–30.

30. Hennes H, Simpson D, Pirrallo R, Rehm J, Sternig K, Szewczuga D, Kim M. PAMPPER: A novel pediatric pain management educational program for EMS providers. Prehosp Emerg Care 2007:(abstract).

10
Preparing Children for Invasive Procedures and Surgery

Ronald L. Blount, Megan L. McCormick, Jill E. MacLaren, and Zeev N. Kain

Abstract: Children undergo numerous medical procedures throughout their lifetime, such as routine needle sticks, and more invasive procedures such as surgery. Common reactions include varying levels of fear and anxiety before the medical event and pain during the actual procedures. Both nonmalleable and malleable variables are predictive of children's medical anxiety and pain, as well as their use of coping behaviors. Nonmalleable correlates of children's fear and anxiety include younger age, negative temperament, high level of distress during prior procedures, and an avoidant coping style. These variables may help identify children in need of intervention, but do little to indicate the best way to intervene. In contrast, the potentially malleable variables that predict children's anxiety and pain include children's training in the use of coping skills and the behaviors of parents and medical staff. Some adult behaviors have been shown to increase child anxiety and pain, while other adult behaviors reduce child distress before and during medical treatments. Generally, parent and medical staff behaviors that are helpful direct children's attention away from their own anxious emotions and the threatening and painful aspects of the medical procedure, to something more pleasant and engaging, In contrast, detrimental adult behaviors enhance children's focus on their own negative emotions and the medical procedure, heightening anxiety and pain.

Techniques that effectively assist children prior to and during invasive procedures include pharmacological agents and a variety of cognitive behavioral interventions. For children undergoing surgery, midazolam is a commonly used sedative to reduce anxiety. In terms of cognitive behavioral interventions, the multicomponent ADVANCE program, explained in detail below, has been shown to effectively reduce children's presurgical anxiety, as well as result in less emergence delirium, postsurgical fentanyl use, and quicker discharge. Health care professionals should consider both pharmacological and psychological interventions, as they have been proven to be effective, noninvasive, and fairly inexpensive options for helping reduce children's pain and anxiety prior to, during, and after medical procedures.

Key words: Anxiety, procedure, pediatric, preoperative, surgery, induction.

Introduction

Children experience multiple medical procedures. These begin at birth and continue beyond adolescence. Common procedures include heel sticks, circumcisions, blood tests, venipunctures, injury treatments, dental procedures, and surgeries [1]. Needle sticks are among the most common painful procedures, with up to 28 immunizations by the age of 6 years [2]. For children with chronic medical conditions, the number of procedures is compounded.

Medical procedures may induce anxiety before the procedures, as well as pain and distress during and after the actual event. Inadequately managed procedural pain may result in long-term adverse consequences, including heightened pain sensitivity and posttraumatic stress symptoms [3]. These reactions may be acquired due to

G.A. Walco and K.R. Goldschneider (eds.), *Pain in Children: A Practical Guide for Primary Care.*
© Humana Press, a part of Springer Science + Business Media, 2008

learning, as well as neurophysiological changes produced by the painful sensations [3–5]. In addition, fear and pain, during pediatric medical procedures predict fear, pain, and avoidance of medical procedures in young adults [6]. Despite these possible outcomes, interventions for reducing pediatric pain are rarely utilized [3].

Up to 40 percent to 60 percent of the four million children who undergo surgery in the United States experience significant preoperative anxiety [7]. Although there are many stressful situations associated with surgery (e.g., separation from parents, unfamiliar hospital procedures), the non-painful event of mask anesthesia induction appears to be the most stressful in the preoperative period [8]. Preoperative anxiety is associated with adverse postsurgical outcomes. Children with high presurgical anxiety were 3.5 times more likely to develop negative postsurgical behavioral reactions [9] such as temper tantrums, separation anxiety and sleep disturbances. Physiological consequences of high presurgical anxiety include increased postoperative emergence delirium and greater need for analgesia [10].

This chapter reviews correlates of pain and anxiety and well-supported interventions for reducing anxiety and pain before and during invasive procedures, and preoperative anxiety associated with surgery.

1. Factors Associated with Pediatric Pain During Invasive Procedures

Knowing the factors that correlate with anxiety and pain can help health care providers identify children who are most likely to need intervention. Consistent with a risk and resiliency framework, these factors can be divided into fixed or nonmalleable factors, versus those that are malleable. Only the malleable factors may be changed to assist the child.

1.1. Nonmalleable Predictors of Children's Pain and Distress

Younger children tend to report higher pain and distress than older children, with overt distress and reports of pain tending to decrease after about age 7 or 8 years [4]. There have been inconsistent findings for gender and little research on racial differences in pain expression in children. Children with a "difficult" temperament generally report higher levels of pain and distress than children with an easier temperamental style [3]. Finally, parents' ratings of their children's distress during prior medical and dental procedures are predictive of distress during upcoming immunizations [11].

Coping style is often studied in this area, and results indicate that children who engage in an information-seeking coping style have better outcomes than those who avoid information [4]. Unfortunately, a review of stress and coping assessment measures indicated that the literature in this area has done little to inform the design of treatment interventions [12]. In contrast to the undesirable effects of information-avoiding coping style, the coping strategy of distraction is associated with lower levels of pain [4]. Distraction differs from information-avoiding in that distraction is a deliberate or prompted refocusing of attention from the threatening situation to more pleasing thoughts, images, objects, or events. In contrast, avoidance is indicative of the patient cognitively or physically escaping or fleeing from the stressor.

1.2. Malleable Predicators of Children's Pain and Distress

High child anticipatory anxiety prior to a medical procedure contributes to greater pain during the procedure. Parental anxiety is also predictive of greater child distress [4]. Similarly, child distress during cleansing and preparation for bone marrow aspirations (BMA) has been found to be highly correlated ($r_s = 0.89$) with distress during the painful BMA [13]. These findings indicate that anxiety and distress should be seen as a chain of behavior that often begins before and continues during painful procedures. Therefore, efforts should be made to intervene early to reduce preprocedural distress.

Children's use of coping behaviors is also malleable, with the potential to be prompted and/or trained. Children who use effective coping behaviors prior to and during procedures have less anticipatory anxiety and subsequent pain and distress than those who do not [1]. Actual performance of coping behaviors is facilitated by adults' prompts to cope while they are in the medical situation.

There are also adult behaviors that have been shown repeatedly in correlational [4, 14] and treatment studies [15] to be counter-therapeutic. There are at least three types of these distress-promoting parent or staff behaviors. These include: reassuring statements, apologies, and empathic statements; giving control to the child; and criticism of the child. Reassurance (e.g., "It's going to be okay, baby") often occurs just prior to a painful event or at the initial signs of child distress. Apologies include statements like, "I'm sorry you have to go through this." Examples of empathic statements are "I know this is hard" or "I know this hurts." These three types of adult behaviors are emotion focusing statements and have the effect of directing the child's attention on his or her own distress and pain, as well as on the threatening aspects of the medical procedure. Focusing on these aspects exacerbates children's anxiety and pain. We have also found that reassurance not only appears to be counterproductive, it was among the most frequent adult vocalizations. In nonacute situations, such as loss of a loved one, these three adult behaviors might be beneficial, but not before or during children's acute medical procedures.

Giving control to the child over the start of the medical procedure appeared to be detrimental in correlational research [14]. A medical staff member may say, "tell me when you're ready…*for this injection.*" Children may be overwhelmed by the responsibility for the start of the frightening and painful medical procedure, and understandably do not want to begin.

Finally, criticism of the child's behavior during medical procedures, although rare, is associated with more distress. However, rather than directly attempting to decrease these adult behaviors, we advocate training adults to more effectively prompt children's coping [16].

2. Assessment of Pain, Distress, and Coping

There are several good observational measures for assessing pain and distress for different age groups [2]. A discussion of pain assessment tools *per se*, can be found in Chapter 3. For assessing children's coping and adults' coping-promoting behaviors, the Child-Adult Medical Procedure Interaction Scale-Revised (CAMPIS-R) is a well-established measure

[12]. However, it is lengthy and not practical for busy clinics. For this reason, a rating scale version has been developed [17] and some researchers have used only select child coping or adult coping-promoting codes from the CAMPIS-R. We strongly advocate monitoring children's coping and adults distracting or coaching their use of coping behaviors. If coping and coping-promoting behaviors occur, anxiety and pain should be less.

3. Interventions for Acute Procedures

Anticipatory anxiety and pain involve sensory, psychological, behavioral, and social influences. Treatment may include medical, behavioral, or combined strategies.

3.1. Pharmacologic Approaches

Interventions for pain associated with major procedures (e.g., BMA, postsurgical) include anti-inflammatory and antipyretic drugs, psychotropic drugs, opiate analgesics, nitrous oxide, and combinations of different medications. For less painful procedures such as injections, topical anesthetics can be used, but they require variable amounts of time to provide sufficient anesthesia [4] (see Chapter 7 for details). Vapocoolant sprays and iontophoresis of lidocaine, as well as counter-irritating the surrounding skin, have also been supported [3]. In addition, thinner needles can help avert some of the sensory aspects of pain [4]. Despite these medical advances, procedures remain a source of anxiety and pain for many children.

3.2. Psychological Interventions for Procedure-Related Pain

Psychological interventions include preparation and treatment [4]. Although preparation programs have been incorporated for brief invasive procedures, they are used more with complex medical stressors, such as surgery, and therefore they will be discussed later.

In a review, Powers [18] concluded that cognitive-behavioral interventions were found to be empirically supported. Within the broad category of cognitive-behavioral interventions, treatment components included relaxation, graduated *in vivo* exposure to the feared stimulus, relaxation, nonprocedural conversation, breathing exercises, reinforcement, rehearsal of coping skills, multiple forms of distraction, making coping statements, and parent and nurse coaching of the child. Some of these coping behaviors require training of the child, while others simply require the distracting stimuli to be present and for the child to be sufficiently prompted to use them. We also note that for infants, sucrose, rocking, pacifiers, and distraction have been shown to be helpful [3, 4].

Blount et al. [4] indicated that the commonality among most of the effective treatments that are listed above is the aspect of distraction, or cognitive refocusing. Distraction always involves directing attention *from* something undesirable and *to* something more pleasant and engaging. Distraction was from the sights, sounds, smells, sensations, negative thoughts and emotions, and even from the pain that accompanies the medical procedure. We should mention that even during medical procedures, some attention by the patient to the medical procedure is understandable, as the patient checks in to see what is happening. However, in most cases it is undesirable for the patient to dwell on painful or frightening procedures.

There are several guidelines for the use of distraction. Distraction should start prior to the medical procedure to reduce anticipatory anxiety and keep the child from enjoining a pathway leading to high procedural distress and pain. During the anticipatory phase and for minor, less painful procedures, more cognitively involved forms of distraction are appropriate and often sufficient. Examples include engaging conversations about nonprocedural topics (e.g., school, pet, vacation, favorite food, and humorous interactions), actively playing with age-appropriate toys or games, watching and perhaps talking with the child about an enjoyable and nonthreatening video and other similar appealing stimuli. Distraction should continue throughout the medical procedure. However, patients who are highly anxious or who are undergoing more painful medical procedures lose the ability to converse or play, even though those coping behaviors might have been useful during the anticipatory period. In those instances, coping behaviors that use less sophisticated cognitive processing, such as deep breathing or use of a party blower, are more appropriate [13, 19]. Deep breathing is a simple coping strategy that may produce therapeutic physiological effects due to

increased oxygen intake, and also serves as a type of distraction [4, 19]. If possible, choose a coping behavior which can be observed and verified. For example, talk with the child about the video rather than just letting the child look at the screen, with perhaps little to no engagement of attention.

It is important that parents and/or medical staff sufficiently prompt the child to encourage the use of coping behaviors. This is particularly important at procedural junctures (e.g., cleansing), or during mild displays of distress. We have found that children undergoing BMAs [14] seldom use deep breathing unless repeatedly coached to breathe during painful medical events. Importantly, when one adult prompts the child to cope, other adults often join in and also prompt the child [14, 20]. Cohen, Blount, and Panopoulos [21] found that one well-trained medical staff member in the room with successive parent-child dyads was a cost-effective way to increase the parents' coping-promoting prompts and the children's coping, and reduce their distress and pain. Examples of coaching children to use coping strategies during painful procedures include repeatedly saying "Breathe" or "Blow into this party blower" for distraction. Effective preprocedural coping–promoting interactions with children lowers anticipatory anxiety, while prompts during the procedure help keep it low or reduce it if it escalates.

4. Interventions to Reduce Presurgical Anxiety

There are three main interventions that have been utilized for treating perioperative anxiety in children: sedatives, parental presence during the induction of anesthesia (PPIA), and preparation programs [10].

4.1. Midazolam

Midazolam is the most common preoperative sedative medication. In randomized trials it has been shown to reduce child anxiety and distress, and to increase cooperation. Further, it yields satisfactory results within 20 minutes of administration [7]. Although effective, side effects may include delay in emergence and discharge, the potential for maladaptive behaviors post-surgery, and amnesia. It appears that the most effective oral dosage with the fewest side effects is 0.50 mg/kg [7].

4.2. Parental Presence

Most parents prefer to be with their children during medical procedures and believe that their presence helps their children, and most children prefer to have their parents present [4]. Potential benefits of parental pressure at induction of anesthesia (PPIA) include reducing child separation anxiety and the amount of sedative premedication that is required, increasing child cooperation, and increasing parent satisfaction and sense of fulfillment in their parental role. Potential drawbacks include increased parental anxiety, higher staff workload due to having to care for parents, and disruption in the usual medical procedures [7].

Piira et al. [22] reviewed 13 studies that examined the effects of parental presence on children's presurgical anxiety. They found no benefit of parental presence on children's anxiety in the studies that included randomized designs. However, in the studies that were not randomized (e.g., parents could select the condition they would be in), parental presence was associated with less anxiety in six of the nine studies. Results of PPIA on parent distress were also mixed. Notably, although less anxious parents were found to benefit most from PPIA [23], the more anxious parents were the ones who reported a greater desire to be present [24]. The general conclusion is that parental presence has not been shown to reliably reduce children's preoperative anxiety [10]. However, the beneficial effects of PPIA may be enhanced if they were adequately trained to coach their child prior to and during induction.

4.3. Preparation Programs

Preparation may include information provision, modeling and teaching coping strategies. Jaaniste, Hayes and von Baeyer [25] indicated that preparation programs inform children what to expect, allowing them to ready themselves for the procedure. They also may reduce anxiety due to exposure to the tolerable aspects of the threatening event, and they facilitate more realistic appraisals of what to expect. Information should include sensory (what will be experienced, expressed in non-threatening terms) as well as procedural (what will happen) components, and should be more detailed rather than general. If a procedure is painful, the

child should be informed of that. As for the format for conveying this information to children, video-taped peer modeling has been studied most in the literature, but is often not a practical alternative in many settings. Medical play using dolls is not considered an adequate method for conveying information. If written information is used, it should be accompanied by illustrations, particularly for less competent readers. Training in coping procedures via instruction and role-play should be included, and adults should be trained to prompt the child [19, 26]. In terms of the timing of information, at least five days advanced notice seems indicated for older children and more involved medical procedures. New procedural information should be kept to a minimum as the time of the medical procedure approaches to avoid overwhelming the child. The focus at that time should shift to distraction-based interventions [4].

Coping skills training has been rated by experts in this area as the most effective method for preparing children for surgery, followed by modeling, play therapy, tours of the OR, and written or printed materials [7, 27]. Kain et al. [10] examined the effectiveness of a multicomponent behavioral coping intervention (ADVANCE program) for 2- to 10-year-olds undergoing mask anesthesia induction for outpatient surgery. The ADVANCE program includes techniques for anxiety reduction, distraction, video modeling and education, incorporating parents, avoiding excessive reassurance, parent coaching of the child in the holding area and throughout induction, and an exposure/shaping component to facilitate children's acceptance of the mask. More detailed information about these procedures is included in the publication. The ADVANCE program took approximately 30 minutes to administer.

Results indicated that the trained children exhibited lower anxiety in the holding area, compared to children in the standard care, midazolam premedication, or PPIA groups. During mask anesthesia induction, children in the ADVANCE condition had lower anxiety than children in the standard care or those in the PPIA condition, and similar anxiety to those children who received midazolam. Parents in the ADVANCE condition were less anxious than the parents in the other three groups while in the holding area and after induction. Following surgery, children in the training condition were less likely than children in the other three conditions to display emergence delirium. Further, in the recovery room they required half as much fentanyl as children in the PPIA group, and one-third as much fentanyl as children in the control and midazolam groups. They were also discharged quicker than children in the other three conditions. This investigation demonstrated that the cognitive-behavioral intervention not only reduced preoperative child anxiety, but also helped parents and resulted in better postsurgical outcomes.

5. When to Refer

Implementing the guidelines in this chapter should improve patients' reactions to invasive medical procedures and surgery. However, children with extreme levels of anxiety and pain, as well as those who seem unresponsive to office-based interventions, may warrant referral to appropriately trained medical and psychological specialists skilled in anxiety and pain management techniques.

5.1. For Further Information

The review articles and chapters by Blount et al. [4], Wright et al. [7] and Young [3] provide additional information on many of the topics covered in this chapter. Articles by Piira et al. [22] and Jaaniste et al. [25] provide additional information on parental presence and preparation programs.

Take-Home Points

For reducing anxiety, pain and associated difficulties:

- Information-based interventions can be used to good effect.
- Most coping skills have a common ingredient of distraction, or attention refocusing, from the fearful and painful aspects of the medical procedure to more pleasant stimuli.
- Children may be trained in coping skills and adults may be trained to coach them to facilitate the use of those coping skills during the times they are most needed.
- The need to train each child and parent is lessened when the medical procedure is less involved and less painful, the child is less anxious, more

engaging stimuli for distraction are used, and effective prompts are provided by medical staff. Non-trained parents will often quickly join in when the medical staff takes the lead in prompting the child to engage in coping behaviors.

- Role play as a means of training coping skills under simulated conditions that approximate the medical procedure may be desirable for more complex situations.
- Training parents and medical staff to better assist children also gives them a genuinely helpful role, thereby reducing their distress and increasing their sense of competence.

References

1. Blount RL, Piira T, Cohen LL, Cheng PS. Pediatric procedural pain. Behav Modif 2006;30:24–49.
2. Cohen LL, Lemanek KL, Blount RL, et al. Evidence-based assessment of pediatric pain. J Pediatr Psychol, in press.
3. Young KD. Pediatric procedural pain. Ann Emerg Med 2005;45:160–171.
4. Blount RL, Piira T, Cohen LL. Management of pediatric pain and distress due to medical procedures. In: Roberts MC, editor. Handbook of Pediatric Psychology, 3rd ed. New York: Guilford, 2003:216–233.
5. Taddio A, Katz J. The effects of early pain experience in neonates on pain responses in infancy and childhood. Paediatr Drugs 2005;7:245–257.
6. Pate JT, Smith AJ, Blount RL, Cohen LL. Childhood medical experience and temperament as predictors of adult functioning in medical situations. Children's Health Care 1996;25:281–296.
7. Wright KD, Stewart SH, Finley GA, Buffett-Jerrott SE. Prevention and intervention strategies to alleviate preoperative anxiety in children: A critical review. Behav Modif 2007;31:52–79.
8. Kain ZN, Mayes LC, O'Connor TZ, Cicchetti DV. Preoperative anxiety in children. Predictors and outcomes. Arch Pediatr Adolesc Med 1996;150:1238–1245.
9. Kain ZN, Wang SM, Mayes LC, Caramico LA, Hofstadter MB. Distress during the induction of anesthesia and postoperative behavioral outcomes. Anesth Analg 1999;88:1042–1047.
10. Kain ZN, Caldwell-Andrews AA, Mayes LC, et al. Family-centered preparation for surgery improves perioperative outcomes in children: A randomized controlled trial. Anesth 2007;106:65–74.
11. Frank NC, Blount RL, Smith AJ, Manimala MR, Martin JK. Parent and staff behavior, previous

child medical experience, and maternal anxiety as they relate to child procedural distress and coping. J Pediatr Psychol 1995;20:277–289.

12. Blount RL, Simons LE, Devine KA, et al. Evidence-based assessment of coping and stress in pediatric psychology. J Pediatr Psychol, in press.

13. Blount RL, Sturges JW, Powers SW. Analysis of child and adult behavioral variations by phase of medical procedure. Behav Ther 1990;21:33–48.

14. Blount RL, Corbin SM, Sturges JW, Wolfe VV, Prater JM, James LD. The relationship between adults' behaviors and child coping and distress during BMA/LP procedures: A sequential analysis. Behav Ther 1989;20:585–601.

15. Manimala MR, Blount RL, Cohen LL. The effects of parental reassurance versus distraction on child distress and coping during immunizations. Children's Health Care 2000;29:161–177.

16. Blount RL, Bunke VL, Zaff JF. Bridging the gap between explicative and treatment research: a model and practical implications. J Clin Psychol in Med Settings 2000;7:79–90.

17. Blount RL, Bunke V, Cohen LL, Forbes CJ. The Child-Adult Medical Procedure Interaction Scale-Short Form (CAMPIS-SF): Validation of a rating scale for children's and adults' behaviors during painful medical procedures. J Pain and Symptom Manage 2001;22:591–599.

18. Powers SW. Empirically supported treatments in pediatric psychology: procedure-related pain. J Pediatr Psychol 1999;24:131–145.

19. Blount RL, Powers SW, Cotter MW, Swan S, Free K. Making the system work: Training pediatric oncology patients to cope and their parents to coach them during BMA/LP procedures. Behav Modif 1994;18:6–31.

20. Blount RL, Bachanas PJ, Powers SW, et al. Training children to cope and their parents to coach them during routine immunizations: Effects on child, parent and staff behaviors. Behav Ther 1992;23:689–705.

21. Cohen LL, Blount RL, Panopoulos G. Nurse coaching and cartoon distraction: an effective and practical intervention to reduce child, parent, and nurse distress during immunizations. J Pediatr Psychol 1997;22:355–370.

22. Piira T, Sugiura T, Champion GD, Donnelly N, Cole AS. The role of parental presence in the context of children's medical procedures: a systematic review. Child: Care, Health and Develop 2005;31:233–243.

23. Kain ZN, Caldwell-Andrews AA, Maranets I, Nelson W, Mayes LC. Predicting which child-parent pair will benefit from parental presence during induction of anesthesia: a decision-making approach. Anesth Analg 2006;102:81–84.

24. Caldwell-Andrews AA, Kain ZN, Mayes LC, Kerns RD, Ng D. Motivation and maternal presence during induction of anesthesia. Anesth 2005;103:478–483.

25. Jaaniste T, Hayes B, von Baeyer CL. Providing children with information about forthcoming medical procedures: A review and synthesis. Clin Psychol Sci Pract 2007;14:124–143.

26. Powers SW, Blount RL, Bachanas PJ, Cotter MW, Swan SC. Helping preschool leukemia patients and their parents cope during injections. J Pediatr Psychol 1993;18:681–695.

27. O'Byrne KK, Peterson L, Saldana L. Survey of pediatric hospitals' preparation programs: Evidence of the impact of health psychology research. Health Psychol 1997;16:147–154.

11
Pain Relief After Outpatient Surgery

Robert T. Wilder and Kenneth R. Goldschneider

Abstract: Day surgery is a common source of significant pain for children. A combination of opioids, NSAIDs, and regional anesthetic techniques are available to provide comfort postoperatively. Regardless of what is provided in the hospital or surgery center, the patients will need pain care at home. Awareness of the techniques available to children in the operating room can help the primary care physician counsel parents to help them better advocate for their child when they arrive for surgery. Knowing the probable pitfalls in postoperative care that can occur at home can help the parents "keep ahead" of the pain, and avoid unnecessary complications. The preoperative visit is an excellent time in which to educate the family for the day of surgery.

Key words: Outpatient surgery, regional anesthesia, postoperative pain, acute pain, day surgery.

Introduction

Day surgery, or outpatient surgery, offers multiple advantages to children, families, and society. These include decreased cost and allowing the child to recover in a familiar, less threatening environment. Day surgery does place an increased burden on the child's primary caregiver, however, as this person now becomes responsible for providing the patient's postoperative medical care, in addition to the usual child care for the patient and any siblings. Since most parents are not trained to deliver medical care, it is important for the health care providers to make this care as simple and efficient as possible. Central is the provision of clear instructions that include not only what to expect in the usual course, but also what can go wrong and how to deal with complications, including whom to call.

Postoperative analgesia is an important aspect of postsurgical care. Importantly, parents generally prefer receiving this information ahead of time, and in written form, citing the stress and fatigue of the day of surgery as impediments to understanding and processing new information [1]. A preoperative visit is the optimal time to review and educate about postoperative pain care with the families, and a postoperative phone call also can be useful and reassuring to parents [2].

The ideal would be to send patients home comfortable and without need for any additional analgesia. The pain regimen would bring no unwanted side effects such as nausea, itching, or respiratory depression. Although this ideal generally cannot be completely achieved in real life, anesthesiologists and surgeons should strive to obtain an analgesic plan as close to this as possible. Generally that includes using appropriate regional anesthesia whenever possible, using scheduled acetaminophen, administering nonsteroidal anti-inflammatory agents when not contraindicated, and considering preemptive or prophylactic analgesia in an effort to minimize the need for opioid analgesics.

Although opioids have been the gold standard in perioperative analgesia, they are more likely to cause side effects than the other techniques mentioned. Intractable nausea and vomiting, in particular, is one of the most frequent causes of admission after day surgery [3]. Since opioids are a frequent

G.A. Walco and K.R. Goldschneider (eds.), *Pain in Children: A Practical Guide for Primary Care.*
© Humana Press, a part of Springer Science + Business Media, 2008

cause of nausea and vomiting, minimizing opioid use may decrease rates of unplanned admission. Anticipating and treating these symptoms is a step toward improved pain control at home after day surgery [4]. It is important to provide appropriate analgesics and clear instructions on their use, including the benefit of scheduled analgesia administration. This avoids the need for parents to decide if their child is in "enough" pain to warrant prn dosing. All of these issues follow on the heels of interventions administered pre-, intra-, and immediately postoperatively, which will be discussed in greater depth.

1. Regional Anesthesia for Outpatient Surgery

Regional anesthetics, in combination with general anesthesia, are frequently used for children undergoing surgical procedures. Advantages of this technique are a smoother intraoperative course, decreased requirements for general anesthetics—often leading to a faster, smoother wake-up, decreased stress response, and excellent pain relief in the immediate postoperative period. Disadvantages include exposing the patient to the risks of two types of anesthesia for a single procedure. In skilled hands the benefits appear to outweigh the risks, although data are still sketchy. There are several guidelines to aid in the placement and intraoperative use of regional blocks that can help maximize the benefit–risk ratio of the combined technique. Several regional anesthesia techniques will be described, so that the primary care physician can better explain to the family what to expect on the day of operation, and better identify side effects or complications in the postoperative period (the reader can find details on these and more advanced regional anesthetic techniques in Chapter 12).

1.1. Caudal Anesthesia

The epidural space can be reached at many levels, including via the caudal canal. This latter route is especially worthy of consideration in very small children, particularly for the practitioner less experienced in epidural catheter placement. The anatomy

of the caudal space makes the caudal route to the epidural space very safe, although it is not without risk. It is possible to reach the dural sac in children and cause an inadvertent high spinal block (this occurs when local anesthetic ascends to the level of the brainstem, and can cause loss of consciousness and cardiopulmonary arrest). This phenomenon is rarely seen after caudal analgesia, however. There are also epidural veins in the caudal space making intravascular injection a possibility. The use of short beveled needles minimizes the chance of puncturing a blood vessel [5]. The caudal approach is the most likely to be used for a single shot, or one-time injection. It is also useful as a site for inserting a continuous catheter, especially in infants.

1.1.1. Single Shot Caudals

Single shot caudals are one of the most useful and most often performed regional blocks in pediatric anesthesia. They are suitable for lower extremity, perineal, inguinal, and lower abdominal surgery. Properly performed, a single shot caudal is a rapid, safe technique that leads to better patient comfort, potentially better outcomes, and should decrease anesthesia time by speeding room turnover. By placing a caudal block at the start of the case, one can minimize inspired concentration of anesthetic gasses and avoid intraoperative opioids, allowing for a rapid, comfortable wake-up at the end of the case.

Bupivacaine is the most commonly used local anesthetic. Its long-lasting effect makes it preferable for single shot caudals, and it tends to produce greater sensory than motor block, which is a nice feature for postoperative analgesia. The significant disadvantage of bupivacaine is its marked cardiotoxicity. The safety margin between the toxic dose and the effective dose is less for bupivacaine than for lidocaine, chloroprocaine, or ropivacaine.

The ideal concentration of bupivacaine for outpatient caudals would give long-lasting pain relief without motor block. It has been shown that, for plain bupivacaine, 0.1875 percent is most ideal [6]. This may vary if clonidine is added. Common practice often seems to come down to bupivacaine 0.25 percent if the block is placed preoperatively, and bupivacaine 0.125 percent when the block is placed postoperatively. Total doses of bupivacaine for pediatric patients are 2.5 mg/kg as a load and 0.4 mg/kg/hr thereafter.

Ropivacaine is similar to bupivacaine, but may have even more selective sensory block and improved cardiotoxicity [7]. Ropivacaine is thought to be less cardiotoxic because it is sold as only the *S* enantiomer. The *R* enantiomer of bupivacaine is more potent than *S*-bupivacaine in blocking the inactivated state of the cardiac sodium and potassium (hKv1.5) channels. Dosing of ropivacaine is similar to bupivacaine.

Clonidine is an excellent addition to a single shot caudal and may be offered by the anesthesiologist. Addition of 1 to 2 mcg/ml clonidine to a single shot caudal appears to significantly prolong the duration of analgesia [8–10]. In children this dose does not appear to cause problems with hemodynamic instability or respiratory depression [8]. A dose of 2 mcg/kg has been associated with respiratory depression in a single case report of a neonate [11].

Parents need to know that a caudal blockade can be expected to cause weakness of the legs. An analogy can be made to the effects of a labor epidural, as many of the same nerve roots are involved. Therefore, the child may need to be carried home, and should be assisted with walking until it is clear that the child has good stability. In babies, the block should wear off in less than 12 hours, but occasionally it will last longer. Blocks that last more than 12 hours, or prolonged numbness or weakness in a single leg, should be reported to the surgeon or anesthesiologist. As with all blocks, the parents should have medication to give immediately as the block wears off, as there will be no medication in the child's system and the pain may be difficult to control if the parents "get behind" the pain (see below).

1.2. Peripheral Nerve Blocks

1.2.1. Fascia Iliaca Block

Dalens et al. first described the fascia iliaca block in 1989 as an alternative to the traditional three-in-one block designed specifically for children [12]. Advantages of the fascia iliaca block include better efficacy, improved safety, and ease of placement. Dalens compared the fascia iliaca block to the three-in-one block performed with a nerve stimulator in sleeping children. He found that both techniques blocked the femoral nerve with a high rate of success, but the fascia iliaca block was better at blocking the lateral femoral cutaneous,

obturator, and genitofemoral nerves. The success rate was about 90 percent for these three nerves using the fascia iliaca block, versus about 15 percent using the three-in-one block. This block is used for muscle biopsies of the quadriceps, femur fracture repairs, or other orthopedic procedures on the upper leg and knee, including ACL repairs.

Safety is also improved with the fascia iliaca block because the needle is inserted away from any major neurovascular structures. As well, it is easier to place because accurate placement is dependent on easily located landmarks and does not require a nerve stimulator. A large volume is used to assist spread to all nerves: 0.8 ml/kg. To avoid injecting a toxic dose of local anesthetic, concentration should be limited to 0.25 percent bupivacaine. This will give a long-lasting block: 12 or more hours of postoperative analgesia. After this or a femoral nerve block, the quadriceps will be weak, and the thigh numb. Use of crutches is not impeded.

1.2.2. Ilioinguinal/Iliohypogastric Nerve Blocks

Ilioinguinal/iliohypogastric nerve blocks are useful for a variety of procedures requiring groin incisions such as herniorrhaphies, orchidopexies, or hydrocele repairs. Although adults will sometimes have these operations performed solely under such blocks, their main use in pediatric anesthesia is to provide postoperative analgesia.

While the anesthesiologist may perform the block percutaneously at the beginning of the case, the surgeon will often perform this block through the incision at the end of the repair. Advantages include the lack of any distortion of tissue planes by local anesthetic that might complicate the repair. The disadvantage is the inability to obtain preemptive analgesia. On the plus side, the nerves can be easily visualized in the wound allowing accurate placement of the local anesthetic.

Of interest, the splash technique [13] has been described because the open technique surprisingly often fails to provide an adequate block. This is the easiest method to obtain these blocks. Bupivacaine is poured into the wound and left for five minutes before aspiration. It is said to be as effective as open infiltration.

The two latter techniques do not provide preemptive analgesia or the anesthetic sparing effect of a combined regional–general technique. If the surgeon prefers to place an ilioinguinal/iliohypogastric nerve block at the end of the case, the anesthesia team may offer to place a single shot caudal at the start. As for any block, the total load of bupivacaine should be no more than 2.5 mg/kg, plus 0.4 mg/kg/hr for the time between the two blocks. It is reasonable to mention to parents and patients ahead of time that the crease of the groin, and sometimes the thigh, rarely can become numb after this block, and the hip flexors and quadriceps may be weak for several hours after this block [14].

1.2.3. Penile Blocks

The distal part of the penis is supplied entirely by the dorsal penile nerves. This is readily blocked with local anesthetic for operations such as circumcision or distal hypospadias repair. Penile blocks have become more commonly used in the newborn nursery for circumcisions. The scrotum and proximal penis derive their nerve supply from the genitofemoral and ilioinguinal nerves. Thus, a dorsal penile block alone is inappropriate for operations involving the scrotum or base of the penis. An advantage of penile blocks over caudal anesthesia is the lack of sensory and motor block to the lower extremities that might interfere with ambulation postoperatively in a day surgery patient.Three techniques are described for penile block.

First, the traditional dorsal penile nerve block is performed by injecting local anesthetic deep to Buck's fascia at the base of the penis. The needle is inserted to the symphysis pubis, then withdrawn and redirected caudally to pass beneath it just until a loss of resistance is felt as Buck's fascia is penetrated. This should be at a distance of about 5 mm. Care must be taken not to advance too far as one may potentially damage the dorsal vein or arteries of the penis or the corpus cavernosum. As with all blocks of the penis, epinephrine-containing solutions must never be used as they may cause vasoconstriction of the end arteries of the penis which could lead to gangrene. The major potential complication of this block is a hematoma caused by piercing the dorsal artery or vein or the corpus cavernosum. This could potentially lead to increased pressure under Buck's fascia with resultant ischemia of the penis. This complication is avoided by the other two techniques.

The second technique is simply to perform a ring block around the base of the penis. The disadvantage is that this requires two or more sticks and can lead to hematomas and swelling around the base of the penis.

The final technique is the subpubic approach described by Dalens [15]. The penis is pulled gently downward to put Scarpa's fascia under tension. The insertion sites are just below the pubic rami, 0.5 to 1 cm on either side of the symphysis pubis. The needle is directed 15 degrees medially and caudally to the skin from each of the two insertion sites. As the needle penetrates Scarpa's fascia there will be a distinct "pop." If the needle is released at this point it will remain fixed in place and not tilt or recoil. Inject 0.1 ml/kg of local anesthetic on each side.

Finally, practitioners have used Eutetic Mixture of Local Anesthetics (EMLA) cream and have dripped solutions of lidocaine onto the wound to provide postoperative analgesia for circumcision. EMLA, while fairly effective, is not presently recommended by the FDA for use on mucus membranes as absorption is unknown in this setting. There is concern that toxic levels of either lidocaine or prilocaine may be absorbed. Solutions of lidocaine on the dressing are clearly inadequate for performing the procedure, but may provide postoperative analgesia if changed frequently. Care must be taken to avoid absorption of toxic levels of lidocaine in this setting as well. Assume that all the lidocaine administered will be absorbed through the wound and mucosa.

1.3. Conclusions

This section has provided practical points on performing some common regional nerve blocks in pediatric patients. For the practitioner with an interest in this subject, an excellent reference is "Regional Anesthesia in Infants, Children and Adolescents" by Bernard Dalens [16]. It provides details on a wide range of nerve blocks, including how the placement of the blocks varies with age.

2. Medication Management of Postoperative Pain

2.1. Acetaminophen

Acetaminophen should not be overlooked as an analgesic! When administered in appropriate doses it is extremely safe in all but a handful of patients, primarily those with preexisting liver disease. Acetaminophen provides significant analgesia in its own right. Its opioid sparing effects have compared favorably to ketorolac in double-blind comparisons [17], and it is a centrally acting analgesic without anti-inflammatory effects. It can thus be co-administered with nonsteroidal anti-inflammatory drugs with additive or synergistic analgesia, but no increase in nonsteroidal side effects [18]. It is commonly co-administered with opioids because of synergistic analgesia. This allows decreased opioid dosing, thus minimizing side effects.

The major caveat for acetaminophen is that, since it is so commonly mixed with other analgesics, it is easy for the unwary or inadequately informed patient (or parent) to administer an excessive dose. One common mechanism is to administer plain acetaminophen every four hours, but then to rescue with a preparation containing additional acetaminophen and opioid. Sometimes a "cold" medicine will be given, not realizing that these may also have acetaminophen. It is important to have a frank discussion with parents or other caregivers regarding both benefits and risks of acetaminophen use.

Route of administration is important for acetaminophen. In the United States there is not an intravenous preparation yet. Propacetamol (a pro-drug of acetaminophen, or paracetamol, as it is known in Europe) is available for intravenous use in Europe. Acetaminophen is thus generally administered either orally or rectally. The pharmacokinetics and pharmacodynamics of oral acetaminophen are fairly well established. Patients often require an initial dose of 20 mg/kg to obtain adequate blood levels. Subsequent doses should be 10 to 15 mg/kg every 4 hours, not to exceed 90 to 100 mg/kg per day, up to a maximum total dose of 4,000 mg per day. Higher doses risk hepatic toxicity.

Rectal dosing of acetaminophen can be problematic. Absorption is slow and variable. Given the variable absorption by the middle hemorrhoidal plexus which drains into the portal system and the lower hemorrhoidal plexus that drains systemically, the final bioavailability of rectally administered acetaminophen is unknown and may vary from patient to patient or even dose to dose, depending on where the suppository is placed. In general, peak plasma levels after rectal administration of acetaminophen occur at least two hours from the time of dosing. The height of the peak is generally lower than would be obtained with oral dosing. Because the bioavailability seems to be half or less than when acetaminophen is given orally, it is reasonable to administer an initial dose of 30 to 45 mg per kg rectally, when the oral route is not practical. Although subsequent dosing is less clear, a conservative approach is to keep subsequent doses at 15 mg/kg every 4 hours, thus staying at 90 mg/kg per day after the initial load. However, rectal doses of 15 mg/kg may not be effective, so transition to oral dosing as soon as possible is recommended, for both efficacy and safety reasons.

2.2. Nonsteroidal Anti-Inflammatory Drugs

Nonsteroidal anti-inflammatory drugs (NSAIDs) also provide useful analgesia. Intravenous ketorolac has been compared to a dose of 5 to 10 mg of morphine in adult patients and demonstrates an opioid sparing effect of 30 to 66 percent in children [19-20]. Oral nonsteroidal agents also decrease the need for opioids, thus decreasing the likelihood of nausea, emesis, and other opioid side effects. Unlike acetaminophen, nonsteroidal anti-inflammatory agents work both centrally and in the periphery. Through inhibition of prostaglandin synthesis, they reduce inflammation. For some procedures this may provide excellent analgesia.

Because they inhibit prostaglandin synthesis, NSAIDs cause certain expected side effects of their own, such as inhibition of platelet function. This can lead to increased bleeding and may be a relative contraindication to their use for surgical procedures where bleeding cannot be easily monitored (e.g., tonsillectomy) or where even a minor amount of bleeding may cause severe complications (e.g., airway compromise from a neck hematoma or loss of a skin graft from bleeding beneath it). NSAIDs also may cause gastric irritation and can lead to acute renal failure in the setting of hypovolemia or other prerenal causes of azotemia. Rarely, NSAIDs have been associated with liver damage.

Although individual patients may clearly tolerate one nonsteroidal drug better than another, it is difficult to show clear efficacy or decreased side effects between these drugs in large populations. It is, therefore, appropriate to choose medication based on pediatric data, cost, ease of administration, and the individual practitioner's familiarity with the drugs. Good data are available for the use of ibuprofen, naproxen, and ketorolac in pediatric patients.

Ketorolac is best used intraoperatively as a single intravenous dose during closure. It is the only nonsteroidal approved as an intravenous analgesic. Doses of 0.5 mg/kg are recommended [19–23].

For home use, ibuprofen is recommended at a dose of 8 to 10 mg/kg three times per day. It is available as a liquid suspension at 20 mg/mL, and also in chewable tablets of 50 mg or 100 mg strength.

For older children who can swallow pills, naproxen is a longer lasting medication that requires only twice daily dosing. The manufacturer only recommends naproxen for children over 12 years of age [24]. The recommended dose for patients with juvenile arthritis is 15 mg/kg/day. The 220 mg tablet size would be appropriate for a 30 kg child given twice per day.

2.3. Opioids

Multiple opioid preparations are available for use in children. Most are reasonably equivalent when used in equipotent doses, but there are a few points worth emphasizing on opioid preparations. First, a fentanyl patch is never indicated for outpatient postoperative analgesia in opioid naïve patients. There are case reports of death with such use. Transdermal fentanyl creates a reservoir in the skin which continues to release fentanyl to the blood even after patch removal [25].

Second, although codeine is a traditional oral opioid for young children, it is perhaps time to rethink that tradition. About 5 to 10 percent of Caucasians and fewer, but still a significant number of patients from other ethic groups, are unable to metabolize codeine to morphine. Thus, these patients will not achieve any analgesia from codeine. For this reason, hydrocodone/acetaminophen or oxycodone/acetaminophen (for more severe postoperative pain) are overall better choices than codeine-containing products.

Third, methadone has had a recent surge in popularity in the United States. Given the very long half-life of methadone, it is also a poor choice for outpatient surgical patients. Initial doses will not bring the drug to steady state and so may pro-

vide inadequate analgesia. If the patient receives repeated doses to achieve analgesia, delayed respiratory depression may appear after the patient's pain has started to resolve. Methadone accounts for a much higher percentage of opioid-related deaths than expected from the percent of opioid prescriptions written.

Fourth, meperidine (Demerol®) is a poor oral analgesic. It is only about 20 percent bioavailable and the remainder is immediately converted to normeperidine, the metabolite responsible for the drug's potential to cause seizures. Meperidine is also a weak analgesic, with only about one-tenth the potency of morphine (when both are given intravenously). Propoxyphene (Darvon®, Darvocet N-100®) is another weak opioid. The analgesia of propoxyphene with acetaminophen is equivalent to acetaminophen alone. It is also associated with a number of adverse effects: seizures, prolongation of the QT interval leading to dysrhythmias, and euphoria [26]. These properties make propoxyphene another poor choice.

Remaining choices include hydrocodone, oxycodone, hydromorphone, and morphine. Chapter 8 provides greater detail, but a few points are worth discussing here. Hydrocodone comes premixed with acetaminophen. Brand names include Lortab® and Vicodin®. Hydrocodone is available in both pill and liquid forms. Exact dosing guidelines are available from the manufacturer, but the recommended dose is approximately 0.15 mg/kg of the hydrocodone, and approximately 10 mg/kg of the acetaminophen every 4 to 6 hours. Hydrocodone is not available separate from acetaminophen, so caution is in order regarding the total acetaminophen load when prescribing it (see above). Oxycodone has approximately twice the oral bioavailability, and roughly 1.5 times the potency of morphine. It is often reserved for more severe postoperative pain. The recommended dose is 0.05 to 0.15 mg/kg every 4 to 6 hours. Morphine is also available as an elixir of 20 mg/mL but this formulation is only recommended for patients who are opioid-tolerant. Dosing is roughly 0.3 mg/kg orally every 4 hours. Many pharmacies can make more dilute solutions of either oxycodone or morphine to allow for easier measurement. Finally, hydromorphone (Dilaudid®) is available in a 1 mg/mL solution. Recommended doses are 0.03 to 0.08 mg/kg. Choosing between these medications is, to some extent, a matter of personal preference of either the clinician or the patient. Clearly, if the patient has a history of severe nausea and vomiting with a particular drug it is wise to avoid it. Otherwise, for postoperative pain that is expected to be mild to moderate, hydrocodone with acetaminophen is a good choice. If the pain is expected to be more severe, oxycodone or hydromorphone may be more appropriate. These are good choices, in particular, because they can be dosed independently of the acetaminophen dosing.

3. The Transition from Recovery Room to Home

An area where the primary care physician can do great good is in educating the parents about safely and effectively maneuvering the child from the hospital or surgery center to home. Several main points are germane. First, information regarding postoperative analgesia should be provided ahead of time as parents may have difficulty processing information on the day of surgery. Next, if there is any history of non-response to codeine in family members, the parents should ask for something else for their child. The alternative is to ask for the first dose to be given at the surgical facility so the effect can be assessed before they leave. This will allow a second prescription to be provided, in case the codeine does not provide adequate analgesia. Third, it is better to stay ahead of pain, rather than to catch up. Therefore, it is reasonable to recommend to the parents that they use a "reverse prn" approach to giving the analgesics for the first 24 hours. For instance, NSAIDs (if allowed by the surgeon) should be given around the clock. Opioid products should be offered to the child on a regular basis, and only withheld if the child is sleepy or has no pain. In that case the parent should check back with the child an hour later. Waiting for the child to ask for medication may lead to undertreatment.

If a child has had a nerve block, two issues arise. First, the child must be helped to monitor that the affected extremity does not sustain injury while the block is effective. That is, having a finger or foot caught in a car door, or leaned against a hot radiator (among other possibilities) may lead to injury, as the usual protective pain response will be blunted by the nerve block. Therefore, it is helpful to counsel the parent to help the child keep visual track of the extremity until the block recedes. Second, it can be tricky to assess when to transition to oral medications, but this is a key point in providing optimal postoperative analgesia. Parents should begin giving NSAIDs as soon as the next dose is possible, even without complaints of pain. As soon as the child complains even a little of pain, dosing of any other medications should begin. The change from numb and comfortable to normal sensation and pain can be abrupt. Lastly, parents should be advised to obtain contact numbers for the surgeon or anesthesia provider in case there are complications or questions regarding any block that was placed or medication prescribed. Unusually severe pain or pain that increases over a few days can be a sign of a complication, and parents should know how to contact the appropriate physician. Of course, having the number of the primary care physician is always a source of security for parents, and the primary physician can advocate for the child if a potential complication (with the nerve block or surgery) is suspected.

In short, analgesia for outpatient pediatric surgery should be obtained with a combined approach including regional anesthesia (whenever applicable), acetaminophen, NSAIDs, and judicious use of opioids. Doing so should minimize side effects and decrease unexpected admissions to the hospital. Providing clear guidelines to the child's parents or other primary caregiver will help assure that he or she receives appropriate analgesia.

Take-Home Points

- Parents can be encouraged to advocate for their child and provide better analgesic treatment during a preoperative visit than on the day of surgery.
- Day surgery is an excellent venue for regional anesthesia, when appropriate to the surgical procedure.
- The transition from a regional blockade to oral medication should be planned ahead of time for best results.

- A "reverse prn" regimen can assist the parents in staying ahead of the pain and should be considered for the first 24 hours after surgery.
- Parents should be educated regarding whom to call for inadequate analgesia or potential surgical complication.

References

1. Kankkunen P, Vehvilainen-Julkunen K, Pietila AM, Halonen P. Is the sufficiency of discharge instructions related to children's postoperative pain at home after day surgery? Scand J Caring Sci 2003;17:365–372.
2. Jonas DA. Parent's management of their child's pain in the home following day surgery. J Child Health Care 2003;7:150–162.
3. Mills N, Anderson BJ, Barber C, et al. Day stay pediatric tonsillectomy–a safe procedure. Int J Pediatr Otorhinolaryngol 2004;68:1367–1373.
4. Finley GA, McGrath PJ, Forwards P, McNeal G, and Fitzgerald P. Parents' management of children's pain following 'minor' surgery. Pain 1996;64:83–87.
5. Dalens B, Hasnaoui A. Caudal anesthesia in pediatric surgery: success rate and adverse effects in 750 consecutive patients. Anesth Analg 1989;68:83–89.
6. Wolf AR, Valley RD, Fear DW, Roy WL, Lerman J. Bupivacaine for caudal analgesia in infants and children: The optimal effective concentration. Anesthesiology 1988;69:102–106.
7. Morrison LM, Emanuelsson BM, McClure JH, et al. Efficacy and kinetics of extradural ropivacaine: comparison with bupivacaine. Br J Anaesth 1994;72:164–169.
8. Dupeyrat A, Goujard E, Muret J, Ecoffey C. Transcutaneous CO_2 tension effects of clonidine in paediatric caudal analgesia. Paediatr Anaesth 1998;8:145–148.
9. Ivani G, De Negri P, Conio A, et al. Ropivacaine-clonidine combination for caudal blockade in children. Acta Anaesthesiol Scand 2000;44:446–449.
10. Klimscha W, Chiari A, Michalek-Sauberer A, et al. The efficacy and safety of a clonidine/bupivacaine combination in caudal blockade for pediatric hernia repair. Anesth Analg 1998;86:54–61.
11. Breschan C, Krumpholz R, Likar R, Kraschl R, Schalk HV. Can a dose of 2microg.kg(-1) caudal clonidine cause respiratory depression in neonates? Paediatr Anaesth 1999;9:81–83.
12. Dalens B, Vanneuville G, Tanguy A. Comparison of the fascia iliaca compartment block with the 3-in-1 block in children. Anesth Analg 1989;69:705–713.
13. Casey WF, Rice LJ, Hannallah RS, Broadman L, Norden JM, Guzzetta P. A comparison between bupivacaine instillation versus ilioinguinal/iliohypogastric nerve block for postoperative analgesia following inguinal herniorrhaphy in children. Anesthesiology 1990;72:637–639.
14. Lipp AK, Woodcock J, Hensman B, Wilkinson K. Leg weakness is a complication of ilio-inguinal nerve block in children. Br J Anaesth 2004;92:273–274.
15. Dalens B, Vanneuville G, Dechelotte P. Penile block via the subpubic space in 100 children. Anesth Analg 1989;69:41–45.
16. Dalens B. Regional Anesthesia in Infants, Children, and Adolescents. London: Williams and Wilkins Waverly Europe, 1995.
17. Rusy LM, Houck CS, Sullivan LJ, et al. A double-blind evaluation of ketorolac tromethamine versus acetaminophen in pediatric tonsillectomy: analgesia and bleeding. Anesth Analg 1995;80:226–229.
18. Qiu HX, Liu J, Kong H, Liu Y, Mei XG. Isobolographic analysis of the antinociceptive interactions between ketoprofen and paracetamol. Eur J Pharmacol 2007;557:141–146.
19. Watcha MF, Jones MB, Lagueruela RG, Schweiger C, White PF. Comparison of ketorolac and morphine as adjuvants during pediatric surgery. Anesthesiology 1992;76:368–372.
20. Carney DE, Nicolette LA, Ratner MH, Minerd A, Baesl TJ. Ketorolac reduces postoperative narcotic requirements. J Pediatr Surg 2001;36:76–79.
21. Pappas AL, Fluder EM, Creech S, Hotaling A, Park A. Postoperative analgesia in children undergoing myringotomy and placement equalization tubes in ambulatory surgery. Anesth Analg 2003;96:1621–1624.
22. Hackmann T. Smaller dose of 0.5 mg/kg IV ketorolac is sufficient to provide pain relief in children. Anesth Analg 2004;98:275–276.
23. Dsida RM, Wheeler M, Birmingham PK, et al. Age-stratified pharmacokinetics of ketorolac tromethamine in pediatric surgical patients. Anesth Analg 2002;94:266–270.
24. Reiff A, Lovell DJ, Adelsberg JV, et al. Evaluation of the comparative efficacy and tolerability of rofecoxib and naproxen in children and adolescents with juvenile rheumatoid arthritis: A 12-week randomized controlled clinical trial with a 52-week open-label extension. J Rheumatol 2006;33:985–995.

25. Grond S, Radbruch L, Lehmann KA. Clinical pharmacokinetics of transdermal opioids: focus on transdermal fentanyl. Clin Pharmacokinet 2000; 38:59–89.

26. Barkin RL, Barkin SJ, Barkin DS. Propoxyphene (dextropropoxyphene): A critical review of a weak opioid analgesic that should remain in antiquity. Am J Ther 2006;13:534–542.

12
Regional Anesthesia

Elliot J. Krane, Artee Gandhi, and R.J. Ramamurthi

Abstract: This chapter identifies the role of regional anesthesia in pediatric pain management, not only for postoperative pain control, but also as a diagnostic and therapeutic tool for chronic pain conditions. The pharmacology of commonly used local anesthetics and adjuvant medications is described with explanations of pediatric physiology, dosing regimens, and toxicity. Various types of nerve blocks with their anatomical descriptions and specific indications are outlined, with reference to regional anesthesia textbooks for further details. By reviewing this chapter, the primary care physician should be able to identify the indications for regional anesthesia, the medications employed, and their function in the management of pediatric pain conditions.

Key words: Pain, child, regional anesthesia, nerve block, local anesthetic.

Introduction

Over the past 20 years, pediatric regional anesthesia has become an important part of patient care [1-3]. Neuraxial and peripheral nerve blocks play a role in both postoperative pain management, treatment of acute pain such as after long bone fractures, in acute pancreatitis and management for chronic painful conditions such as headaches, abdominal pain, complex regional pain syndromes (CRPS), and cancer pain. A review by Giaufre et al. that comprised a 12-month prospective review of pediatric regional anesthesia in their institution demonstrated both the utility and the safety of regional anesthesia in children [4]. Regional anesthesia provides an alternative to or augmentation of opioid-based pain control, thus eliminating or minimizing opioid-induced side effects of nausea, vomiting, somnolence, respiratory depression, pruritus, and constipation, while providing generally better quality pain relief by interrupting nociceptive pathways and more profound inhibition of endocrine stress responses. Further clinical benefits of regional techniques for patients may be earlier ambulation, prevention of atelectasis, and earlier discharge from the hospital [2]. Therefore, regional anesthesia has become widely used both for intraoperative anesthesia and postoperative analgesia in children.

Regional anesthesia has most commonly contributed to superior analgesia in the postoperative milieu. In order to perform these procedures successfully, cooperation must exist between the anesthesiologist, surgeon, and family members. Contributing to the success and ease of these techniques has been the recent use of peripheral nerve stimulators to identify the target nerve structures, and ultrasound to visualize the target nerves and assure correct needle placement.

The purpose of this chapter is not to give the pediatrician, family practitioner, or other professional instruction in how to perform regional anesthetic blocks in children. That, of course, requires specific training and supervision. Rather the purpose of this chapter is to familiarize the reader with the range of blocks available so that the reader may request specific therapeutic or analgesic blocks as part of consultation requests, and to have the reader understand the pharmacology and toxicity of local anesthetics when they are administered to children.

1. Local Anesthetic Pharmacology

Table 12-1 lists the commonly used local anesthetics in the United States, and the safe maximum doses for infants and children as boluses and as infusions [5]. Systemic toxicity is the most frequent complication of regional anesthetics [6], and doses should be carefully calculated based on weight [7].

One of the most important factors in utilizing regional anesthesia in children is recognizing the difference between pediatric and adult pharmacology that may lead to an increased risk of local anesthetic toxicity [2].

There are several differences in local anesthetic pharmacology to take into account in children [1, 3, 4, 7-10]. The steady state volume of distribution (Vd_{ss}) is larger in children than in adults. While this factor results in the advantageous effect of lower peak blood levels of local anesthetics after bolus administration, it also means that less anesthetic is presented to the liver for metabolism per unit of time, decreasing drug clearance. Also mitigating the effect of Vd_{ss} on anesthetic blood levels is that the increased

cardiac output and regional blood flow in infants and children increase local anesthetic uptake from areas of injection into the blood, resulting in more rapid and higher blood levels, compared with adults.

Amide local anesthetics are metabolized in the liver. The immature liver demonstrates a reduced ability to metabolize the "amino amides." Furthermore, the fact that young infants have decreased serum levels of the proteins that bind to local anesthetics in the blood, alpha-1-acid glycoprotein (AAG) and albumin, increases their susceptibility to the risk of toxicity due to the increased availability of "free" unbound drug (Table 12-2) [11]. Protein binding is also pH-dependent, so that metabolic acidosis or hypocapnea will decrease the protein affinity to local anesthetic molecules, and will increase the free unbound fraction of the drug.

Finally, infants have decreased serum levels of choline esterases, decreasing their ability to metabolize the "ester" based local anesthetics. In practice, though, this is not a major factor in the use of this class of local anesthetics.

Symptoms of local anesthetic toxicity (tinnitus, dizziness, taste alterations) usually alert the clinician to impending complications of systemic toxicity, but cannot be reported by infants or young children. Thus, the first manifestations of toxicity in children may be alterations in consciousness, seizures, and cardiovascular arrhythmias or collapse (Table 12-2) [7].

TABLE 12-1. Local anesthetic doses.

Drug	Class	Concentration: skin infiltration	Concentration: nerve block	Onset of action	Duration of action	Maximum dose without epinephrine	Maximum dose with epinephrine
Procaine (Novacaine®)	Ester	1–2%	0.25–1%	5–15 min	45–60 min	7 mg/kg	9 mg/kg
Tetracaine (Pontocaine®)	Ester	0.05–0.1%	*	10–20 min	1½–3 hr	*	*
Lidocaine (Xylocaine®)	Amide	0.5–1%	1–2%	3–5 min	1–1½ hr	4.5 mg/kg	7 mg/kg
Bupivacaine (Marcaine®)	Amide	0.25%	0.25–0.5%	5–10 min	1½–8 hr	2 mg/kg	3 mg/kg
Ropivacaine (Naropin®)	Amide	0.1%	0.10–0.2%	5–10 min	1½–8 hr	2 mg/kg	3 mg/kg
Levobupivacaine (Chirocaine®)	Amide	0.1%	0.10–0.2%	5–10 min	1½–8 hr	2 mg/kg	3 mg/kg

Note: Tetracaine is not used for peripheral nerve and epidural blocks; its use is limited to topical and intrathecal (spinal) anesthesia, for which the dose is not limited based on toxicity. The maximum safe dose for topical skin administration has not been established. Use of trade names is for example only and does not imply brand preference.

TABLE 12-2. Toxicity of local anesthetics.

Central nervous system	Mild: Visual disturbance, tongue numbness, lightheadedness, apprehension, restlessness
	Moderate: Perioral paresthesia, muscle twitching, slurred speech, excitability, drowsiness
	Severe: Seizures, cardiorespiratory depression, coma
Cardiovascular	Mild: Palpitations, vasodilation
	Moderate: Hypertension, dysrhythmias, myocardial depression, hypotension
	Severe: Bradycardia, ventricular arrhythmias, Torsade de Pointes, cardiovascular collapse, asystole
Respiratory	Mild/Moderate: Hypoventilation
	Severe: Respiratory arrest
Immunologic	Anaphylaxis: Only with ester anesthetics (e.g., tetracaine)
Hematologic	Methemoglobinemia: Only with prilocaine

2. Regional Anesthetic Nerve Blocks and their Indications in Children

With the proper training, equipment and understanding of pediatric pharmacology and anatomy, peripheral nerve blocks can be performed safely and effectively. While most of these nerve blocks are frequently within the province of the anesthesiologist or pain management physician, a few may be performed by non-anesthesiologists with appropriate training. Further, the practicing pediatrician should be aware of these nerve blocks, both because their patients may be so treated by anesthesiologists, and also so that they may request their colleagues in anesthesiology or pain management to perform an appropriate nerve block in specific clinical circumstances. Several textbooks of regional anesthesia provide detailed illustration of techniques and discussions of pitfalls and complications for the reader who wishes further detail [1, 12–16].

The following section will divide the available nerve blocks by anatomic areas.

2.1. Head and Neck Blocks

Primary pain syndromes of the head, such as trigeminal neuralgia, are distinctly unusual in the pediatric population. Few surgical conditions of the head and neck are amenable to regional anesthesia—for example, pain following tonsillectomies has not been found to be amenable to nerve blockade—and neurosurgical incisional pain is usually mitigated by local infiltration of local anesthetic into the wound margins by the surgeon. Headache disorders, however, are very common in the pediatric age group, and many chronic headache disorders will be responsive to occipital nerve block.

2.1.1. Occipital Nerve Block

Indications: Cervicogenic headache (whiplash), migraine, skull fracture, scalp laceration. Where pharmacologic and nonpharmacologic modalities are unsuccessful in treating headache, nerve blocks as such may be beneficial [17–19].

Anatomy: The greater and lesser occipital nerves provide sensation to much of the scalp, from the vertex down to the cervical region. The greater occipital nerve is found adjacent to the occipital artery, which can often be palpated at the occipital ridge midway between the occipital prominence and the mastoid process. The lesser occipital nerves emerge from deeper layers midway between the greater occipital nerve and the mastoid process, where subcutaneous infiltration is effective.

Technique: The occipital arterial pulse can often be palpated, or the occipital artery can be visualized using common ultrasound devices. Alternatively, the needle can be inserted at the point where the artery is expected to be. The needle is inserted just below the occipital ridge and directed toward the ridge until bone is contacted; it is then withdrawn slightly and the local anesthetic is injected. By deliberately contacting the bone and withdrawing, one can be certain the anesthetic has not been injected into the subarachnoid space. The lesser occipital nerves are anesthetized by inserting the needle at the same point as for the greater nerves, but directing it laterally toward the mastoid process, injecting in a subcutaneous fan-like distribution from midway toward the mastoid to the mastoid process.

Drug and Dose: 0.25 percent bupivacaine or 0.2 percent ropivacaine is most often used for maximal duration of the block. A total of 2 to 4 ml of local anesthetic is sufficient on each side to produce the desired block. The local anesthetic is often combined with methylprednisolone (Depo-Medrol®) if a component of occipital neuritis is suspected. If chronic headache responds well, although transiently, to occipital nerve block, the block may be repeated with botulinum toxin, or the nerve can be ablated by pulsed radiofrequency.

Assessment: This block is fairly straightforward with low morbidity.

2.2. Upper Extremity Blocks

Brachial plexus blocks provide postoperative pain control for surgical procedures of the upper extremities, as well as to protect the extremity from movement, and reduce arterial spasm. Brachial plexus block also provides blockade of the sympathetic outflow to the upper extremity. Depending on the location of pain, the brachial plexus may be blocked above the clavicle (roots and trunks) or below the clavicle (cords) corresponding to procedures proximal or distal to the elbow.

The brachial plexus is an arrangement of nerve fibers originating from spinal nerves C5, C6, C7, C8, and T1 that extend into the neck, axilla, arm, and hand. The brachial plexus is responsible for cutaneous and motor innervation of the entire upper limb except for the trapezius muscle and an area of skin near the axilla. The roots merge to form three trunks: Superior (C5–6), middle (C7), and inferior (C8–T1). Each trunk then splits into two to form six divisions: anterior division of the superior, middle and inferior trunks, and posterior division of the superior, middle and inferior trunks. The six divisions then form three cords that are named by their position in relation to the axillary artery. The posterior cord is formed from the three posterior divisions of the trunks (C5–T1), the lateral cord from the anterior divisions of the middle and upper trunks (C5–C7), and the medial cord as a continuation of the lower trunk (C8–T1). The terminal branches include the musculocutaneous nerve (from the lateral cord), the median nerve (from the lateral cord), the axillary nerve (from the posterior cord), the radial nerve (from the posterior cord), and the ulnar nerve (from the medial cord).

2.2.1. Interscalene Brachial Plexus Block

Indications: Pain in the shoulder or upper arm; surgery of the shoulder or upper arm [1, 2, 20, 21].

Anatomy: The interscalene block anesthetizes the nerves at the level of the trunks, with the injection at the level of the cricoid cartilage.

Technique: Electrical nerve stimulation and/or ultrasound are used to direct the needle to the appropriate location. The technique is technical and generally best performed by an anesthesiologist or interventional pain physician. Interested readers may refer to several textbooks of regional anesthesia for further instruction and detail. This and the following brachial plexus blocks may be performed as a single injection technique, or with placement of a continuous infusion catheter for prolonged maintenance of anesthesia.

Drug and Dose: 0.25 percent bupivacaine or 0.2 percent ropivacaine are most frequently used. If there is a desire to anesthetize only sensory and sympathetic fibers and spare motor fibers, a more dilute solution may be used (e.g. 0.16% or 0.08% bupivacaine). The typical dose is 0.3 ml/kg to establish a block, and 0.05 ml/kg/hr as a continuous infusion.

Assessment: This is an advanced block, with higher potential morbidity, best performed by an anesthesiologist or pain physician.

2.2.2. Infraclavicular Brachial Plexus Block

Indications: Surgery or pain of the arm or forearm.

Anatomy: The infraclavicular block is performed at the level of the divisions of the brachial plexus, inferior to the clavicle.

Technique: Electrical nerve stimulation and/or ultrasound are used to direct the needle to the appropriate location. Interested readers may refer to several textbooks of regional anesthesia for further instruction and detail.

Drug and Dose: 0.25 percent bupivacaine or 0.2 percent ropivacaine are most frequently used. If there is a desire to anesthetize only sensory and sympathetic fibers and spare motor fibers, a more dilute solution may be used (e.g. 0.16% or 0.08% bupivacaine). The typical dose is 0.3 ml/kg to establish a block, and 0.05 ml/kg/hr as a continuous infusion.

Assessment: This is an advanced block, with higher potential morbidity, best performed by an anesthesiologist or pain physician.

2.2.3. Axillary Brachial Plexus Block

Indications: Surgery or pain in the wrist or hand.

Anatomy: The brachial plexus exists as cords in the axillary fossa, running with and around the axillary artery. Controversy exists regarding whether the structures of the plexus and the axillary artery and vein exist within a fascial sheath.

Technique: Electrical nerve stimulation and/or ultrasound are used to direct the needle to the appropriate location. Interested readers may refer to several textbooks of regional anesthesia for further instruction and detail.

Drug and Dose: 0.25 percent bupivacaine or 0.2 percent ropivacaine are most frequently used. If there is a desire to anesthetize only sensory and sympathetic fibers and spare motor fibers, a more dilute solution may be used (e.g., 0.16% or 0.08% bupivacaine). The typical dose is 0.3 ml/kg to establish a block, and 0.05 ml/kg/hr as a continuous infusion.

Assessment: This is a moderate level block, with moderate potential morbidity and failure rate, better left to experienced practitioners.

2.2.4. Intravenous Regional (Bier) Block

Indications: Surgery of the wrist or hand; management of complex regional pain syndromes of the hand.

Technique: An intravenous cannula is inserted into the distal extremity, and after exsanguination of the extremity by wrapping it in an elastic bandage and/or elevating it, a double pneumatic tourniquet is applied and the proximal cuff is inflated. Local anesthetic is then injected into the intravenous cannula, filling the exsanguinated vasculature. Anesthesia for the extremity below the double pneumatic tourniquet is limited only by the duration of the tourniquet inflation, which is in turn limited by the occurrence of pain underneath the tourniquet after 30 to 60 minutes of ischemia. The tourniquet must remain inflated for at least 15 minutes to allow fixation of local anesthetic to tissues, which reduces peak blood concentration and toxicity on tourniquet deflation. Incremental tourniquet deflation is also recommended to slow the entry of local anesthetic into the circulation. Readers may refer to textbooks of regional anesthesia for further instruction and detail.

Drug and Dose: 0.5 percent lidocaine is most frequently used, and bupivacaine is generally never used because of the increased cardiovascular toxicity associated with release of the large local anesthetic dose into the circulation on tourniquet deflation. The typical lidocaine dose for the upper extremity is 3 mg/kg, and 6 mg/kg for the lower extremity. Phentolamine 2.5 to 5 mg and/or ketorolac 0.75 mg/kg may be added for prolonged analgesic effect in regional pain syndromes.

Assessment: This is a low morbidity, high success block, but usually the very indication for the block requires that the child be sedated or anesthetized, thus limiting general use.

2.3. Truncal Somatic and Visceral Blocks

Truncal blocks provide somatic and visceral analgesia and anesthesia for surgery of the thorax and abdominal area. Sympathetic, motor and sensory blockade may be obtained. These blocks are often used in combination to provide optimal relief. Intercostal and paravertebral blocks may be beneficial in those patients for whom an epidural injection or catheter is contraindicated; for example, in the presence of a coagulopathy. Respiratory function is usually well maintained and the side effects of opioid therapy are eliminated.

2.3.1. Intercostal Nerve Block

Indications: Surgery or pain of the chest wall such as from injury, chest tube, rib fractures, and rib lesions; surgery or pain associated with thoracotomy, gastrostomy, cholecystectomy, or other upper abdominal surgery [22].

Anatomy: The intercostal nerves are the anterior rami of the thoracic nerves from T1–T11 with the following branches: 1) rami communicantes to and from the sympathetic trunk; 2) posterior cutaneous branch to the intercostal muscles and pleura; 3) lateral cutaneous branch to the lateral wall skin and muscles; and 4) anterior cutaneous branch to the anterior wall skin and muscles. T1 and T2 supply the upper limbs and upper thorax, T3–T6 the thorax, and T7–T11 the abdominal wall and skin of the front part of the gluteal region. The intercostal nerves lie inferior and posterior to the rib with their corresponding vein and artery.

Technique: In order to obtain adequate analgesia and anesthesia, the two dermatomes above and below the site of pain must be blocked. The landmarks for the block are identified by palpation, generally without the use of ultrasound or electrical nerve stimulation. There is an obvious risk of pneumothorax and this block should not be performed in a patient who already has respiratory compromise (especially if an ipsilateral chest tube is not in place). Interested readers may refer to several textbooks on regional anesthesia for further instruction and detail.

Drug and Dose: 0.25 to 0.5 percent bupivacaine, 1 to 2 percent lidocaine, or 0.5 to 0.75 percent ropivacaine, with epinephrine 1:100,000 to 1:400,000. Since this block requires multiple injections, local anesthetic toxicity is a concern. Because uptake of local anesthetic from injection site to blood is very rapid with intercostal blocks, epinephrine should always be used and the maximum safe doses of local anesthetics should be observed (Table 12-1). The maximum allowable dose of epinephrine is 4 mcg/kg.

Assessment: This is an advanced block, with higher potential morbidity, best performed by an anesthesiologist or pain physician.

2.3.2. Paravertebral Block

Indications: Surgery or pain associated of the chest as above, unilateral upper abdominal surgery such as nephrectomy or splenectomy, as an alternative to intercostal nerve block.

Anatomy: The thoracic paravertebral space is lateral to the vertebral column, containing the sympathetic chain, rami communicantes, and dorsal and ventral roots of the spinal nerves. Since it is a continuous space, local anesthetic injection will provide sensory, motor, and sympathetic blockade to these structures in several dermatomes. The paravertebral block is essentially a technique that provides multiple intercostal blocks using a single injection. As for many blocks, it may be performed as a single injection, or for a very prolonged effect a catheter can be left in the paravertebral space for a continuous infusion over several days or weeks.

Technique: Interested readers may refer to several textbooks of regional anesthesia for further instruction and detail.

Drug and Dose: 0.25 percent bupivacaine and 0.2 percent ropivacaine are most commonly used, 0.25 ml/kg, and then 0.001 to 0.1 ml/kg/hr as a continuous infusion of bupivacaine 0.125 percent or ropivacaine 0.1 percent.

Assessment: This is an advanced block, with higher potential morbidity, best performed by an anesthesiologist or pain physician.

2.3.3. Rectus Sheath Nerve Block

Indications: Surgery or pain around the umbilical area; parumbilical and umbilical hernia repair.

Anatomy: The umbilicus divides the abdomen into upper and lower, right and left quadrants and is innervated by dermatome T10. The tenth thoracoabdominal intercostal nerve from each side provides cutaneous sensation to the skin of the umbilical area. The nerve runs between the rectus sheath and the posterior rectus abdominus muscle. The rectus sheath itself contains the rectus abdominus muscle, the superior and inferior epigastric vessels, the terminal branches of the intercostal nerves, T7–11 and the subcostal vessels and nerves.

Technique: The umbilicus and linea semilunaris are identified. The linea semilunaris is the tendinous line on either side of the rectus abdominus muscle. A 23 g needle is inserted perpendicularly 0.5 cm above or below the umbilicus, medial to the linea semilunaris. The needle is advanced until it encounters the posterior rectus sheath, which is usually at a depth of 0.5 to 1.5 cm. The goal is to be between the rectus muscle and the posterior aspect of its sheath. Therefore, a "blunt" bevelled needle that will not easily penetrate the sheath is useful. After aspirating, local anesthetic is injected. Ultrasound is quite helpful for this block since the muscle is easily identified and one can visualize the space between the muscle and the posterior aspect of the sheath as it expands with local anesthetic. Accidental puncture of the posterior sheath and needle entry into the peritoneum is the most common complication. For umbilical pain, bilateral rectus sheath blocks are necessary.

Drug and Dose: 0.25 percent bupivacaine or 0.2 percent ropivacaine, 2 to 5 ml.

Assessment: This is a simple block, with low morbidity, but is most often used in the operating room.

2.3.4. Ilioinguinal and Iliohypogastric Nerve Block

Indications: Surgery for inguinal hernia repair, hydrocele, or orchiopexy repair [16].

Anatomy: The first lumbar nerve divides into the iliohypogastric and ilioinguinal nerves which emerge from the lateral border of the psoas major muscle. The iliohypogastric nerve supplies the suprapubic area as it pierces the internal oblique muscle and runs deep to the external oblique. The ilioinguinal nerve supplies the upper medial thigh and superior inguinal region as it also pierces the internal oblique muscle (but lies deeper to the muscle) and runs across the inguinal canal.

Technique: The anterior superior iliac spine is identified and a 23 to 25 g needle is inserted perpendicular to the skin approximately 2 to 3 cm along a line from the anterior superior iliac spine to the umbilicus. Local anesthetic is injected as the needle is advanced through each layer of muscle fascia. Infiltration is performed in both directions along this line. Ultrasound guidance is useful in identifying the muscle planes in which the nerve is located and confirmation of correct anatomic injection of local anesthetic, although the nerves themselves may be too small for ultrasonic visualization.

Drug and Dose: 0.25 to 0.5 percent bupivacaine or 0.2 percent, 0.3 ml/kg.

Assessment: This is a simple block, with low morbidity, but is most often used in the operating room.

2.3.5. Penile Block

Indications: Circumcision or hypospadias repair [16].

Anatomy: The dorsal nerves of the penis arise from the pelvic plexus and pudendal nerve providing sensory enervation to the shaft of the penis.

Technique: The penis is retracted downward and injections are made on each side of the base, 0.5 to 1 cm lateral to the midline and inferior to the symphysis pubis.

Drug and Dose: 0.25 percent bupivacaine or 0.2 percent ropivacaine. Epinephrine should never be used for penile nerve blocks. The typical dose is 1 to 2 ml on each side.

Assessment: This is a simple block, with low morbidity.

2.3.6. Celiac Plexus Block

Indications: Surgery or pain of the pancreas and/or upper abdominal viscera.

Anatomy: The celiac plexus contains one to five ganglia and is located on each side of L1. The aorta lies posterior, the pancreas anterior, and the inferior vena cava lateral. It receives sympathetic fibers from the greater, lesser, and least splanchnic nerves,

as well as parasympathetic fibers from the vagus nerve. Autonomic fibers from the liver, gallbladder, pancreas, stomach, spleen, kidneys, intestines, and adrenal glands originate from the celiac plexus.

Technique: CT guidance or fluoroscopy is required for this procedure to provide direct visualization of the appropriate landmarks and to confirm correct needle placement. The close proximity of structures such as the aorta and vena cava make this a high-risk procedure and that is generally best performed by an anesthesiologist, interventional pain physician, or radiologist. Interested readers may refer to several textbooks of regional anesthesia for further instruction and detail.

Assessment: This is an advanced block, with high potential morbidity, best performed by an anesthesiologist, interventional radiologist or pain physician.

2.4. Lower Extremity Blocks

Lumbosacral plexus blocks provide pain control for painful conditions or surgical procedures of the lower extremities, with the benefit of providing analgesia to only one extremity while preserving motor and sensory function of the opposite leg. In contrast to some caudal or lumbar epidural blocks, the patient may still bear weight [16, 23].

The lumbosacral plexus is an arrangement of nerve fibers originating from spinal nerves L2–L4, and S1–S3. The lumbar plexus arises from L2–L4 and divides into the lateral femoral cutaneous, femoral, and obturator nerves. These nerves supply the upper leg with a sensory branch of the femoral nerve extending below the knee to innervate the medial aspect of the ankle and foot (saphenous nerve). The sacral plexus arises from L4–S3 and divides into the major branches of the sciatic nerve, the tibial and common peroneal nerves. These nerves supply the lower leg and foot. Unlike brachial plexus blocks, the entire lower extremity cannot be anesthetized with a single injection because the lumbosacral sheath is not as accessible as is the brachial plexus sheath in the neck or axilla. Separate injections are necessary for the posterior (sciatic) and anterior (lumbar plexus) branches.

All the lower extremity blocks described below may be performed as a single injection, with analgesia limited to the duration of the anesthetic injected, or catheters can be placed for continuous infusion of local anesthetic to provide analgesia over periods of days or weeks.

2.4.1. Lumbar Plexus Block

Indications: Surgery or pain of the hip, femur, knee, and/or surrounding soft tissues [23].

Anatomy: The lumbar plexus arises from spinal roots L2–L4 to form the lateral femoral cutaneous, femoral, and obturator nerves. These roots are located in a fascial plane between the quadratus lumborum muscle and the psoas muscle.

Technique: Electrical nerve stimulation is used to direct the needle to the appropriate location deep to or within the psoas muscle in the back. Interested readers may refer to several textbooks of regional anesthesia for further instruction and detail.

Drug and Dose: 0.25 percent bupivacaine or 0.2 percent ropivacaine, 0.3 ml/kg to establish a block, and then 0.1 to 0.2 ml/kg/hr as a continuous infusion of bupivacaine 0.125 percent or ropivacaine 0.1 percent.

Assessment: This is an advanced block, with moderate potential morbidity and higher technical requirement, best performed by an anesthesiologist or pain physician.

2.4.2. Femoral Nerve Block

Indications: Surgery or pain of the thigh including the femur and quadriceps muscle.

Anatomy: The femoral nerve arises from the lumbar plexus L2–L4 and descends between the psoas muscle and iliacus in the lumbar plexus, and below the inguinal ligament it lies lateral to the femoral artery.

Technique: Electrical nerve stimulation and/or ultrasound are used to direct the needle to the appropriate location. Interested readers may refer to several textbooks of regional anesthesia for further instruction and detail.

Drug and Dose: 0.25 percent bupivacaine or 0.2 percent ropivacaine, 0.5 ml/kg to establish a block, and then 0.3 ml/kg/hr as a continuous infusion of bupivacaine 0.125 percent or ropivacaine 0.1 percent.

Assessment: This is a moderately advanced block, with moderate potential morbidity and technical requirements, best performed by an anesthesiologist or pain physician.

2.4.3. Sciatic Nerve Block

Indications: Pain of the lower leg, tibia/fibula, posterior thigh, ankle and foot, except the medial ankle.

Anatomy: The sciatic nerve arises from the sacral plexus L4–S3 at the piriformis muscle. It leaves the pelvis through the greater sciatic notch of the ischium, and lies deep to the gluteus maximus muscle as it descends between the ischial tuberosity and the greater trochanter of the femur. The sciatic nerve courses along the posterior aspect of the thigh until it divides into the common peroneal nerve (laterally) and tibial nerve (medially) above the knee in the popliteal fossa.

Technique: The sciatic nerve may be approached in several ways, depending on the location of surgery or pain, and the patient's position. Use of electrical nerve stimulation and/or ultrasound directs the needle to the appropriate location. Interested readers may refer to several textbooks of regional anesthesia for further instruction and detail.

Drug and Dose: 0.25 percent bupivacaine or 0.2 percent ropivacaine, 0.5 ml/kg to establish a block, and then 0.05 ml/kg/hr as a continuous infusion of bupivacaine 0.125 percent or ropivacaine 0.1 percent.

Assessment: This is a more advanced block, with modest potential morbidity, but higher technical requirements, best performed by an anesthesiologist or pain physician.

2.4.4. Saphenous Nerve Block

Indications: Surgery or pain of the medial calf or medial ankle.

Anatomy: The saphenous nerve is the largest branch of the femoral nerve. It runs down the medial border of the tibia, anterior to the medial malleolus and terminates in branches that supply the medial aspect of the foot. At the knee the saphenous nerve lies under the sartorius muscle, which runs from the anterior superior crest of the ilium to the medial condyle of the femur. It is a purely sensory nerve.

Technique: The nerve can be injected "blindly" under the sartorius muscle, or identified using ultrasound. Interested readers may refer to several textbooks of regional anesthesia for further instruction and detail.

Drug and Dose: 0.25 percent bupivacaine and 0.2 percent ropivacaine are most frequently used. The typical dose is 0.1 to 0.2 ml/kg.

Assessment: This is a straightforward block, with low potential morbidity.

2.4.5. Intravenous Regional (Bier) Block

Indications: Surgery or pain of the lower leg below the knee or foot; management of complex regional pain syndromes of the foot.

Technique: The technique is similar to that of the upper extremity, but requires a larger tourniquet.

Drug and Dose: 0.5 percent lidocaine is most frequently used. The typical dose for the lower extremity is 5 to 6 ml/kg. Phentolamine 2.5 to 5 mg and/or ketorolac 0.5 mg/kg may be added for enhanced analgesic effect in regional pain syndromes.

Assessment: This is a low morbidity, high success block, but usually the very indication for the block requires that the child be sedated or anesthetized, thus limiting general use.

2.5. Sympathetic Blocks

The peripheral sympathetic trunk is formed by the branches of the thoracic and lumbar spinal segments, extending from the base of the skull to the coccyx. The sympathetic chain consists of separate ganglia containing nerves and autonomic fibers with separate plexuses which can be differentially blocked. These centers include the stellate ganglion in the lower neck and upper thorax, the celiac plexus in the abdomen, the second lumbar plexus for the lower extremities, and the ganglion impar for the pelvis. Sympathetic blocks may be useful in the diagnosis and treatment of sympathetically mediated pain, complex regional pain syndrome, and some neuropathic pain conditions [23]. By performing these blocks, a sympathectomy is obtained without attendant motor or sensory anesthesia.

The analgesia produced by peripheral sympathetic blocks usually outlives the duration of the local anesthetic, often persisting for weeks or indefinitely. However, if analgesia is transient, the blocks may be performed with catheter insertion for continuous local anesthesia of the sympathetic chain over a period of days or weeks.

2.5.1. Stellate Ganglion Block

Indications: Pain in the face or upper extremity, complex regional pain syndrome, phantom limb pain or amputation stump pain, circulatory insufficiency of the upper extremities [23].

Anatomy: The stellate ganglion arises from spinal nerves C7–T1 and lies posterior to the first rib. It contains ganglionic fibers to the head and upper extremities. Structures in close proximity include the subclavian artery and vertebral artery anteriorly, the recurrent laryngeal nerve and the phrenic nerve. Chassaignac's tubercle, which is the transverse process of the C6 vertebral body, and which is superior to the stellate ganglion, is a useful and easily palpable landmark for the block. However, most of the stellate ganglion lies inferior to C6; therefore fluoroscopy allows more accurate needle placement than palpation of bony landmarks.

Technique: The patient is placed in the supine position with the head rotated to the side away from the procedure. The cricoid cartilage is identified and the carotid artery palpated at that level between the sternocleidomastoid muscle and the trachea. The skin is retracted laterally and the transverse process of C6 palpated. A 22 g needle is directed perpendicular to the skin until bone is contacted and then withdrawn approximately 2 mm. After aspiration and test dose, local anesthetic is injected. Fluoroscopy with contrast can be used to confirm correct needle placement or to aid in needle placement opposite C7 or T1. Cervical ganglion block commonly causes an ipsilateral Horner's syndrome (ptosis, miosis, anhidrosis) and is not an unexpected consequence. Risks include recurrent laryngeal nerve block, phrenic nerve block, intravascular injection of local anesthetic, intrathecal, subdural, or epidural injection and pneumothorax.

Drug and Dose: 0.25 percent bupivacaine is most frequently used. The typical dose is 5 to 20 ml.

Assessment: This is an advanced block, with high potential morbidity/mortality, best performed by an anesthesiologist or pain physician.

2.5.2. Lumbar Sympathetic Block

Indications: Pain in the lower extremity, complex regional pain syndrome (CRPS), phantom limb pain or amputation stump pain, circulatory insufficiency of the lower extremities [23]. Patients with CRPS may benefit from an indwelling catheter and hospital admission for aggressive physical therapy.

Anatomy: The lumbar sympathetic chain contains ganglionic fibers to the pelvis and lower extremities. It lies along the anterolateral surface of the lumbar vertebral bodies and is most often injected between the L2 and L4 vertebral bodies.

Technique: CT guidance or fluoroscopy is required for this procedure to provide direct visualization of the appropriate landmarks to confirm correct needle placement. Interested readers may refer to several textbooks of regional anesthesia for further instruction and detail.

Drug and Dose: 0.25 percent bupivacaine is most commonly used. The typical dose is 0.25 ml/kg.

Assessment: This is an advanced block, with high potential morbidity, best performed by an anesthesiologist or pain physician.

2.6. Neuraxial Nerve Blocks

Neuraxial blocks such as epidural and spinal blocks provide analgesia for a variety of conditions including postoperative pain control and acute and chronic pain conditions. Either single injection or continuous catheter techniques may be employed. Local anesthetic is injected into the epidural or subarachnoid space, as well as adjuvants, such as opioids or alpha-2 agonists to enhance the analgesic effect. Depending on the circumstance, local anesthetic can be more or less concentrated if both motor and sensory blocks are required, or just sensory blockade alone. Precise radiographic-guided placement of the epidural needle or catheter will provide analgesia targeted to specific dermatomes.

2.6.1. Epidural Anesthesia (Thoracic, Lumbar)

Indications: Surgery or pain below the clavicles, management of complex regional pain syndromes, cancer pain unresponsive to systemic opioids or limited by side effects, sciatica.

Anatomy: The three layers of the spinal meninges protect the neural tissue. These layers are the dura mater (outermost), the arachnoid mater (middle) and the pia mater (innermost). The subdural space is a potential space between the dura and arachnoid mater. The subarachnoid space is an actual space containing CSF between the arachnoid mater and pia mater. The epidural space which contains fat, lymphatics, and blood vessels, separates the dura mater from the periosteum. The epidural space extends from the foramen magnum to the sacral hiatus. Anatomically, the conus medullaris ends at L3 in infants and L1 in adults. The fat in the epidural space is not as dense in children, thereby facilitating the spread of the local anesthetic.

Technique: Interested readers may refer to several textbooks of regional anesthesia for further instruction and detail.

Drug and Dose: 0.25 percent bupivacaine and 0.2 percent ropivacaine are most frequently used for a single injection. 0.062 percent to 0.125 percent bupivacaine, or 0.05 percent to 0.1 percent ropivacaine are used as a continuous infusion. The typical dose is 0.5 to 1 ml/kg to establish neuraxial blockade, and then 0.25 to 0.4 ml/kg/hr as a continuous infusion to maintain analgesia. The epidural space in the thoracic region is generally smaller and requires a smaller volume of local anesthetic. Adjuvants to epidural anesthesia include epinephrine, 1:200,000 to 400,000, which is most helpful in recognizing accidental intravascular catheter insertion by the resultant tachycardia; opioids such as fentanyl, preservative-free morphine (Duramorph®, Astramorph®) and hydromorphone, and clonidine, an alpha-2 agonist that improves and prolongs the effect of local anesthetics (Table 12-3).

Epidural anesthesia and analgesia produces blockade of both sensory and sympathetic fibers and, if the local anesthetic is of sufficient concentration, motor fibers. Because sympathetic blockade occurs, mild hypotension may occur although it is distinctly unusual in children less than 8 years of age. Epidural injection high in the thoracic spine may also anesthetize the sympathetic nerves to the heart (the cardiac accelerator fibers), producing bradycardia.

Other side effects associated with epidural opioid administration include delayed respiratory depression, particularly when hydrophilic opioids such as morphine are used. The risk of delayed respiratory depression requires that children receiving epidural opioids by intermittent injection or continuous infusion be monitored. Typically this monitoring consists of continuous pulse oximetry and nursing observation, particularly during the first 24 hours of therapy. Respiratory depression occurring after the first 24 hours of epidural opioid administration is unusual.

Epidural clonidine is associated with minimal risk and side effects. Although product labeling

TABLE 12-3. Drugs used in epidural blocks; typical dosing for naïve patients, side effects and signs of toxicity.

Drug class	Drug name	Bolus dose	Infusion dose	Side effects	Toxicity
Local Anesthetic	Lidocaine (Xylocaine®)	1–2%, 0.5 ml/kg	0.25%, 0.25–0.5 ml/kg/hr	Motor weakness	Arrhythmia
	Bupivacaine (Marcaine®)	0.25%, 0.5 ml/kg	0.08–0.1%, 0.25–0.4 ml/kg/hr	Hypotension	Seizure
	Ropivacaine (Naropin®)	0.2%, 0.5 ml/kg	0.1%, 0.25–0.5 ml/kg/hr		
	Levobupivacaine (Chirocaine®)	0.25%, 0.5 ml/kg	0.1%, 0.25–0.5 ml/kg/hr		
Opioids	Morphine (preservative-free: Duramorph®, Astramorph®)	3 mcg/kg	0.25 mcg/kg/hr	Sedation	Respiratory depression
	Hydromorphone	1 mcg/kg	0.1 mcg/kg/hr	Pruritus	
	Fentanyl	0.5 mcg/kg	0.1 mcg/kg/hr	Urinary retention	
Alpha-2-agonists	Clonidine (Duraclon®)	1–2 mcg/kg	0.1 mcg/kg/hr	Sedation	Hypotension Bradycardia

Note: Trade names are used for example only, and do not imply brand preference.

indicates its use only for children with severe cancer pain, it is commonly used for routine postsurgical pain, and pain syndromes such as complex regional pain syndrome. The most common side effect is mild and dose-related sedation. It does not cause nausea, urinary retention or pruritus.

Assessment: These are advanced blocks, with high potential morbidity, best performed by an anesthesiologist or pain physician.

2.6.1.1. Caudal (Sacral) Epidural Anesthesia

Indications: Surgery or pain below the diaphragm such as circumcision, inguinal herniorrhaphy, orchiopexy, hydrocele repair, club foot repair, and regional pain syndromes [16].

Anatomy: The landmarks for caudal epidural include the posterior–superior iliac spines and the fifth sacral cornua. The sacral hiatus is easily palpated between these two cornua and the sacrococcygeal ligament between is pierced, resulting in needle placement in the sacral epidural space ("caudal" space). In infants, the conus medullaris of the spinal cord may extend as low as L3 and the sacral sac as low as S3. Caudal blocks are performed below this level, but accidental intrathecal injection is still possible in infants if needles are inserted to an excessive distance after piercing the sacrococcygeal ligament.

Technique: Interested readers may refer to several textbooks of regional anesthesia for further instruction and detail.

Drug and Dose: 0.25 percent bupivacaine or 0.2 percent ropivacaine with 1:200,000 epinephrine is the most frequently used. The typical dose is 0.5 to 1 ml/kg, followed by a continuous infusion of 0.3 ml/kg/hr of bupivacaine 0.062 percent to 0.1 percent, or ropivacaine 0.05 percent to 0.1 percent. As for thoracic and lumbar epidural analgesia, opioids and/or clonidine can be used in the same doses, with the same monitoring precautions.

Assessment: This is an advanced block, with high potential morbidity, best performed by an anesthesiologist or pain physician.

2.6.1.2. Intrathecal (Spinal) Anesthesia

Indications: Intrathecal catheters infused with opioids, clonidine, ziconotide, and local anesthetics are occasionally applicable to pediatric patients suffering from intractable cancer pain or other forms of intractable chronic pain.

Technique: Interested readers may refer to several textbooks of regional anesthesia for further detail.

Assessment: This is an advanced block, with high potential morbidity and mortality, best performed by an anesthesiologist or pain physician.

Take-Home Points

- Regional anesthetic techniques are available to children for a variety of procedures and painful conditions.
- Local anesthetic dosing requires attention to weight and age, especially in infants.
- Risks of regional anesthesia are generally very low. Some interventions require a certain expertise. However, there are some that can be learned and applied outside the operating room.
- Parents often do not expect that their child may be offered a block as part of their anesthetic. Hearing that such interventions are available and have potential benefits prior to arriving at the hospital may reduce child and parent stress on the day of operation.

References

1. Dalens BJ. Regional anesthesia in infants, children, and adolescents. Baltimore: Williams & Wilkins, 1995.
2. Ross AK, Eck JB, Tobias JD. Pediatric regional anesthesia: beyond the caudal. Anesth Analg 2000;91:16–26.
3. Gunter JB. Benefit and risks of local anesthetics in infants and children. Paediatr Drugs 2002;4: 649–672.
4. Giaufre E, Dalens B, Gombert A. Epidemiology and morbidity of regional anesthesia in children: a one-year prospective survey of the french-language society of pediatric anesthesiologists. Anesth Analg 1996;83:904–912.
5. Yaster M. Pediatric Pain Management and Sedation Handbook. St. Louis: Mosby, 1997.
6. Naguib M, Magboul MM, Samarkandi AH, Attia M. Adverse effects and drug interactions associated with local and regional anaesthesia. Drug Saf 1998;18: 221–250.
7. Berde CB. Toxicity of local anesthetics in infants and children. J Pediatr 1993;122:S14–20.
8. Hansen TG, Ilett KF, Lim SI, Reid C, Hackett LP, Bergesio R. Pharmacokinetics and clinical efficacy of long-term epidural ropivacaine infusion in children. Br J Anaesth 2000;85:347–353.
9. Ingelmo PM, Fumagalli R. Central blocks with levobupivacaine in children. Minerva Anestesiol 2005;71:339–345.
10. McCann ME, Sethna NF, Mazoit JX, et al. The pharmacokinetics of epidural ropivacaine in infants and young children. Anesth Analg 2001;93:893–897.
11. Kakiuchi Y, Kohda Y, Miyabe M, Momose Y. Effect of plasma alpha1-acid glycoprotein concentration on the accumulation of lidocaine metabolites during continuous epidural anesthesia in infants and children. Int J Clin Pharmacol and Therapeutics 1999;37:493–498.
12. Brown DL. Atlas of Regional Anesthesia, 3rd ed. Philadelphia: Saunders Elsevier, 2006.
13. Hadzic A, New York School of Regional Anesthesia. Textbook of Regional Anesthesia and Acute Pain Management. New York: McGraw-Hill Medical, 2007.
14. Jankovic D, Harrop-Griffiths W, Jankovic D. Regional Nerve Blocks and Infiltration Therapy: Textbook and Color Atlas, 3rd ed. Malden, Mass: Blackwell Publishing, 2004.
15. Meier G, Bèuttner J. Peripheral Regional Anesthesia: An Atlas of Anatomy and Techniques, 2nd ed. Stuttgart, New York: Thieme, 2007.
16. Mulroy MF. Regional Anesthesia: An Illustrated Procedural Guide, 3rd ed. Philadelphia: Lippincott, Williams & Wilkins, 2002.
17. Naja ZM, El-Rajab M, Al-Tannir MA, Ziade FM, Tawfik OM. Repetitive occipital nerve blockade for cervicogenic headache: A double-blind randomized controlled clinical trial. Pain Pract 2006;6:278–284.
18. Naja ZM, El-Rajab M, Al-Tannir MA, Ziade FM, Tawfik OM. Repetitive occipital nerve blockade for cervicogenic headache: Expanded case report of 47 adults. Pain Pract 2006;6:278–284.
19. Suresh S, Voronov P. Head and neck blocks in children: An anatomical and procedural review. Paediatr Anaesth 2006;16:910–918.
20. Cooper K, Kelley H, Carrithers J. Perceptions of side effects following axillary block used for outpatient surgery. Reg Anesth 1995;20:212–216.
21. Ecoffey C. Pediatric regional anesthesia - update. Curr Op Anaesth 2007;20:232–235.
22. Matsota P, Livanios S, Marinopoulou E. Intercostal nerve block with bupivacaine for post-thoracotomy pain relief in children. Eur J Pediatr Surg 2001;11:219–222.
23. Benzon HT. Essentials of Pain Medicine and Regional Anesthesia, 2nd ed. Philadelphia: Elsevier Churchill Livingstone, 2005.

Part III
Recurrent and Chronic Pain Management

13

How to Talk to Parents about Recurrent and Chronic Pain

Tonya M. Palermo and Carl L. von Baeyer

Abstract: Children and adolescents frequently present to the pediatric office-based practitioner with complaints of recurrent and chronic pain. The majority of these children will have no easily treatable physical cause for the pain. A biopsychosocial framework is useful for considering the interrelationships among physical, cognitive, affective, and social factors that influence the child's experience of pain and the extent of pain-related functional impairment. Parents play an integral role in the treatment of children's chronic pain. Communicating with parents in a sensitive manner is essential to facilitate understanding and acceptance of a biopsychosocial perspective on chronic pain. Counseling by the primary care physician can help to prevent and relieve children's pain. Guiding the child in a return to normal activity and aiding parents in encouraging adaptive coping in their child are critical aspects of the counseling. Children with complex pain problems, comorbid psychiatric disturbances, or excessive disability may need referral for specialized pain or psychological treatment. The primary care pediatrician can facilitate such referrals and help the parents and child understand the focus and goals of these treatments.

Key words: Chronic pain, children, parents, biopsychosocial model.

Case Illustration

Emma is a 15-year-old female who is accompanied by her mother to the primary care office with a chief complaint of headache. For over 3 months she has been experiencing persistent headache from when she wakes in the morning until she falls asleep at night. Over-the-counter analgesics do not provide any pain relief. There are no red flags in her history to suggest a structural problem in the brain (e.g., tumor, traumatic brain injury), chemical (e.g., MSG reactions), or other identifiable "causes" that can be readily treated if diagnosed (e.g., sinus infection, poor vision). There are no unusual symptoms or signs such as fever, morning vomiting, visual disturbances, paralysis, or any sudden changes in alertness, speech, or thinking. The headaches are beginning to interfere significantly with Emma's ability to attend school, complete school work, and participate in her usual physical and extracurricular activities. Emma describes some recent stressors at school and a high level of general worry. Emma's mother is very upset and wants to do whatever is necessary to get pain relief for her daughter.

Some pertinent questions stemming from this case are: How does the primary care physician understand and explain this pain problem? How can the physician explore the onset of symptoms, and inquire about any apparent association with a life change or accident in his or her clinical evaluation? What steps can the physician take to ensure that the parent engages in effective strategies to help this teen cope with the pain problem? Should the teen be referred for specialty pain care? What barriers might be encountered in managing the teen's pain problem?

Introduction

Evaluating the child with recurrent or chronic pain complaints often falls on the office-based pediatric practitioner, and it can be a complex

G.A. Walco and K.R. Goldschneider (eds.), *Pain in Children: A Practical Guide for Primary Care.*
© Humana Press, a part of Springer Science + Business Media, 2008

and time-consuming effort. Physicians often fear that they are missing an organic explanation, despite lengthy, expensive, and sometimes invasive workups. It can be difficult to identify the red flags in the history, physical, and laboratory investigations that may suggest additional investigation is needed. Moreover, parents are often quite distressed and may experience frustration and anger, particularly when they fear that their child's problems are misunderstood or are not being thoroughly investigated. The parents of a child with recurrent and chronic pain do not just want a diagnosis; they want the clinician to reduce their child's pain and suffering.

However, chronic pain often occurs without a clear and easily treatable physical explanation. Thus, it is important for the pediatrician to understand possible etiological factors that contribute to children's recurrent and chronic pain, and how to communicate these in a sensitive manner to parents. In addition, because recurrent and chronic pain complaints can be successfully managed in the primary care pediatrician's office for many children, parents must be effectively engaged in the treatment of their child's pain complaint.

In this chapter, we review possible etiological factors for recurrent and chronic pediatric pain, present a framework for discussing recurrent and chronic pain complaints with parents, and identify critical issues in referring patients for specialized pain services.

1. Significance of Recurrent and Chronic Pain

An estimated 15 to 25 percent of children and adolescents suffer with recurrent or chronic pain conditions [1, 2]. Recurrent and chronic pain can lead to significant interference with daily functioning for some children and adolescents [3] and increases their risk of having a chronic pain syndrome in adulthood [4]. Despite physicians' reassurance children will "outgrow" recurrent pain complaints, the symptoms of many children with pain complaints persist. Although the overall base of knowledge of the natural history and course of pain is limited, the data that are available suggest that early exposure to pain may alter later pain response and that initial pain complaints often

persist over time and may occur in another part of the body, or other somatic symptoms may develop in the child [4].

Of concern for many children with recurrent and chronic pain are the associated decrements in their ability to function in important life roles. Children may experience limitations in their ability to attend school and complete academic work, as well as in their participation in physical, social and peer activities [3]. Repeated absence from school can directly affect academic performance and school success, and impact a child's socialization and maintenance of peer relationships. Chronic pain can have a negative impact on family life, including increased restrictions on parental socialization, high parental stress levels, anger and hostility. Parents also experience the financial burden of evaluation and management of recurrent and chronic pain, including direct costs of pain treatment such as hospitalization, visits to doctors, and costs of medications. Indirect costs include parental time off from work, transportation costs, child care, and incidental costs [5].

2. A Biopsychosocial Framework

A number of models have been developed to understand children's recurrent and chronic pain that fall under biobehavioral or biopsychosocial frameworks. Central to these models are interrelationships among physical, cognitive, affective, and social factors that influence children's pain and disability. Many studies have articulated important individual child and parent factors that appear to predict the extent of pain and disability experienced by children. There are central nervous system pain mechanisms that may play a role in the persistence of pain. For example, in understanding functional bowel disorders, current theories suggest that the pain or symptoms are caused by abnormal brain-intestinal neural signaling that create intestinal or visceral hypersensitivity [6]. Parental response to a child's pain is one of several familial factors that have been identified as potentially important in the etiology of pain-related disability [7, 8]. Positive behaviors demonstrated by a parent can be related to better child coping behaviors and less pain, while solicitous or overly reinforcing responses to the child's pain can be related to increased child functional impairment. Working with parents on methods to promote positive coping behaviors is, therefore, an important aspect of treatment.

However, in clinical practice, a biopsychosocial framework is not implemented as often as it could be and parents are rarely helped to understand their child's pain from this multidimensional perspective. Unfortunately, this lack of understanding impedes engaging the parents and children in effective forms of treatment. For the office-based practitioner deciding whether to pursue more diagnostic testing to workup a chronic pain complaint, he or she may find that it is difficult to move beyond the question of whether the pain problem has an organic or physical etiology that is treatable. Most primary care practitioners have very limited training in the biopsychosocial model of recurrent and chronic pain. Below we discuss some practical tips in explaining the biopsychosocial framework to children and parents.

2.1. Explaining the Biopsychosocial Framework to Children and Parents

The initial evaluation and explanation to the child and family sets the stage for effectively addressing the pain problem. The simplest explanation of the biopsychosocial framework is that all pain has physical and psychological contributors. An example is when a person is distracted from a painful injury (such as during a sporting game) and he or she may not feel the physical sensation of pain strongly until he or she is alone and the game is over. It is important to explain to the family that any comprehensive evaluation and treatment plan for recurrent and chronic pain should address both physical and psychological contributors. Parents need to "buy into" the evaluation and treatment plan because they play a critical role in decreasing pain and improving function for their child. Therefore, clear, empathetic communication with the parents is crucial.

Once treatable physical causes are ruled out, most parents need, and are willing to accept, an explanation based on both physical and psychological factors. It is often helpful to describe pain in terms of pain receptors becoming very sensitive, sometimes as a result of an earlier illness that has since resolved, and sometimes as a result of stress or worry. This can help parents understand why diagnostic tests have not revealed any answers since the physical reason that initiated the pain may be long gone. Either way, the important question now is how to help, rather than determining the original cause. Therefore, a variety of physical and psychological treatment strategies are important for altering these pain patterns to address physical actions and changes in emotion and thinking.

3. Clinical Evaluation of Recurrent and Chronic Pain

A biopsychosocial framework should guide clinical evaluation of the recurrent or chronic pain problem. Therefore, a comprehensive clinical evaluation includes assessing the following: pain and pain history; other physical symptoms; physical, social, academic, family, emotional, and cognitive functioning; coping style and problem-solving capacity; perceived stressors; major life events; and pain consequences. For example, evaluating a child who presents with headaches includes assessment of all of the above factors, and should not be aimed just at "ruling out organic pathology." Several resources are available that provide detailed interview questions for evaluating recurrent and chronic pain in children [9–11].

One productive way to initiate the history is to elicit the patient's and parents' narrative about the pain, rather than beginning with targeted questions. Further prompts about the pain can then be provided. It is important to communicate to the parents that evaluation of the child's functioning is just as critical as evaluation of the pain itself. The next part of the history should bring forth how the pain has interfered with functioning, including sleep (onset and maintenance), eating, school attendance and performance, and physical, social, and family activities. By highlighting the impact of the child's pain on their ability to function in important life roles, management strategies can be discussed with the parents that are directed toward an increase in function. Throughout the initial evaluation, communication that establishes reassurance, rapport, and a belief in the significance of the pain problem will be best received by the parents and child.

3.1. Communicating about Psychological Contributors and Interventions

Psychological or behavioral interventions can help the child with recurrent or chronic pain in two different ways. Psychological intervention can help children cope with the pain and improve function by teaching self-management strategies, and changing the consequences that occur around the child's behaviors. This type of intervention is relevant for any child who is experiencing recurrent pain that is interfering with their daily functioning. In contrast, for some children there are primary psychological etiologies of their pain, and psychological interventions are focused around a particular issue. For instance, the primary care physician may have uncovered significant untreated anxiety in the child or clear problems in school that seem to be limiting the child's desire to be in that setting. In either case, it can be helpful to reinforce to the parents and child that all children with recurrent or chronic pain can benefit from attention to the psychosocial, as well as the biomedical aspects of their pain.

Unfortunately, parents may not be ready to hear specific psychological contributors to their child's pain problem. In clinic, we have found that parents often reject psychological diagnoses and interpretations, which may lead to even more invasive medical testing to find a physical cause of the child's pain problem. As one parent relayed, when physicians suggested very early in the workup of her 8-year-old daughter that she had a conversion disorder, she did not want that to be the first possibility explored. She sought a variety of opinions from other physicians so that all medical explanations would be considered and explored. It is important to convey to this parent that, although a primary psychological etiology was being explored, medical attention (through regular visits and monitoring by the primary care physician) to the child's symptoms would continue alongside psychological evaluation. Another way to convey this idea is to assure the parents that the patient is being approached as a whole person, not just a hurting body part; pain affects thoughts, feelings, and actions and is influenced by them as well. The biopsychosocial approach allows complete evaluation and treatment, which most parents desire in the first place, even if they are more used to thinking

of tests, X-rays, and medications as "complete" as opposed to psychological evaluation or physical therapy-based treatments.

It takes increased sensitivity to communicate to parents about specific psychological contributors that require treatment and/or referral. Often parents are more receptive when a biopsychosocial framework has been described early on. However, parents are living with a suffering child and can become frustrated if they feel the physician is minimizing the significance of the pain. It is useful to recognize that parents need an explanation that matches their level of concern. Psychological explanations should not downplay the significance of the child's pain. It is important to remind parents that you appreciate the significant suffering of their child. You may need to explicitly state that psychological explanations do not imply that the child's pain is "in their head." You should compliment the parents on their tremendous efforts to help the child, and let them know it is no longer necessary to treat the pain as an acute problem, and that the good news is further diagnostic tests are not needed for now. Reassure the parent and child, however, that you will continue to monitor for changes in symptoms on a routine basis. It is sometimes be helpful to set up routine follow-up visits with the child (every 2 weeks or so) to continue to monitor and provide counseling.

4. Engaging the Parent in Counseling by the Physician

Management usually starts with counseling by the physician and may include referral for other services if these are needed and available. It is wise to limit unnecessary referrals because it can help to reduce cure-seeking and can discourage multiple medical investigations of unclear benefit. Brief counseling from a physician can be of great help to children with recurrent pain and to their parents. Because parents play a crucial role in the treatment of the child's pain problem, it is important to focus elements of the counseling on how parents can promote more effective child coping.

Time should be spent with the parents to help reduce the amount of attention paid to pain symptoms in favor of increased attention paid to functional improvement. Physicians can help parents change their focus away from worry and distress over their suffering child by recognizing that positive attention can be a great motivator for their child to use more adaptive coping methods.

Perhaps the most important element of treatment that can be provided in counseling is a return to normal activity. Parents are critical in this endeavor. Clear, graded plans for increasing activity should be constructed with the child and parents. It can be explained to children and parents that functional improvement often precedes, rather than follows, pain relief. It is important to set concrete goals and expectations around activities like school, as many parents struggle and feel ineffective in trying to push their child to do more. It is helpful to be frank with parents about the difficulty of balancing how much to push the child with feeling guilt over not being sympathetic to their child's pain. Having the child hear this message about return to normal activity from the physician can be extremely helpful. Parents can be encouraged to provide incentives for the child's efforts toward functional improvement such as earning special privileges or rewards for reaching a school attendance goal. A partnership between parents and physicians can set the stage for a successful pain management plan.

5. Guidelines in Making Referrals

Children with complex pain complaints, excessive disability or comorbid psychiatric disturbance may require referral for specialized care. In general these options will typically include referral to a pediatric pain clinic, mental health provider, for physical therapy, and/or complementary or alternative therapies.

Children who receive care in a multidisciplinary pediatric pain clinic are typically offered a multicomponent treatment involving psychological therapies, physical therapy, complementary or alternative therapies, and medication management under the philosophy of a rehabilitation approach to treatment. In this approach, pain is accepted as a symptom that might not be eradicated, and efforts are directed toward improving function. As functioning and coping skills are improved, pain often remits as well. The specific structure of each program differs with some providing inpatient rehabilitation and other programs exclusively treating children on an outpatient basis. For example, the effectiveness of an inpatient residential pediatric pain program involving physiotherapy and psychological therapy was recently evaluated in a group of adolescents with chronic pain and pervasive disability, finding good support for this multicomponent treatment [12]. We refer the reader to Zeltzer and Schlank [9] for a listing of pediatric pain and gastrointestinal pain programs in the United States, Canada, and internationally. There are many regions of the country, however, in which a specialized pediatric pain clinic will be unavailable.

Referring the patient for psychological intervention can supplement the primary care physician's management of the pain problem. Some clinicians have recommended that psychological intervention begin as soon as functional impairment is noted, meaning a child begins to miss school or curtail participation in regular activities due to pain. The process of how the physician makes the referral for psychological intervention is critical to the subsequent acceptance of psychological management approaches and thus should be done with appropriate care. Patients and their families are more likely to accept a psychological referral and not feel abandoned by their physician if it is presented early and as a routine procedure in all cases of persistent pain causing disruption of normal activities. Referrals that are presented early on may be received more readily than waiting for psychological intervention as a last resort after all other physical attempts to understand and treat the problem have failed. Early involvement of psychology also underscores the idea that the pain is a complicated, serious problem, rather than being relegated to an emotional or behavioral problem. This can be the message heard when a psychology referral is made only after a long, organically-based pain workup has been completed.

Referral for psychological treatment is often very helpful, but may be difficult to arrange in many communities. It can be useful to talk with physician colleagues about their relationships with mental health care providers to identify recommended clinical psychologists, psychiatrists, social workers, or counselors. Many mental health professionals do not have adequate training in pain management or in a biopsychosocial model of care. Useful questions for identifying appropriate mental health providers are to inquire about their experience with children and adolescents, with treating children with medical problems, and in using cognitive-behavioral therapy. The best referral options will have affirmative responses to each of these areas of inquiry. Once psychological treatment has been initiated, communication between the mental health provider and the primary care physician is essential for ensuring work toward consistent treatment goals and for allowing a shared view of the child's pain problem. The primary care physician may reinforce elements of psychological treatment with the parents to ensure their understanding of the importance of the treatment for addressing the child's pain problem.

Take-Home Points

- Recurrent and chronic pain in childhood is a frequent presenting problem and is often due to functional etiologies. Daily functioning is impaired for some children as demonstrated by inability to attend school or participate in physical, social, and peer activities.
- The vast majority of children will have no life threatening or easily treatable physical cause for the pain. Instead, a biopsychosocial understanding of the pain is needed to evaluate and manage the problem. This framework describes interrelationships among physical, cognitive, affective, and social factors that influence children's pain and pain-related functional impairment. The simplest explanation is that all pain has physical and psychological contributors.
- Familial factors are important to consider. Positive behaviors demonstrated by a parent can be related to better child coping behaviors and less pain, while solicitous or overly reinforcing responses to the child's pain can be related to increased child functional impairment.
- If families hear an explanation of the biopsychosocial nature of chronic pain from their primary care physician, who they know and trust, that may facilitate understanding and acceptance of this view.
- Communicating with parents about possible psychosocial and family factors that may contribute

to problems in coping with pain must be done with care. Counseling by the physician should focus on guiding the child to return to normal activity and aiding parents in encouraging adaptive coping in their child.
- Referral for specialized psychological treatment or multidisciplinary pain treatment may be considered for children with complex problems, comorbid psychiatric disturbances, or excessive disability. However, in many communities these services will be difficult to access. The primary care physician plays an important role in communicating with providers and helping parents to understand the goals of treatment.

References

1. Perquin CW, Hazebroek-Kampschreur AA, Hunfeld JA, Bohnen AM, van Suijlekom-Smit LW, Passchier J, van der Wouden JC. Pain in children and adolescents: a common experience. Pain 2000;87:51–58.
2. Roth-Isigkeit A, Thyen U, Stoven H, Schwarzenberger J, Schmucker P. Pain among children and adolescents: Restrictions in daily living and triggering factors [Electronic version]. Pediatrics 2005;115:e152–162.
3. Palermo TM. Impact of recurrent and chronic pain on child and family daily functioning: A critical review of the literature. J Dev Behav Pediatr 2000;21:58–69.
4. Fearon P, Hotopf M. Relation between headache in childhood and physical and psychiatric symptoms in adulthood: National birth cohort study. BMJ 2001;322:1145.
5. Sleed M, Eccleston C, Beecham J, Knapp M, Jordan A. The economic impact of chronic pain in adolescence: Methodological considerations and a preliminary costs-of-illness study. Pain 2005;119:183–190.
6. Drossman DA. What does the future hold for irritable bowel syndrome and the functional gastrointestinal disorders? J Clin Gastroenterol 2005;39:S251–256.
7. Palermo TM, Chambers CT. Parent and family factors in pediatric chronic pain and disability: an integrative approach. Pain 2005;119:1–4.
8. Walker LS, Garber J, Greene JW. Psychosocial correlates of recurrent childhood pain: A comparison of pediatric patients with recurrent abdominal pain, organic illness, and psychiatric disorders. J Abnorm Psychol 1993;102:248–258.
9. Zeltzer L, Schlank C. Conquering Your Child's Chronic Pain: a Pediatrician's Guide for Reclaiming a Normal Childhood. New York: Harper Collins Publishers, 2005.
10. Palermo T, Krell H, Janosy N, Zeltzer L. Pain and somatoform disorders. In: Wolraich M, Dworkin P, Perrin

E, Drotar D, editors. Developmental and Behavioral Pediatrics. Philadelphia: Mosby, Inc, in press.

11. von Baeyer CL. Understanding and managing children's recurrent pain in primary care: a biopsychosocial perspective. Paediatrics and Child Health, in press.

12. Eccleston C, Malleson PN, Clinch J, Connell H, Sourbut C. Chronic pain in adolescents: evaluation of a programme of interdisciplinary cognitive behaviour therapy. Arch Dis Child 2003;88: 881–885.

14
Multidisciplinary Approaches to Chronic Pain

Steven J. Weisman

Abstract: Many chronic pain conditions in children are complex and patients can benefit most when an integrated care plan can be brought to bear on the problem. Multidisciplinary pain centers (MPC) and clinics aim to coordinate evaluation and treatment of complex pain problems. Disciplines that are routinely part of these centers include medicine, physical therapy, psychology, and advanced practice nursing. As fiscal constraints have limited the number and availability of comprehensive centers, partnerships between these tertiary care facilities and primary care offices can bring many of the benefits of the MPCs to children who live a distance from them. This chapter describes the goals and functions of MPCs, and how they can integrate with primary care practice for children with chronic pain.

Key words: Chronic pain, multidisciplinary approach, multidisciplinary pain center.

Introduction

Chronic pain is a major problem in the pediatric population that affects, conservatively, an estimated 10 to 15 percent of the population [1]. In the past, chronic pain was usually defined as pain present for more than 6 months. The International Association for the Study of Pain (IASP) classifies chronic pain as less than 1 month, 1 to 6 months and greater than 6 months in duration [2]. Today chronic pain can be recognized much earlier. Unfortunately, signs of sympathetic nervous sys-tem arousal, which are quite common in the acute pain setting, are rarely present in chronic pain processes. This lack of objective findings may lead the inexperienced clinician to say the patient "does not look like he or she is in pain" or that "the pain is in the patient's head" [3, 4]. Chronic pain must be assessed, managed and treated with the same high priority that one would treat any ongoing illness.

Chronic pain conditions most commonly seen in large pediatric pain centers include headache, abdominal pain, myofascial pain, arthritis, back pain, complex regional pain syndrome, phantom limb pain, cancer pain, sickle cell pain, and cerebral palsy-related pain. By the time many of these patients reach a tertiary care pain center, they will have seen at least four physicians. This process of referrals and evaluations will take, on average, 4 to 6 months, even though, all the while, these patients have significant alterations in their lifestyles. They commonly have poor school attendance, there has been major family restructuring to accommodate the pain, and the patients have experienced social withdrawal. Many primary care child health specialists have limited experience treating patients with chronic pain. Invariably, almost all patients have undergone extensive medical testing that has been costly and often revealed little or no insight into what the cause or treatment of the painful problem may be (Fig. 14-1) [5].

Chronic pain may start out as an acute event, but continues beyond the normal time expected for recovery. What, specifically, leads to the development of chronic pain in children remains elusive in some patients. In others, of course, there is a direct link to a clearly definable ongoing disease process. In

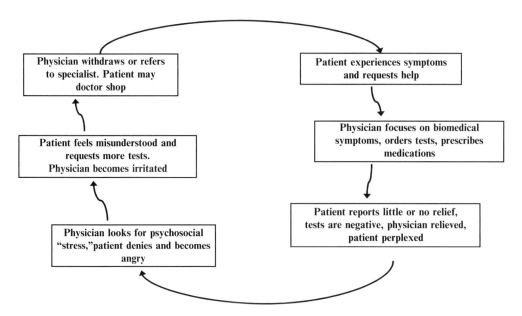

FIGURE 14-1. Somatically-fixated physician–patient interaction. McDaniel, S.H., et al. 1992 created this model to illustrate the nonproductive loop of overemphasis of somatic explanations of a variety of medical conditions [5]

both situations chronic pain results from a dynamic integration of biological processes with contributing psychological factors, sociocultural factors, and developmental and family dynamics. Through these mechanisms, pain becomes the illness, rather than being a symptom of an illness or injury. To be able to effectively evaluate and treat chronic childhood pain, a multidisciplinary approach is essential.

Treatment teams should incorporate physicians, nurses, psychologists, psychiatrists, physical therapists (PT), occupational therapists (OT), and social workers (Table 14-1). The driving principles behind effective development of a multidisciplinary approach to the treatment of chronic pain must leave behind the mind–body dualism that drives much of medical practice. To continue to think that chronic pain is likely to be associated with a single physical cause can often result in aggressive repeated invasive testing, laboratory tests, procedures, and the over-prescription of medications. One needs to acknowledge that patients with chronic pain have a multidimensional experience, and treatment of the condition will require a multidimensional approach by a multidisciplinary team.

TABLE 14-1. Multidisciplinary pain management team members.

Pain specialist physician
Pediatric psychologist/therapist
Consulting psychiatrist
Advanced practice nurses
Pediatric physical/occupational therapist
Social worker
Administrative assistants

1. Models of Care

Just after World War II ended, Dr. John J. Bonica developed pain management as a specialty within his department of anesthesiology. Dr. John Loeser reviewed the history of the development of multidisciplinary pain programs in the text, *Bonica's Management of Pain* [6]. Dr. Bonica first published his ideas about and description of such programs in 1974 [7]. In the 1970s through the1990s, pain management programs erupted across the globe [8]. By the 1980s there were a handful of pediatric pain management programs, as well.

TABLE 14-2. Types of pain management facilities.

Multidisciplinary pain center
Multidisciplinary pain clinic
Pain clinic
Modality-oriented clinic

Programs can exist in a variety of forms (see below). In 1990, Dr. Loeser led a task force for the International Association for the Study of Pain and issued a report on the "Desirable Characteristics for Pain Treatment Facilities" [9, 10] (Table 14-2).

1.1. Multidisciplinary Pain Center

This is an organization of health care professionals and basic scientists which includes research, teaching, and patient care related to acute and chronic pain. This is the largest and most complex of the pain treatment facilities and, ideally, would exist as a component of a medical school or teaching hospital. Clinical programs must be supervised by an appropriately trained and licensed clinical director; a wide array of health care specialists is required, including physicians, psychologists, nurses, physical therapists, occupational therapists, vocational counselors, social workers, and other specialized health care providers.

The spectrum of health care disciplines is required to effectively serve the variety of patients seen and maximize the health care resources of the community. The members of the treatment team must communicate with each other on a regular basis, both about specific patients and about overall development. Health care services in a multidisciplinary pain center must be integrated and based upon multidisciplinary assessment and management of the patient. Inpatient and outpatient programs are offered in such a facility.

1.2. Multidisciplinary Pain Clinic

This is a health care delivery facility staffed by physicians of different specialties and other non-physician health care providers who specialize in the diagnosis and management of patients with chronic pain. This type of facility differs from a multidisciplinary pain center only because it does not include research and teaching activities in its regular programs. A multidisciplinary pain center may have diagnostic and treatment facilities which are outpatient, inpatient, or both.

1.3. Pain Clinic

This is a health care delivery facility focusing upon the diagnosis and management of patients with chronic pain. A pain clinic may specialize in specific diagnoses or in pains related to a specific region of the body. A pain clinic may be large or small, but it should never be a label for an isolated solo practitioner. A single physician functioning within a complex health care institution which offers appropriate consultative and therapeutic services could qualify as a pain clinic, if chronic pain patients were suitably assessed and managed. The absence of interdisciplinary assessment and management distinguishes this type of facility from a multidisciplinary pain center or clinic. Pain clinics can, and should, be encouraged to carry out research, but it is not a required characteristic of this type of facility.

1.4. Modality-Oriented Clinic

This is a health care facility which offers a specific type of treatment and does not provide comprehensive assessment or management. Examples include nerve block clinic, transcutaneous nerve stimulation clinic, acupuncture clinic, biofeedback clinic, etc. Such a facility may have one or more health care providers with different professional training; because of its limited treatment options and the lack of an integrated, comprehensive approach, it does not qualify for the term, multidisciplinary.

2. Multidisciplinary Centers for Children

While the multidisciplinary pain center (MPC) is the ideal, resource limitations have dictated that only a few such pediatric centers exist in the United States, with a couple dozen multidisciplinary clinics and a few pain clinics rounding out the specialty pain clinics. Most programs are almost exclusively for outpatients. On rare occasions patients are admitted for interventional therapy, sometimes in conjunction with rehabilitation specialists, neurologists, or general pediatricians as collaborators. Although the specialty clinics are relatively few, they offer help both directly, and by establishing models of care that can be extrapolated to other practice situations.

The MPC model of care is a family-centered interventional model (Fig. 14-2). This model views chronic pain as a biopsychosocial phenomenon that involves the patient, family, and the social construct in which the patient functions. Chronic pain symptoms are considered in the context of the medical pathology and findings, but viewed in the framework of the family, relationships, and social milieu (Fig. 14-3).

Assessment of the family includes a careful medical and mental health history. We search for family stressors and appraise the vulnerability and threat these pose to the family. How has the fam-

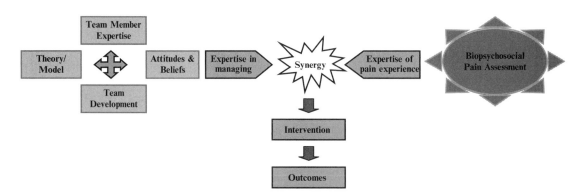

FIGURE 14-2. Chronic pain interventional model (personal communication, Ladwig, R.) The skilled pain management team offers varied expertise to create a synergistic treatment plan with the patient and family that is grounded in a complete biopsychosocial assessment.

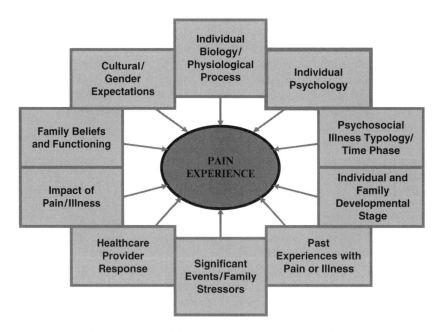

FIGURE 14-3. Biopsychosocial pain assessment (personal communication, Ladwig, R.) The pain experience of the patient reflects multiple influencing factors.

ily accommodated to the patient's pain problem? Does the family perceive these stressors and the threat they pose to the patient and/or the family?

Children and adolescents with chronic pain may have confounding school avoidance as well [11]. School absenteeism has been a common presenting feature of pediatric chronic pain [12]. It frequently results in poor academic performance, accusations of truancy, and dismissal of pain complaints by the school teachers and administrators [13]. It is important to carefully assess academic functioning, school accommodations, and presence or lack of an individualized educational plan. Invariably, direct contact with school administrators is a crucial, productive step in organizing a structured return to regular school functioning or in the implementation of an alternative educational plan (e.g., computer-based learning or home schooling).

Feedback from our patients reveals that the initial extended interview is often the first time that the patient and family feel that their "whole" story has been told and heard. After so many prior tests and interventions, it is tedious, but important, to tease out all the details of prior medical treatment and not rely upon written reports from prior health care providers. Often this discussion reveals distrust or disbelief in prior medical relationships. It enables our team to acknowledge the perceived threat of the pain problem and to sensitively develop a plan with implied trust and open communication. Families appreciate the clinic team's ability to coordinate care despite the socially dysfunctional results of the pain condition.

Patients with chronic pain have a high concordance of psychosocial factors that may reflect comorbidity or concordance with their pain problem [14–18] (Table 14-3). For example, poor family functioning or family hostility are associated with increased headaches and physical

TABLE 14-3. Vulnerability factors.

Marital, work or financial strains
Significant school absences
Major family accommodation
School transitions
High performance demands
Relationship rejection or loss

symptoms [19–20]. Significant school absenteeism is a major predictor for challenging treatment outcomes [11]. Patients present more frequently at nodal school epochs, such as eighth grade or during their first year of high school. It is also common to see patients in their junior year of high school, when many of the pressures of career planning and challenging academic curricula surface. Many MPC pain patients not only are enrolled in demanding academic course loads, but they frequently are engaged in multiple extracurricular activities including music, sports, religious groups, and social volunteerism. All of these activities place a high demand on the student to perform. If parents have made direct lifestyle accommodations, such as quitting jobs or taking family medical leave, this may also predict refractoriness of the pain. Lastly, recent relationship loss, including family, peers or friends, should be viewed as another vulnerability factor.

3. Organization of the Multidisciplinary Evaluation

The initial evaluation at an MPC or pain clinic should be extensive. The evaluation of a patient with chronic pain should begin with a complete history. The history taking in an MPC is sometimes conducted with all team members present. Alternatively, separate members of the team meet with the patient sequentially. The initial evaluation can last one to two hours or might encompass the better part of an entire day. As yet, there are no evidence-based guidelines to establish the most effective model for assessing a patient.

During the initial interview, the presenting pain symptom is discussed including: onset, triggers, quality, region, severity, functional limitations, sleep, and alleviating factors. It is critical to determine what therapies have been tried and which, if any, have afforded some degree of relief. Family history of chronic pain problems should be investigated. Often families will refrain from sharing their use of complimentary and alternative treatment modalities. However, the team should be open to gathering information about and, possibly supporting, the use of these modalities. Comorbid psychopathology is usually not disclosed with the entire team present. Instead, this is often revealed to the mental health practitioner by the parent(s). Social history of how the pain problem has affected the family structure, including who lives at home, how the patient is doing in school, and the parents' vocations and work status is also clarified at the first visit. Recent stressors should be identified including a death in the family, change in school, parental separation or divorce, or a move. Frequently, the chronic pain patient has missed a considerable amount of school and extracurricular activities. Details on psychological evaluation, treatment and thoughts on how to present the role of the mental health providers can be found in Chapters 13 and 15.

3.1. Initial Physical Exam

Although the pain complaint is often localized, there are a number of systemic diseases that can present with focal symptoms. Therefore, the first examination at an MPC is often quite complete. Physical exam points are discussed in more detail in the chapters on particular diagnoses. The primary goal is to discern overlooked etiologies (such as myofascial trigger points in abdominal pain or back pain), and to reassure the patient and family that the child has been examined carefully and thoroughly.

3.2. Initial Physical/Occupational Therapy Exam

A functional evaluation is done by or with a physical or occupational therapist (OT/PT) to identify areas that would be appropriate for physical rehabilitation intervention. Pain often leads to altered body mechanics, disturbed posture, and deconditioning. The power of simultaneous evaluations by the OT/PT and the physician is that the physician rules out signs of danger or potential threats to safety, while the OT/PT begins to guide the family and patient toward enhanced physical function. One consistent observation is that physical function often improves before pain remits, and the OT/PT will educate the family regarding this point at the first visit. As rapport is gained, it is often within dialogues between the patient and the OT/PT that the patient reveals psychosocial

issues which can be shared with the rest of the treating team.

3.3. The Feedback Session

The plan is then presented to the family and patient by the entire team. Multifaceted in nature, the plan incorporates therapies including pharmacological, physical and occupational therapy, cognitive behavioral pain strategies including meditation, deep relaxation, guided imagery techniques, mindfulness meditation and individual, and family counseling. Sleep hygiene is always reviewed, as it is common for patients to have very abnormal sleep habits [12]. Treatment recommendations may include massage therapy and acupuncture. A discussion of the use of dietary supplements, counseling about nutrition, and the impact of obesity on chronic pain issues takes place. Finally, if possible, general suggestions for regular exercise or treatment-specific activities are recommended as part of the daily treatment plan.

Major goals are established to improve psychological functioning (decreased school absences and return to extracurricular activities), psychological support for the entire family, and communication between the patient's school and physician can occur. The plan focuses on modulating the pain to tolerable levels, so that the patient can consider a return to school (even if part-time) and a return to participation in activities with friends and family. The initial evaluation can require one and one-half to six hours, but families usually appreciate the efficiency of the "one-stop-shop" approach. The fact that all team members communicate immediately and directly, with a resultant integrated specific treatment plan, is very attractive to many families.

3.4. The MPC and Primary Physicians

Long distances from MPCs impede, but do not prevent, success. In these cases empowerment and reorientation of the medical resources closer to home, so that they can support an integrated model of improvement, can yield positive outcomes. Members of the MPC view primary practitioners as members of an extended team, and realize that resources will vary from location to location. With the easy interaction provided by e-mail and phone calls, coordination and follow-up care between the MPC and the primary physician or local providers should be reasonably straight-forward. Complex pain treatment at a distance is further discussed in Chapter 5.

As with any medical encounter, not all patients will be satisfied with the results of an MPC visit. About 10 to 15 percent of the families we evaluate remain fixed in a dichotomous view of the patient's pain problem. Most commonly they maintain a viewpoint that the correct diagnosis has been missed, despite numerous tests and exams. Many times these families continue to pursue medical procedures or evaluations by their primary care or other subspecialist physicians. The primary care physician can strengthen the therapeutic plan by underscoring the theme of "de-medicalizing" the pain. It appears that until aggressive investigations are discontinued and the medical providers begin to acknowledge the integrated family-centered approach to care, these patients will make very slow progress, if any.

3.5. Treatment and Cost-Effectiveness of MPCs

Engaging an MPC to address chronic pain may appear, on the surface, to be an expensive endeavor. Although specific outcome data on clinical outcomes and cost-effectiveness are lacking in the pediatric population, a very strong argument has been made for these approaches to chronic nonmalignant pain in adults. Gatchel and Okifuji conducted a substantial review of studies reporting treatment outcomes for patients with chronic pain [21]. Their results clearly showed that comprehensive pain programs offer the most efficacious and cost-effective means of addressing these problems. They also point out, however, that the short-sighted cost containment policies of third party payors often limit the prevalence of these models.

4. Specific Disease Examples

Several chapters in this book are devoted to some of the more prominent pain conditions. What follows is an introduction to several conditions whose treatment might include working with an MPC.

4.1. Complex Regional Pain Syndrome (CRPS) Type I

CRPS type I, formerly known as reflex sympathetic dystrophy (RSD), is a syndrome of persistent neuropathic pain associated with nondermatomal autonomic dysfunction [22, 23]. It occurs after minor injury and patients have symptoms including spontaneous pain, allodynia (pain to light touch), temperature and color changes (including cyanosis), edema, trophic changes of the skin, and significant loss of bone density. The pain is out of proportion to the inciting event, and is not limited to the expected distribution of a nerve [24]. This latter characteristic often leads to accusations of faking or malingering, as the stocking or glove distribution of symptoms is non-anatomic.

The cause of pain is not completely understood, but is thought to be related to abnormal discharges in sympathetic afferent nerves, along with nociceptive effects produced by the incidental trauma. Sensitivity of nerve receptors, spontaneous neuronal ectopy, and psychological components of the pain are always present. As early as 1982 Ruggeri et al. suggested that CRPS in pediatrics is benign and will respond to physical therapy [25]. Others suggest that a subset of patients will continue to have severe pain and disability [23, 26, 27].

In an early article on CRPS, Wilder et al. published a series of 70 patients who were predominately female, with involvement of the lower extremity disease [23]. This was one of the early papers describing multidisciplinary treatment of pain in children. Treatments included physical therapy, transcutaneous electrical nerve stimulation (TENS), tricyclic antidepressants (TCAs), cognitive behavioral therapies, and relaxation therapies. In a more recent report from the same group of investigators, a 6-week course of intensive physical therapy and cognitive behavioral therapies reduced pain and improved functioning without the need for sympathetic blockade [22]. Neuromodulating drug therapy (TCAs with gabapentin or other antiepileptic agents) with intensive physical therapy, administered on a 3-day-per-week regimen up to even twice per day, plus cognitive behavioral therapy, was successful in most patients. Psychotherapy included a focus on cognitive-behavioral interventions, plus intensive decatastrophizing of the illness.

CRPS is a disorder that can be disabling and requires evaluation of physical, psychosocial, and functional impact, followed by comprehensive and coordinated treatment. Although nerve blocks might bring relief, pain often returns. It is a fairly uniform finding that refractory or migratory CRPS symptoms signal unrecognized or unresolved psychosocial issues. Although it is likely that many patients have self-limited disease that will respond quickly to over-the-counter pain medications and increased physical activity of the involved extremity, after 1 to 2 weeks of symptoms, patients with suspected CRPS Type I should be referred to a pediatric pain management center.

4.2. Musculoskeletal Pain and Fibromyalgia

Most everyday musculoskeletal pain is effectively treated with nonsteroidal anti-inflammatory drugs (NSAIDs), massage, muscle stretches, and reassurance. It is important, in children with persistent musculoskeletal pain, to rule out other major illnesses as a cause of the pain. Evaluating musculoskeletal pain tends to be straightforward, with attention to "red flags" such as fever, rash, swelling and weight loss (see Chapter 19 for details). Clearly, patients with rheumatologic, infectious, or orthopedic conditions will need focused evaluation. Even though treatments for some rheumatologic and orthopedic etiologies may include specific immunomodulatory and surgical interventions, a biopsychosocial approach is still worthwhile.

One should explore functional factors, such as athletics, inactivity, sleep habits, and stressors, as well as traditional components of the medical history and physical examination. Once major illness has been ruled out, the treatment plan incorporates lifestyle changes, including sleep, diet, exercise, and structuring of social activities. Anti-inflammatory drugs and muscle relaxants can be beneficial. Occasionally, TCAs, trigger point injections, and topical treatments are useful. Aerobic exercises and strength training not only have a localized effect, but also have a more generalized beneficial effect on mood, sleep, appetite, and general well-being.

Acute-onset back pain in children and adolescents is usually associated with new-onset pathology [28-30]. Back pain in children is rarely due to the common causes of low back pain in adults, such as discogenic pain or arthropathy. Children with scoliosis will rarely have back pain that needs to be treated aggressively with NSAIDs or opioids. Myofascial pain involving single or multiple muscle groups is the more common cause of back pain in the otherwise healthy pediatric population, especially in the adolescent and early adult years. Myofascial pain is characterized by widespread pain, trigger points on examination, referred pain, generalized fatigue, sleep-related problems, and mood disturbances, and may be associated with headaches and abdominal pain. For the more common myofascial syndromes, as well as nonspecific low back pain, localized heat application, regular aerobic exercise, physical conditioning, improved sleep hygiene, cognitive-behavioral techniques, massage therapy, muscle relaxants, NSAIDs, and low dose TCAs have been known to afford success, improving both pain and sleep disturbances [29, 31]. Acupuncture on a regular basis has been successful in children with myofascial pain and fibromyalgia [32, 33].

4.3. Headache

The incidence of headaches is around 10 to 20 percent in children less than 10 years of age [34–39]. The common causes of headache in children are migraine, tension-type headaches, psychogenic headaches, and those related to refractive errors, dental braces, sinusitis, sleep apnea, viral illnesses, and temporomandibular joint dysfunction. Migraine headaches become more common around puberty in both boys and girls, and about 60 percent of these patients will continue to have migraines as adults. The incidence of tension-type headaches usually increases from early school-age into adolescence. Children sometimes have the fear that they could have a brain tumor and certainly any headache with signs of elevated intracranial pressures or focal neurological signs warrants further investigation and imaging (see Chapter 18 for "warning signs" and further discussion). Headaches can be quite disabling and evaluation and treatment planning must consider the level of social and scholastic functioning, as well as situational triggers (e.g., academic stress, lighting, bullies, institutional noise, etc.). Headache treatment may be preventative or abortive and includes acetaminophen, NSAIDs, TCAs, selective serotonin reuptake inhibitors, beta blockers, anticonvulsants, and abortive drugs such as the triptans and ergotamines. Nonpharmacologic treatment is invaluable in the management of pediatric headaches. This includes biofeedback, relaxation techniques, cognitive reframing and a variety of standard psychotherapeutic interventions. Acupuncture and TENS may also be options.

4.4. Abdominal and Pelvic Pain

Abdominal pain is a common complaint in school-age children and a common cause of school absenteeism. Recurrent abdominal pain is usually periumbilical, varied in duration and severity, and may be associated with nausea, vomiting, changes in food intake and disturbances in sleep and bowel movements. It is often difficult to find a specific cause for the pain and most patients presenting to a pain clinic have undergone a battery of tests, including imaging and endoscopies by GI specialists before referral.

Pelvic pain is seen in older adolescents and can be secondary to endometriosis, pelvic inflammatory disease, ovarian cysts, musculoskeletal injury, psoas abscesses, or constipation (see Chapter 17). It is often useful to have the female patients be seen by a gynecologist to rule out pathology and to consider hormonal means of treatment, if indicated.

It is then important to communicate to the patient and family that, although an organic cause cannot be found, the pain is real and referral to a MPC will lead to improvement. Management incorporates dietary changes to avoid constipation and lactose exposure in intolerant patients. Attention to sleep hygiene, learning biofeedback, coping skills and relaxation techniques in conjunction with medications such as NSAIDs, TCAs, gabapentin, tramadol or selective serotonin reuptake inhibitors will usually lead to improvement or resolution of symptoms. Regional and lytic blocks are almost never performed in children, unless for cancer-related pain in a child with limited life expectancy.

5. Conclusion

Chronic pain in children and adolescents should be managed by a skilled team of practitioners from a variety of medical disciplines. Care models exist that use inpatient treatment programs, as well as outpatient or community-based treatment. Unfortunately, such comprehensive pain programs are very labor- and cost-intensive. Many organizations will not have the resources and commitment to provide this type of care. Nonetheless, the principles of integrated, multidisciplinary, non-dualistic care that includes attention to mind–body interactions should be considered for children with chronic pain disorders.

Take-Home Points

- The complex nature of many pain conditions requires a thorough, multidisciplinary evaluation.
- MPCs offer the most comprehensive evaluation and treatment, although the cost and labor-intensity of such programs limits their number and availability.
- Medical, psychological, occupational and physical therapy, and nursing are the basic disciplines involved in pain evaluation and treatment.
- The principles of multidisciplinary evaluation and treatment can be assembled in the local communities, although often with difficulty.
- MPC members consider primary care providers as team members, and will be happy to help coordinate care from a distance.

References

1. Goodman JE, McGrath PJ. The epidemiology of pain in children and adolescents: a review. Pain 1991;46:247–264.
2. Merskey H, Bogduk N. Classification of Chronic Pain, IASP Task Force on Taxonomy. Seattle: IASP Press 1994.
3. McGrath PJ, Finley GA. Chronic and recurrent pain in children and adolescents. In: McGrath PJ, Finley GA, editors. Chronic and Recurrent Pain in Children and Adolescents. Seattle: IASP Press, 1999:1–4.
4. American Pain Society. Principles of analgesic use in the treatment of acute pain and cancer pain, 2003.
5. McDaniel SH, Hepworth J, Doherty WJ. Medical Family Therapy: A Biopsychosocial Approach to Families with Health Problems. New York: Basic Books, 1992.
6. Loeser JD, Bonica JJ. Bonica's Management of Pain. Philadelphia: Lippincott, Williams & Wilkins, 2001.
7. Bonica JJ. Organization and function of a pain clinic. In: Bonica JJ, editor. Advances in Neurology

International Symposium on Pain. New York: Raven, 1974:433–443.

8. McQuay HJ, Moore RA, Eccleston C, Morley S, Williams AC. Systematic review of outpatient services for chronic pain control. Health Technol Assess 1997;1:1–135.

9. Loeser JD. Desirable characteristics for pain treatment facilities. Pain 1990;41:S479.

10. Loeser JD. Desirable characteristics for pain treatment facilities, 2007. *http://www.iasp-pain.org/ AM/Template.cfm?Section=Home&template=/CM/ HTMLDisplay.cfm&ContentID=3011*

11. Ladwig RJ, Khan KA. School avoidance: implications for school nurses. J Spec Pediatr Nurs 2007;12:210–212.

12. Palermo TM. Impact of recurrent and chronic pain on child and family daily functioning: a critical review of the literature. J Dev Behav Pediatr 2000;21:58–69.

13. Campo JV, Jansen-McWilliams L, Comer DM, Kelleher KJ. Somatization in pediatric primary care: Association with psychopathology, functional impairment, and use of services. J Am Acad Child Adolesc Psychiatry 1999;38:1093–1101.

14. Palermo TM, Chambers CT. Parent and family factors in pediatric chronic pain and disability: An integrative approach. Pain 2005;119:1–4.

15. Eccleston C, McCracken LM, Jordan A, Sleed M. Development and preliminary psychometric evaluation of the parent report version of the Bath adolescent pain questionnaire (BAPQ-P): A multidimensional parent report instrument to assess the impact of chronic pain on adolescents. Pain 2007;131:48–56.

16. Gauntlett-Gilbert J, Eccleston C. Disability in adolescents with chronic pain: Patterns and predictors across different domains of functioning. Pain 2007;131:132–141.

17. Jordan AL, Eccleston C, Osborn M. Being a parent of the adolescent with complex chronic pain: An interpretative phenomenological analysis. Eur J Pain 2007;11:49–56.

18. Hunfeld JA, Perquin CW, Hazebroek-Kampschreur AA, Passchier J, van Suijlekom-Smit LW, van der Wouden JC. Physically unexplained chronic pain and its impact on children and their families: the mother's perception. Psychol Psychother 2002;75:251–260.

19. Wickrama KA, Conger RD, Wallace LE, Elder GH, Jr. Linking early social risks to impaired physical health during the transition to adulthood. J Health Soc Behav 2003;44:61–74.

20. Anttila P, Sourander A, Metsahonkala L, Aromaa M, Helenius H, Sillanpaa M. Psychiatric symptoms in children with primary headache. J Am Acad Child Adolesc Psychiatry 2004;43:412–419.

21. Gatchel RJ, Okifuji A. Evidence-based scientific data documenting the treatment and cost-effectiveness of comprehensive pain programs for chronic nonmalignant pain. J Pain 2006;7:779–793.

22. Lee BH, Scharff L, Sethna NF, et al. Physical therapy and cognitive-behavioral treatment for complex regional pain syndromes. J Pediatr 2002;141:135–140.

23. Wilder RT, Berde CB, Wolohan M, Vieyra MA, Masek BJ, Micheli LJ. Reflex sympathetic dystrophy in children. Clinical characteristics and follow-up of seventy patients. J Bone Joint Surg Am 1992;74:910–919.

24. Stanton-Hicks M, Janig W, Hassenbusch S, Haddox JD, Boas R, Wilson P. Reflex sympathetic dystrophy: changing concepts and taxonomy. Pain 1995;63:127–133.

25. Ruggeri SB, Athreya BH, Doughty R, Gregg JR, Das MM. Reflex sympathetic dystrophy in children. Clin Orthop 1982;163:225–230.

26. Tong HC, Nelson VS. Recurrent and migratory reflex sympathetic dystrophy in children. Pediatr Rehabil 2000;4:87–89.

27. Malleson PN, al-Matar M, Petty RE. Idiopathic musculoskeletal pain syndromes in children. J Rheumatol 1992;19:1786–1789.

28. Feldman DS, Straight JJ, Badra MI, Mohaideen A, Madan SS. Evaluation of an algorithmic approach to pediatric back pain. J Pediatr Orthop 2006;26: 353–357.

29. Malleson P, Clinch J. Pain syndromes in children. Curr Opin Rheumatol 2003;15:572–580.

30. de Inocencio J. Musculoskeletal pain in primary pediatric care: analysis of 1,000 consecutive general pediatric clinic visits. Pediatrics 1998;102:E63.

31. Eccleston C, Malleson PN, Clinch J, Connell H, Sourbut C. Chronic pain in adolescents: evaluation of a programme of interdisciplinary cognitive behaviour therapy. Arch Dis Child 2003;88: 881–885.

32. Tsao JC, Meldrum M, Bursch B, Jacob MC, Kim SC, Zeltzer LK. Treatment expectations for CAM interventions in pediatric chronic pain patients and their parents. Evid Based Complement Alternat Med 2005;2:521–527.

33. Lin YC, Bioteau AB, Lee AC. Acupuncture for the management of pediatric pain: a pilot study. Medical Acupuncture 2002;14:45–46.

34. Anttila P, Metsahonkala L, Sillanpaa M. Long-term trends in the incidence of headache in Finnish school children. Pediatrics 2006;117:e1197–1201.

35. Petersen S, Brulin C, Bergstrom E. Recurrent pain symptoms in young school children are often multiple. Pain 2006;121:145–150.

36. Annequin D, Tourniaire B. Migraine and headache in childhood. Arch Pediatr 2005;12:624–629.

37. Ramchandani PG, Hotopf M, Sandhu B, Stein A, ALSPAC Study Team. The epidemiology of recurrent abdominal pain from 2 to 6 years of age: results of a large, population-based study. Pediatrics 2005;116:46–50.

38. Larsson B, Zaluha M. Swedish school nurses' view of school health care utilization, causes and manage-ment of recurrent headaches among school children. Scand J Caring Sci 2003;17:232–238.

39. Aromaa M, Sillanpaa M, Rautava P, Helenius H. Pain experience of children with headache and their families: a controlled study. Pediatrics 2000;106:270–275.

15
Psychological Interventions for Chronic Pain

Susmita Kashikar-Zuck and Anne M. Lynch

Abstract: Recurrent and chronic pain conditions such as headaches, abdominal pain, back pain or other musculoskeletal pains, are common problems encountered in pediatric primary care settings. Primary care physicians are well aware that psychological stress, family context, and lifestyle factors can have a strong influence on pain symptoms and children's ability to cope with pain. In these situations behavioral pain management interventions are a very useful complement to usual medical care. This chapter introduces empirically supported treatments for chronic pediatric pain, including biofeedback training and pain coping skills training with parental guidance in behavior management techniques. Other clinically relevant approaches such as family intervention, school consultation, and assessing the need for more intensive psychiatric care are also discussed. Behavioral principles discussed in this chapter are implemented most successfully when the entire health care team provides a consistent message that promotes active and adaptive coping by patients and their families.

Key words: Coping skills, biofeedback, chronic pain, multidisciplinary treatment, behavior management.

Introduction

Behavioral interventions are an integral component of multidisciplinary care for chronic pediatric pain. The objective of this chapter is to familiarize primary care physicians with the range of psychologically based treatments available for children with chronic pain. Although behavioral pain management interventions are best implemented by trained psychologists, the principles behind behavioral techniques have broad utility for the entire health care team and can often be integrated into the overall care and management of pediatric pain patients. In the last decade research evidence has accumulated from increasingly well-designed pediatric studies that demonstrate the efficacy of behavioral treatments for pediatric chronic pain conditions such as chronic migraines, recurrent abdominal pain, and juvenile fibromyalgia [1–3]. In this chapter, the description of treatments is based upon the best available evidence from current research, but we also include explanations of the full range of psychological services that are often needed for the clinical management of complex pain patients.

As in the treatment of any chronic condition, it is crucial for the health care team to educate the patient and family early in the course of treatment to create realistic expectations. This is especially true in the case of behavioral treatment, where misconceptions about the nature of treatment may deter a family from seeking appropriate care. Among pain patients, early education about the nature of behavioral treatment prevents excessive focus solely on immediate pain reduction, and broadens the scope of treatment to deal with lifestyle issues which may in fact be maintaining the problem. Specific clinical outcomes that can be expected to improve as a result of behavioral intervention are: gradual return to functional activities, improved self-confidence in managing pain, lowered pain-related anxiety and depressive symptoms, and pain reduction. Contrary to what

G.A. Walco and K.R. Goldschneider (eds.), *Pain in Children: A Practical Guide for Primary Care.*
© Humana Press, a part of Springer Science + Business Media, 2008

most parents (and sometimes physicians) expect of pain management treatment, we have found that reduction in pain intensity is often a "lagging indicator" of improvement. The most commonly held belief is that the child will return to usual activities and begin to feel more cheerful *after* their pain is completely relieved. In fact, we have observed that the reverse is actually more typical. As the child (and their parents) gain more confidence in self-management strategies and actively engage in the treatment process, they begin to experience improvement in functional and emotional well-being, which is then followed by reduction in pain intensity.

The following sections describe the most commonly used behavioral interventions for pediatric pain management. The sections are organized roughly in order of what interventions might be recommended given the complexity of the presenting problem, or become necessary as new issues emerge during the course of treatment. We begin with the most straightforward and well-studied approaches that are widely used for children and adolescents with chronic pain. These include biofeedback and coping skills training (also known as cognitive-behavioral therapy) which are useful in situations where the child's activities and/or mood are impaired by pain, but in which the patients have a reasonably stable psychosocial environment. More intensive interventions may be added in situations where dysfunctional psychosocial environments are causing or maintaining the child's coping difficulties. These may involve interventions at the family level and consultation with school personnel. Finally, we discuss situations in which serious psychiatric problems may require referral for more intensive mental health services.

1. Biofeedback-Assisted Relaxation Training

For many children with pain, the pain itself or subsequent pain-related anxiety results in an elevated stress response in the body, increased tension, or postural adjustments (guarding) to compensate for pain. These changes may not be noticeable to the child or associated with pain in the short-term. However, when pain becomes chronic, these physiological responses may be sustained for a lengthy period of time and lead to additional problems. For example, children with low back pain may experience increased muscle tension and pain that spreads to their upper back and shoulders, or engage in compensatory postures (e.g., leaning, slouching) to reduce pain while unwittingly straining other muscles repetitively over time.

Biofeedback is a modality used to help patients gain volitional control over physiological processes in the body, previously believed to be unchangeable. Computer equipment is utilized to provide electronic monitoring of autonomic functions such as heart rate and blood pressure, muscle tension, peripheral blood flow, and respiration. Monitoring muscle tension through electromyography (EMG biofeedback) and peripheral blood flow (thermal biofeedback) are the most common biofeedback modalities used in the treatment of chronic pain. They have also been the most well-studied in the pediatric pain literature [4]. Information is typically relayed back to the child in auditory (sounds, tones, music) and/or visual displays (bars, lines, pictures) providing immediate "feedback" about how the child's body is reacting in real time.

Biofeedback is a clinically valuable and generally well-liked complementary treatment because: 1) it is noninvasive; 2) it promotes body awareness; 3) it can be used in conjunction with medications without worry of side effects; and 4) it provides immediate and easily understandable information to a child as he or she engages in strategies to enhance relaxation [5]. Biofeedback has been used for a number of different pain conditions, but has been found to be particularly effective for children with migraine and tension-type headaches and Raynaud's disease [4]. Although less well-studied, biofeedback has also been utilized in the treatment of fibromyalgia, irritable bowel syndrome, and other chronic pain problems [6].

Biofeedback equipment can be used alone to promote physiological changes, but more commonly, relaxation strategies are introduced simultaneously to enhance the process and promote success [6, 7]. Diaphragmatic breathing is a technique designed to shift patients from taking rapid, shallow breaths (or holding their breath) when in pain, to instead inhaling slowly and deeply so that the abdomen rises and falls ("belly breathing"). While most children acknowledge that their parents have encouraged them to "take a deep breath" to relax, they rarely engage in the technique for longer than a minute or two. Consistent use of this style of breathing reduces anxiety, produces a calming effect and provides the child with an inconspicuous strategy to cope with pain in public (school, church). Children report that they spontaneously generalize the use of this technique to test or exam-related anxiety, control of moodiness, and sleep onset. Thus, children often describe this technique to be the easiest and most effective.

Guided imagery techniques involve developing detailed mental images of special, comforting places or objects (e.g., the beach on vacation). Descriptions of the image are first elicited from the child focusing on aspects of the five senses (e.g., What do you see at the beach? What do you hear at the beach?), and then presented back to "guide" them through the mental creation of the image. Guided imagery encourages distraction from pain and promotes increased relaxation.

Finally, progressive muscle relaxation is a strategy that combines deliberate tensing, then relaxing, of muscle groups in the body to reduce muscle tension and increase body awareness [7]. For children who experience tension-related pain flare-ups, this strategy provides relief in a way that common relaxing activities like watching TV do not. Children learn these techniques, paying particular attention to post-relaxation readings of reduction in EMG activity and/or increase in surface skin temperature at the extremities.

When deciding whether or not to refer for biofeedback services, the following aspects should be considered. Age or developmental level are important in terms of treatment efficacy. A child has to possess sufficient attention and cognitive awareness to engage in relaxation strategies. Our experience suggests that children age 7 or older can benefit from this technique [8], while younger children or children diagnosed with Attention Deficit Hyperactivity Disorder (ADHD) need to be considered on an individual basis in terms of their degree of insight and activity level. Children with a low IQ are often unable to generalize their experiences from biofeedback training, or do not adequately comprehend the goals of treatment. Patients with untreated posttraumatic stress disorder (PTSD) may experience intrusive flashbacks when attempting to relax, be inattentive and fidgety

due to anxiety, and be markedly sensitive to physical contact by unfamiliar individuals (when attaching electrodes). Finally, regular home practice is critical to skill mastery and without it, frustration will arise and likely compromise the helpfulness of biofeedback-assisted relaxation training. Thus, the patient's motivation to devote at least a few minutes per day of time and energy to the practice of relaxation skills is essential and must be considered. It can be helpful to explain to the patient that a whole-hearted effort and consistent practice of the "homework" they will be given is required for the psychological therapies to work. Also, phrasing the referral in terms of tutoring or training in a skill set can defuse some of the initial resistance that may arise when a referral to a psychologist is discussed with families.

Biofeedback provides intangible benefits in addition to addressing autonomic arousal. Patients learn better self-monitoring, improve their sense of self-efficacy, increase hopefulness for pain management, and improve their coping skills [4]. These benefits may be as reinforcing as the direct effects of treatment. Biofeedback seems to be more effective in children compared to adult chronic pain patients, who have typically suffered for years and may possess more significant psychopathology and entrenched responses to stress that may hinder meaningful change [8].

2. Pain Coping Skills Training

Many children and adolescents with chronic pain present with increased functional disability, poor coping, and increased anxiety and depression related to persistent pain symptoms [9]. Often, children and their parents report that pain-related disability is more devastating than the pain intensity by itself. Children describe numerous school absences, stacks of uncompleted homework, decreased athletic participation, and reduced social and recreational activities. In many respects, every aspect of their normal life has been compromised by pain. Their faith in the medical system is often shaken as many chronic pain conditions have unclear origins and have not responded well to medication management. Thus, addressing the thoughts, feelings and behaviors associated with persistent pain is a significant component of treatment.

Pain coping skills training is based on a cognitive-behavioral approach to pain management, and focuses on common maladaptive thoughts ("If I hurt, I cannot go to school.") and behaviors ("Only resting or sleeping takes away my pain.") that may accompany pain. The goals of pain coping skills training are to: 1) resume normal functioning despite pain; 2) decrease functional disability; 3) improve independent pain management; 4) improve pain-related anxiety and depression; and 5) increase self-efficacy [3].

The first component of coping skills training is providing a rationale for the behavioral management of pain, rather than solely a medication management approach. Patients benefit from a developmentally-appropriate explanation of the physiological mechanisms of pain (Gate Control Theory of Pain), including how behavioral strategies such as relaxation and distraction can reduce pain intensity. This information demystifies the pain experience, reducing the fear and panic associated with pain flare-ups. Additionally, it may dispel the common patient or family perception that the child has been sent to a psychologist because she is "making up" the pain or because the pain is "not real" and "in her head."

Coping skills training also involves regular monitoring through daily diaries of pain intensity, stress-related antecedents to flare-ups, and activity level [2, 3]. Self-monitoring can lead to better awareness of pain patterns and may improve the child's sense of control and knowledge about pain [2]. Because pain frequently compromises activity level, increasing pleasant activities is targeted with training in activity pacing. Pleasant activities serve as a distraction from pain, and also improve mood. However, children and adolescents tend to take an "all or nothing" attitude—either becoming completely sedentary or resuming levels of activity or exercise that are too intense given the lack of endurance and deconditioning that may have developed over the course of their pain problems. This mentality is particularly notable for athletes who have been forced to stop sports participation and who use pain reduction as an indicator that previous strength and flexibility have returned. Activity pacing emphasizes a graduated approach to activities, with frequent use of rest breaks during the activity to prevent overexertion ("too much, too soon") that could lead to a pain flare-up.

Many pediatric pain patients become progressively more frustrated, irritable, withdrawn, anxious, or depressed. Negative cognitions often coexist with maladaptive coping efforts. Children catastrophize about the pain never going away, or are convinced that they are unable to cope with pain outside the home or away from their parents. While understandable and natural emotions, the nature of chronic pain requires the child to attempt to engage in normal functioning despite pain. Improving positive self talk addresses this discouragement, promotes adaptive coping, and coaches the child through stressful situations that the child has to endure because of pain (e.g., friends who do not understand pain-related limitations; unpredictable flare-ups). Finally, training in problem solving increases the child's ability to creatively use relaxation techniques and coping skills to tackle difficult situations that arise at home or school.

Pain coping skills training places considerable emphasis on patient independence and home practice of skills. While the skills are intuitive and logical, the application of coping skills "in the moment" is considerably more difficult. For younger children, parental coaching and cueing of skills is necessary, while older teenagers tend to balk at excessive parental interference. In our experience, children and teenagers who are more concrete in their thinking, display rigid problem solving, or who fixate on their pain have the most difficulty generalizing the skills. In addition, children with developmental disorders such as Asperger's Disorder or mental retardation derive limited benefits from this treatment method. Research studies have found promising results for cognitive behavioral intervention used for the treatment of pediatric abdominal pain [3], fibromyalgia [2], and pediatric chronic pain patients in an inpatient program [10].

3. Parental Guidance in Behavior Management Techniques

Parenting a child with chronic pain is often challenging, and many parents feel unequipped to handle behavioral issues (e.g., changes in mood, school refusal, withdrawal from usual activities) that commonly occur in children with persistent pain symptoms. Research shows that parental behavior in response to children's pain plays an important role in creating a context that can favor either adaptive or maladaptive coping in the child [11, 12]. Some parents may inadvertently reinforce passive or dysfunctional coping by taking control and discouraging self-management by the child. Education and training of parents in age-appropriate behavior management strategies can go a long way toward helping a child develop and maintain active coping strategies for pain management. Therefore, parental guidance is often conducted along with coping skills training for the child, so that consistent use of behavioral strategies is implemented in the home and treatment gains are maintained.

Parents are trained in five basic coaching skills [13]. First, parents are taught how to encourage their child to manage the pain independently. This means that they make greater efforts to notice and praise the child when the child is actively coping, distracting him or herself from pain, or maintaining a cheerful attitude despite the pain. Unfortunately, in many families, children get more attention and reassurance when they are highly distressed, seeking assistance, or complaining about severe pain than when they are calm, engaged in activities or otherwise contentedly occupied. The goal is, therefore, to redirect the parents to provide more positive attention towards the child when the child is coping well.

Second, parents are asked to maintain their usual family routines and encourage normal activities for the child, even during pain episodes. Having a child in chronic pain can be highly disruptive to families (e.g., the child staying home from school and the parent having to take time off work, withdrawing from social and recreational activities, and spending a good deal of time in doctors' offices). These disruptions can lead to exacerbation of pain-related distress due to changes in a child's usual activities and relationships. Young patients who have missed a lot of schoolwork or other activities due to pain can become very anxious about returning to school, even after the pain starts to improve, because they are worried that they will be unable to catch up, or they fear teasing from peers about their absence from school. For these reasons we emphasize to parents that, although some lifestyle modifications may be necessary, it is essential to maintain a normal routine, including school attendance and keeping up with schoolwork.

Third, parents are asked to refrain from frequent "status checks;" that is, asking the child how bad the pain is several times a day. This inquiry may be necessary during the acute phase of pain to determine the nature of the problems. However, for pain that has become chronic and when diagnostic tests have ruled out serious underlying medical conditions, repetitive parental checks often become a habit rather than a necessity. Instead, the child should be encouraged to independently communicate about pain to the parent. This ensures that the parent is not constantly reminding the child about their symptoms, allowing the child to self-monitor and take greater responsibility for communicating about pain. This technique works well among children of all age groups, but especially in teenagers, who often say they would prefer that their parent did not frequently ask about pain.

Fourth, guidelines for how medication is to be used are reviewed and it is emphasized that following instructions provided by the health care team is important. While physicians sometimes worry that pain medication may be overused by patients, it is also the case that parents sometimes withhold medication until the pain becomes very severe—because parents fear that their child might become "addicted" to pain medicine. In either case, it is useful to educate the parent about the type of medicine being used to treat their child's pain, and how it is to be used, to ensure medications are used appropriately.

Finally, parents are encouraged to treat pain flare-ups just as they would any other illness. When the pain flares up, the child should be allowed to go to bed or rest in a quiet place for a period of time. Watching TV or playing video games for an extended time is not a substitute for rest. Although these activities can be useful to distract a child from pain for short periods, these can in fact become passive strategies for coping with pain when used by themselves and can reinforce avoidance of more difficult activities like school.

While these guidelines may appear intuitively obvious, many parents of children with chronic pain find it extremely difficult to consistently put these into practice. Therefore, the therapist works with parents to apply these guidelines in their specific situations and helps them troubleshoot barriers to implementing these strategies in the home. The guidelines are also adjusted based upon what is appropriate for the developmental level of the child, with progressively higher levels of independence (and associated responsibility for self-management) being recommended based upon increasing age and maturity level. The primary care physician can positively reinforce parents as they adopt more productive approaches to handling their child's pain.

4. Family-Based Intervention

In working with children with chronic pain and their families, it is important to understand that pain symptoms and pain expression always occur in a psychosocial context. For example, chronic pain is known to aggregate in families and children with chronic pain often have a parent with chronic pain [14-16]. How a parent deals with their own pain often provides insight into how the child copes with pain and their expectations for functioning despite pain, because parents are their most significant role models. If a parent is disabled by their pain or has a catastrophic style of thinking about their pain, it is easy to imagine that this is a completely different environment than one where a parent has pain, but copes actively and effectively. Although parents are not the focus of therapy in this case, integrating parents into the treatment can often help minimize the effects of maladaptive parental pain coping and maximize the effects of adaptive patterns that parents may have developed on their own.

A second situation that perhaps requires even greater attention is the current level of stress in the family system. Family stress or dysfunction should be suspected when a variety of pain management approaches (medication, physical therapy, and coping skills training) have failed to produce any improvement, and a child shows persistent mood difficulties, school avoidance, or prolonged disability in excess of what might be expected. In these cases we have found that some significant source of stress or worry (such as an impending divorce or separation of parents, serious illness in another family member, domestic violence, substance use in the family, etc.) may be an underlying reason why improvement in pain and functioning is difficult to achieve. This information often becomes more evident only later in the course of treatment, when trust and rapport have developed between the patient and the health care team. Maintaining rapport with patients and families, even in some cases

where frustration builds, is probably the best way to enhance trust and help families feel comfortable in providing important information. Only too often, a child or adolescent complains of being "scolded" by his or her physician to push through the pain, get on with life and resume normal activity. Unfortunately, this may only serve to increase resistance to treatment recommendations. While essentially the same underlying message is promoted in behavioral pain management, we have found that a firm but supportive approach, with training in specific coping strategies, yields far better results than a stern lecture that alienates the family and child from the physician. In cases where family stress or dysfunction is present, specialized psychological care should be sought to evaluate and treat underlying issues that may be maintaining the child's disability and distress.

5. Consultation with School Personnel

Similar to the above situation, school-related stressors, such as academic worries or social difficulties in school (test anxiety, social anxiety, being teased or bullied), can often be associated with pain-related disability. Identifying the sources of school avoidance can help the health care team in treatment planning. We have found that simple interventions can dramatically change a child's willingness to remain in school despite pain and physical discomfort. For example, an adolescent male with inflammatory bowel disease and abdominal pain reported that he was missing a great deal of school. Further inquiry revealed that he needed to use the bathroom frequently in school, but he was embarrassed about having to use the public bathrooms. A phone call to his school nurse requesting that he be allowed to use a more private bathroom close to the nurse's office was sufficient to allay his discomfort about going to school.

In other cases where school anxiety, perfectionism about grades, or peer difficulties are revealed, interventions are targeted towards these psychological barriers (e.g., anxiety management or social skills training), in addition to basic pain management skills training. There is little research at this time into the effectiveness of behavioral approaches to school consultation and intervention, but from a clinical perspective, it still forms an essential component of treatment for children with chronic pain.

6. Psychiatric Consultation

As in other chronic medical conditions, psychiatric comorbidity can become a complicating factor in the treatment of chronic pediatric pain if it is not properly addressed. Psychiatric conditions, especially mood and anxiety disorders, are known to have increased prevalence in chronic pain populations [17] and, not surprisingly, are also prevalent in the pediatric age range. Some of the more serious psychiatric conditions that may be encountered in pediatric pain management clinic settings are depression (including suicidal ideation and/or self-injurious behavior), bipolar disorder, panic disorder, substance use, and posttraumatic stress disorder. These psychiatric symptoms may be accompanied by significant behavioral and adherence issues that may interfere with the patient's successful engagement in the multidisciplinary program. Often, pain symptoms are the purported reason for seeking medical care, while psychiatric issues may remain unaddressed, possibly due to the perceived stigma of seeking mental health care. In these cases appropriate consultation with a psychiatrist for medication issues, along with collaborative work with other mental health providers trained in the treatment of severe psychiatric problems, can be of enormous benefit to the patient, and crucial to the success of the pain management treatment.

Take-Home Points

- Behavioral interventions are an essential component in the multidisciplinary management of pediatric chronic pain, and research evidence supports the efficacy of behavioral treatments such as biofeedback and cognitive-behavioral treatment.
- Interventions can range from straightforward approaches, such as biofeedback-assisted relaxation training, to relatively complex psychosocial approaches, including family and school interventions.
- Pediatric primary care providers are in the unique position of having an array of information about the patient's medical, developmental, and psychosocial history. As such, they can play an important role in the early identification, management and referral of pediatric chronic pain patients for specialized behavioral services when indicated.

References

1. Eccleston C, Yorke L, Morley S, Williams AC de, Mastroyannopoulou K. Psychological therapies for the management of chronic and recurrent pain in children and adolescents. The Cochrane Database of Systematic Reviews 2004;1:CD003968.
2. Kashikar-Zuck S, Swain NF, Jones BA, Graham TB. Efficacy of cognitive-behavioral intervention for juvenile primary fibromyalgia syndrome. J Rheumatol 2005;32:1594–1602.
3. Robins PM, Smith SM, Glutting JJ, Bishop CT. A randomized controlled trial of a cognitive-behavioral family intervention for pediatric recurrent abdominal pain. J Pediatr Psychol 2005;30:397–408.
4. Hermann C, Blanchard EB. Biofeedback in the treatment of headache and other childhood pain. Appl Psychophysiol Biofeedback 2002;27:143–162.
5. Gatchel R, Robinson RC, Pulliam C, Maddrey AM. Biofeedback with pain patients: evidence for its effectiveness. Sem Pain Mgmt 2003;1:55–66.
6. Allen KD. Using biofeedback to make childhood headaches less of a pain. Pediatr Ann 2004;33:241–245.
7. Gerik SM. Pain management in children: developmental considerations and mind-body therapies. South Med J 2005;98:295–302.
8. Powers SW, Spirito A. Relaxation training. In: Noshpitz JD, editor. Handbook of Child and Adolescent Psychiatry, vol 6. Basic Science and Treatment. New York: Wiley, 1998:411–422.
9. Kashikar-Zuck S, Goldschneider KR, Powers SW, Vaught MH, Hershey AD. Depression and functional disability in chronic pediatric pain. Clin J Pain 2001;17:341–349.
10. Eccleston C, Malleson PN, Clinch J, Connell H, Sourbut C. Chronic pain in adolescents: Evaluation of a programme of interdisciplinary cognitive behaviour therapy. Arch Dis Child 2003;88:881–885.
11. Peterson CC, Palermo TM. Parental reinforcement of recurrent pain: the moderating impact of child depression and anxiety on functional disability. J Pediatr Psychol 2004;29:331–341.
12. Walker LS, Zeman JL. Parental response to child illness behavior. J Pediatr Psychol 1992;17:49–71.
13. Allen KD, Shriver MD. Role of parent-mediated pain behavior management strategies in biofeedback treatment of childhood migraines. Behavior Therapy 1998;29:477–490.

14. Groholt EK, Stigum H, Nordhagen R, Kohler L. Recurrent pain in children, socio-economic factors and accumulation in families. Eur J Epidemiol 2003;18:965–975.

15. Kovacs FM, Gestoso M, Gil del Real MT, Lopez J, Mufraggi N, Mendez JI. Risk factors for non-specific low back pain in schoolchildren and their parents: a population based study. Pain 2003;103:259–268.

16. Lynch AM, Kashikar-Zuck S, Goldschneider KR, Jones BA. Psychosocial risks for disability in children with chronic back pain. J Pain 2006;7: 244–251.

17. McWilliams LA, Cox BJ, Enns MW. Mood and anxiety disorders associated with chronic pain: An examination in a nationally representative sample. Pain 2003;106:127–133.

16
Complementary and Alternative Approaches for Chronic Pain

Subhadra Evans and Lonnie K. Zeltzer

Abstract: Chronic pain in children and adolescents can be difficult to treat. Many parents and children are turning to complementary and alternative medicine (CAM) to gain relief for conditions as varied as migraines, juvenile arthritis, sickle cell disease, and functional abdominal pain (FAP). This chapter highlights some of the more well-known, safe, and efficacious CAM treatments for children and adolescents, including acupuncture, hypnotherapy, biofeedback, yoga, massage, and meditation. A review of the literature is presented, as well as guidelines for parents and clinicians who are interested in pursuing CAM for pain relief in young people.

Key words: Chronic pain, complementary and alternative medicine, children and adolescents.

Introduction

Complementary and alternative medicine (CAM) has been used successfully to treat a variety of chronic pain conditions in adults and children. By the time pain has reached the point of being classified as chronic, treatment becomes challenging. Although traditional pain management approaches, including the use of drugs and physical therapy, typically meet with some success, the high prevalence of chronic pain regardless of these treatments has led many parents and clinicians to a wider search for pain relief. Estimates of CAM use range from 2 percent in a healthy sample of children [1], to as high as 73 percent in children with cancer [2], with figures pointing to substantial increases across pediatric populations. CAM use often goes unreported to physicians; as many as half of all adults using CAM do so without consulting a practitioner [3] and the figure may be even higher for children [4]. This is despite the desire of many parents to discuss their child's use of CAM with the family pediatrician [5]. Given the popularity of CAM treatments and their often hidden use, those clinicians armed with a more complete understanding of CAM therapies are better served in managing pediatric chronic pain and gaining the trust of patients open to such therapies. In this chapter, we provide a summary of efficacious and safe CAM therapies that can be used for chronic pain in children and adolescents.

It is worth noting that various CAM terms have been used inconsistently in the medical literature. For example, the terms "complementary," "alternative," "holistic," and "integrative" have all been used interchangeably. In addition, the boundary between complementary and alternative medicine and conventional medicine has become blurred. Therapies once considered unconventional in Western medicine are increasingly accepted as scientific evidence mounts in their favor as effective, safe treatments. In order to address these disparities, a working definition of CAM has been devised by the National Center for Complementary and Alternative Medicine at the National Institutes of Health. Here, *complementary* therapies are those techniques used in conjunction with conventional medicine, while *alternative* medicines are those used instead of conventional medicine. Complementary and alternative medicine

G.A. Walco and K.R. Goldschneider (eds.), *Pain in Children: A Practical Guide for Primary Care.*
© Humana Press, a part of Springer Science + Business Media, 2008

can further be identified as those interventions not usually provided by United States hospitals and clinics, and which are typically not taught in medical schools [3].

The National Center for Complementary and Alternative Medicine groups complementary and alternative medicine therapies into five categories: biologically based therapies, manipulative and body-based therapies, energy therapies, mind–body interventions, and alternative medical systems. Biologically based therapies include herbal remedies that employ plant preparations for therapeutic effects, as well as vitamins and other dietary supplements. Manipulative and body-based methods include, for example, chiropractics, osteopathic manipulations, and massage. Energy therapies include reiki and the unconventional use of electromagnetic fields, such as pulsed fields, alternating current or direct current fields. Mind–body interventions relate to a variety of techniques that aim to increase the mind's capacity to enhance bodily function and reduce symptoms, such as mental healing, expressive therapies such as music, art or dance therapy, and spiritual practices such as meditation and prayer. The medical uses of hypnosis and relaxation are also included here. Alternative medical systems are built upon complete systems of theory and practice and may make use of therapies from the biological, body-based, mind–body, and energy modalities. Examples are homeopathic medicine, naturopathic medicine, and traditional Chinese medicine, which includes acupuncture. Although CAM clearly encompasses a variety of techniques from various schools of thought, this chapter will focus on those techniques that have been found to successfully alleviate pediatric chronic pain symptoms.

The use of CAM therapies as outlined above fits with a biopsychosocial definition, which sees pain—particularly chronic pain—as resulting from a complex interplay of central nervous system functioning. Psychological factors include motivation, past experience of pain, anxiety and depression, and the social environment, including social support. On the whole, CAM interventions attempt to restore balance and harmony in the mind and body, not unlike the goal of Western medicine: to restore homeostasis or balance to the bodily functions. Under a biopsychosocial definition, the integration of CAM with more traditional psychological and pharmacological therapies may be the most effective way of dealing with chronic pain in children. Indeed, the National Institutes of Health are increasingly recognizing the potential of CAM interventions by funding a number of large-scale randomized clinical trials assessing the benefits of humor, massage, and energy therapies. Although much of the CAM literature is based on adults, or includes pain that is not typically classified as chronic, such as acute pain (e.g., burn pain) or procedural pain (such as immunizations or post-surgical pain), there is nevertheless sufficient evidence to recognize the value of CAM in treating child and adolescent chronic pain.

1. CAM Treatments for Children and Adolescents

A review of randomized clinical trials using CAM reported that therapies as diverse as aromatherapy, reflexology, hypnotherapy, yoga, and massage are effective in reducing headache, migraine and back pain in adults [6]. The research for children is much more scant and typically limited in design and participant numbers. The treatments reviewed below and presented in Table 16-1 are based on empirical and clinical tests of efficacy as previously reported [7, 8]. The list is by no means exhaustive and, in coming years, we are likely to see further CAM therapies emerging as scientifically supported pain treatments for children.

1.1. Acupuncture

Many CAM practitioners believe an energy force flows through the body which, if blocked, causes imbalance and sickness. Different traditions call this energy "Qi" (pronounced "chi"), "prana," and "life force." Acupuncture is intended to restore natural energy (Qi) through the insertion of needles into points along energy pathways (meridians) in the body. The needles help stimulate the energy flow. Usually, needles are inserted into the skin from one-fourth to one inch deep. The patient often reports light cramping, heaviness, distention, tingling or electric sensation either around the needle or traveling up or down the energy pathway.

TABLE 16-1. CAM interventions for chronic pain.

CAM modality	Description	Where to go for more information*
Acupuncture	Involves insertion of fine sterile needles just under the skin at specific sites of the body—also known as energy pathways—to relieve pain	American Academy of Medical Acupuncture: *www.medicalacupuncture.org* The medical board web page for your state should have a list of licensed acupuncturists
Hypnotherapy	Altered state of consciousness that induces the modification or enhancement of perceptions/ sensations often leading to a feeling of relaxation	Society for Clinical and Experimental Hypnosis (SCEH): *http://www.sceh.us/*
Biofeedback	Electronic feedback of physiological functioning including heart rate, blood pressure, and muscle tension to allow awareness and control over stress and pain	Contact your state biofeedback society and ask for practitioners with certification and specialization in pediatric pain
Therapeutic Yoga	Physical poses intended to correct health-related problems, both in body structure and in internal organ function	The Iyengar Yoga National Association Web page at *www.iynaus.org* Local yoga studios may also be able to provide information about certified yoga teachers on staff
Massage	Manipulation of the body by combining tactile and kinesthetic stimulation often through kneading and stroking of the body's soft tissues	American Massage Therapy Association website: *http://www.amtamassage.org*
Meditation	The discipline of self-regulation of attention by focusing on the present moment regardless of distractions	Mindfulness Awareness Research Centre at UCLA: *http://www.marc.ucla.edu/* For commentary, podcasts and descriptions of practices and references to recent research: *www.innerkids.org and www.ikwiki.org*
Music Therapy	Use of music activities to produce relaxation and desired changes in emotions, behavior, and physiology	Website for the non-profit Children's Music Fund for hospitalized children: *www.ChildrensMusicFund.org* Website for the certification board of music therapists: *http://www.cbmt.org*
Art Therapy	The process of understanding the internal world of the child through exploration of artwork	American Art Therapy Association website: *http://www.arttherapy.org*
Laughter and Humor	The therapeutic process of the use of positive emotions associated with laughter	For the latest findings from laughter and humor research: *www.RXLaughter.org*

*The following resources provide additional information for pediatricians, patients and families considering using CAM for child pain:
Zeltzer, L.K, & Schlank, C.B. (2005). Conquering your child's chronic pain. New York: Harper Collins [ref. 7].
Website for the National Children's Pain Center (NCPC): *http://www.pediatricpain.org*.

Although the precise analgesic mechanisms have not been identified, it is likely that the body's nervous system, neurotransmitters and endogenous substances are involved in needle stimulation [9].

In adults, acupuncture is one of the most popular CAM modalities, effectively treating a variety of chronic pain problems. The lack of research with children is perhaps due to perceptions that children are afraid of needles; therefore, researchers and physicians may be averse to recommending acupuncture. Although preliminary research indicates that adolescents find the experience acceptable [10], it is unknown whether younger children are as accepting. Nevertheless, existing research suggests that acupuncture is an effective treatment for a variety of chronic pain conditions.

Pediatric migraines have been examined in two studies: Pintov and colleagues [11] found that acupuncture resulted in child self-reported pain reduction and an increase in panopioid activity and β-endorphin levels as measured in children's blood samples, while Kemper and colleagues found parent and child reported reduced pain for migraine, endometriosis, and reflex sympathetic dystrophy [10]. Headaches, abdominal pain, fibromyalgia, and complex regional pain syndrome type I have also been reported to benefit from acupuncture [12]. This study included acupuncture and hypnotherapy together, supporting the efficacy of multimodal CAM interventions. Of interest is the evaluation of the effects of acupuncture for chronic pain relief in children when pain is diagnosed and treated through more traditional Chinese medicine [13]. Acupuncture practitioners are licensed and regulated health care professionals in about half the states in the United States. In states that do not currently require licensing, patients should ask their practitioner if he/she is certified by the National Commission for the Certification of Acupuncturists.

1.2. Hypnotherapy

Hypnotherapy used for chronic pain is based upon a mind–body approach to healing. Children with chronic pain often require a calming of the nervous system. The use of hypnotherapy and guided imagery influences this process and is thought to influence the immune system and release stress and pain in the child. During hypnosis, modification or enhancement of sensation and perception often occurs, and children are especially susceptible to these effects. Recent neuroimaging-based research shows that hypnosis is associated with activation of brain areas consistent with decreased arousal, visual imagery, and the likely reinterpretation of perceptual experiences [14].

A number of studies have reported the use of hypnosis (sometimes referred to as hypnotherapy, guided imagery, imagery) to effectively deal with pain in children (see Chapter 15). Although many of these examine procedural pain often in oncology patients or for postoperative pain, a review of 11 studies testing the use of hypnosis for pediatric headaches indicated relaxation/self-hypnosis to be a well-established and efficacious treatment [15]. Moreover, the gains were reported to maintain over time.

1.3. Biofeedback

Biofeedback uses a computer or other feedback device to assist children in managing symptoms by becoming aware of and learning to voluntarily control physiological changes associated with the stress response. These monitored changes may include muscle tension, skin temperature, sweat gland response, brain wave activity, or breathing rate, with the goal of increasing relaxation in the body. Using biofeedback for chronic pain management teaches children to be aware of how their body reacts to experiences and to gain physiologic control of the branch of the nervous system that is activated by pain or stress—essentially breaking the stress–pain cycle. Biofeedback is especially popular for the treatment of migraines and headaches in children. Although gains using biofeedback are less consistent for children than adults, a number of studies have nevertheless reported at least a 50 percent reduction in children's symptoms of headache and migraine pain [8].

There is no license for biofeedback. Most practitioners have other licenses such as R.N. (Registered Nurse), M.F.T (Marriage and Family Therapist), or are physical therapists or psychologists (please see Chapter 14). There is, however, biofeedback certification. Most states have their own certification process and there is national certification as well. To find a biofeedback therapist, contact your state biofeedback society and ask for certified practitioners that specialize in pediatric pain.

1.4. Therapeutic Yoga

Many forms of yoga exist. In therapeutic yoga, the yoga series is matched to the health care needs of the child and changes as the child progresses. The yoga poses are intended to correct health-related problems, both in body structure and in internal organ function, and to develop a sense of mastery. The poses allow children to look at the underlying causes and habits that may contribute to their pain problems and learn how to change them.

A number of positive effects have been reported for yoga. Children's practice of Iyengar yoga, in particular, appears to be beneficial, improving mood and function and reducing stress hormones [16]. One randomized trial also demonstrated that regular home practice of yoga assisted with pain and disability related to irritable bowel syndrome in adolescents [17].

It is best for children to learn yoga, at least initially, with a qualified teacher. Iyengar yoga teachers must have a minimum of 5 years of training before they are certified. It is important that a yoga exercise program is developed by someone who knows human physiology and can tailor the yoga program to the needs of the child with chronic pain. For this reason, private lessons rather than group classes may be most beneficial until the child is familiar with the poses.

1.5. Massage

Massage therapy is one of the oldest methods of health care in practice and continues to be a highly popular CAM treatment. A massage therapist primarily uses his or her hands to manipulate muscles and tissues. Massage therapy is based on the belief that when muscles are overworked, waste products can accumulate in the muscle, causing soreness and stiffness. The therapy aims to improve circulation in the muscle, increasing flow of nutrients and eliminating waste products. Although the underlying mechanisms are unknown, it is likely that massage involves increased parasympathetic activity and a relaxed physiologic state [18].

Again, studies assessing the efficacy of this CAM technique for treating chronic pain in children are few. However, one study examining children with juvenile rheumatoid arthritis compared the effects of a daily 15-minute massage by their parents to a daily 15-minute relaxation session. The massage group experienced less parent and child reported pain, as well as less physician reported pain and morning stiffness (the physician was blind to group assignment). In another study examining children with lymphoblastic leukemia, daily massages for one month resulted in decreased negative affect and increased white blood cell count [19].

1.6. Meditation

Mindfulness meditation involves the conscious monitoring of one's attention and focuses the individual to be "present" and "in the moment." Although many forms of meditation exist, mindfulness mediation involves a concentrated focus on the breath with the goal of stabilizing the mind and promoting calmness. It is likely that mindfulness meditation minimizes pain through the individual's acceptance of pain and a reduction in stress. Mindfulness meditation has been found to decrease pain symptoms in adults living with a wide variety of chronic pain conditions [20]. Meditation also benefits blood pressure and heart rate in adolescents [21]. At the present time there are no empirical studies documenting the use of meditation for children with chronic pain, although case studies suggest that mindfulness mediation is effective in dealing with nausea and epigastric pain in children.

Depending on the developmental teaching style used, mindfulness meditation can be taught to children of all ages. It is likely that meditation practiced by parents and children together is most useful. Parenting a child in pain can be exceedingly difficult, and meditation can provide parents with the resources and patience to deal with their child's pain. When parents are able to reduce their stress levels, children often learn from this strength and cope better with their own stress.

1.7. Other CAM Treatments

A variety of other CAM modalities are likely to benefit children with chronic pain, although empirical research examining their efficacy is wanting. A review of randomized trials of energy therapy and reiki—a system of non-touch (or light touch) healing treatments believed to work on blocks or depletions within the patient's body leading to pain—found "distant healing" to be effective for a variety of chronic illnesses in adults [22]. It is likely that these benefits extend to children [23]. Laughter or humor therapy and the creative arts also hold potential for reducing chronic pain in children. Laughter and humor have been linked to pain control in adults and children [24] and likely have a positive effect on immune function. Art, music, and dance therapy may also be beneficial. Laughter, as well as the creative arts, appears to be effective in reducing pain through distraction, which helps the child to habituate quickly to pain.

Herbal medicine represents another CAM modality worth considering. Although research indicates the potential of certain herbs for certain conditions, such as naturopathic herbal extracts for ear pain related to acute otitis media in children [25], unstudied substances should be treated with caution. Herbal medicines such as megavitamins, herbs, and other botanicals are potent substances and could impact a child's developing organs; they may also interfere with the metabolism of prescribed medications or interact with these drugs to create a toxic effect. Parents should be encouraged to discuss the use of such treatments with their primary physician.

Many CAM treatments are relatively acceptable to parents and children; difficult pain conditions such as fibromyalgia and a lengthy pain experience increase the parents' and children's willingness to try CAM [26]. Although parents and children dealing with chronic pain may find the idea of CAM acceptable, expectations of the benefits of CAM interventions—apart from relaxation—may be relatively low [27]. It is worth noting that treatment expectations for CAM are often no lower than expectations for conventional medicine to treat pediatric chronic pain.

2. Guidelines for Clinicians and Parents

In treating pediatric pain we must rely on many treatments that have not been studied in children, otherwise we would have very little to offer families. This does not mean that such therapies are not safe and effective—many are—but caution

must be exercised when finding a qualified CAM therapist who is experienced in treating children. A CAM therapist must relate well to children and be able to communicate with parents about treatment specifics and goals. The following are some pointers for clinicians and families that may assist with selecting bona fide CAM therapies and practitioners:

- What is the therapist's training/certification/license?
- How long has the therapist been practicing?
- Has the therapist worked with children before? If so, for what conditions?
- What are the expected benefits of the therapy?
- How long before the child can expect to see benefits and how often does the child need to attend before benefits can be seen, on average?
- What are the risks and side effects, if any?
- Will the therapy interfere with conventional treatment?
- Will the therapy be covered by insurance?
- Is the therapist willing to review plans and treatment with the physician?

Ideally, the relationship between the child, parents, and the physicians and therapists treating the child should be based on mutual respect and trust with a sense that everyone is working together to relieve the child's pain. It is preferable if everyone involved understands the strengths and limitations of both conventional medicine and CAM, and recognizes that both methods combine to more completely treat the mind and body aspects of chronic pain.

Take-Home Points

- CAM use is common and growing in popularity.
- Disclosure of CAM use to physicians is limited, so direct questioning on this topic during history taking is important.
- CAM definitions are provided by The National Center for Complementary and Alternative Medicine at the National Institutes of Health.
- Many parents and children with chronic pain are amenable to trying CAM.
- Successful mind-based CAM treatments for children with chronic pain include hypnotherapy, meditation, and biofeedback.

- Successful body-based CAM treatments include yoga, massage, and acupuncture.
- Evidence from other populations indicates the benefits of energy healing, laughter or humor therapy, and the creative arts.
- Further randomized clinical studies of CAM interventions involving children with chronic pain are needed.
- Greatest benefits are seen when families, pediatricians, and CAM therapists work together to relieve the child's chronic pain.

Acknowledgement. Research by the authors is supported in part by R01 MH63779 awarded by the National Institute of Mental Health (PI: Margaret Jacob).

Recommended Reading

Zeltzer LK, Schlank CB. Conquering Your Child's Chronic Pain. New York: Harper Collins, 2005
Website for the National Children's Pain Center (NCPC): *http://www.pediatricpain.org*

References

1. Davis MP, Darden PM. Use of complementary and alternative medicine by children in the United States. Arch Pediatr Adolesc Med 2003;157:393–396.
2. Neuhouser ML, Patterson RE, Schwartz SM, Hedderson MM, Bowen DJ, Standish LJ: Use of alternative medicine by children with cancer in Washington state. Prev Med 2001;33:347–354.
3. Eisenberg DM, Kessler RC, Foster C, Norlock FE, Calkins DR, Delbanco TL: Unconventional medicine in the United States. Prevalence, costs, and patterns of use. N Engl J Med 1993;328:246–252.
4. Spigelblatt L, Laine-Ammara G, Pless IB, Guyver A. The use of alternative medicine by children. Pediatrics 1994; 94:811–814.
5. Sibinga EM, Ottolini MC, Duggan AK, Wilson MH. Parent-pediatrician communication about complementary and alternative medicine use for children. Clin Pediatr 2004;43:367–373.
6. Long L, Huntley A, Ernst E. Which complementary and alternative therapies benefit which conditions? A survey of the opinions of 223 professional organizations. Complement Ther Med 2001;9: 178–185.
7. Zeltzer LK, Schlank CB. Conquering Your Child's Chronic Pain. New York: Harper Collins, 2005.
8. Tsao JC, Zeltzer LK. Complementary and alternative medicine approaches for pediatric pain: a review of the state-of-the-science. Evid Based Complement Alternat Med 2005;2:149–159.
9. Ma SX. Neurobiology of acupuncture: Toward CAM. Evid Based Complement Alternat Med 2004;1: 41–47.
10. Kemper KJ, Sarah R, Silver-Highfield E, Xiarhos E, Barnes L, Berde C. On pins and needles? Pediatric pain patients' experience with acupuncture. Pediatrics 2000;105: 941–947.
11. Pintov S, Lahat E, Alstein M, Vogel Z, Barg J. Acupuncture and the opioid system: implications in management of migraine. Pediatr Neurol 1997;17: 129–133.
12. Zeltzer LK, Tsao JC, Stelling C, Powers M, Levy S, Waterhouse M. A phase I study on the feasibility and acceptability of an acupuncture/hypnosis intervention for chronic pediatric pain. J Pain Symptom Manage 2002;24:437–446.
13. Waterhouse M, Stelling C, Powers M, Levy S, Zeltzer L. Acupuncture and hypnotherapy in the treatment of chronic pain in children. Clinical Acupuncture and Oriental Medicine 2000;1:139–150.
14. Rainville P, Hofbauer RK, Bushnell MC, Duncan GH, Price DD. Hypnosis modulates activity in brain structures involved in the regulation of consciousness. J Cogn Neurosci 2002;14:887–901.
15. Holden EW, Deichmann MM, Levy JD. Empirically supported treatments in pediatric psychology: Recurrent pediatric headache. J Pediatr Psychol 1999;24:91–109.
16. Woolery A, Myers H, Sternlieb B, Zeltzer L. A yoga intervention for young adults with elevated symptoms of depression. Altern Ther Health Med 2004;10: 60–63.
17. Kuttner L, Chambers CT, Hardial J, Israel DM, Jacobson K, Evans K. A randomized trial of yoga for adolescents with irritable bowel syndrome. Pain Res Manag 2006;11:217–223.
18. Ireland M, Olson M. Massage therapy and therapeutic touch in children: state of the science. Altern Ther Health Med 2000;6:54–63.
19. Field T, Cullen, C., Diego, M., Hernandez-Rief, M., Sprinz, P., Kissell, B., Beebe, K. & Bango-Sanchez, V. Leukemia immune changes following massage therapy. Journal of Bodywork and Movement Therapy 2001;5:271–274.
20. Ott MJ. Mindfulness meditation in pediatric clinical practice. Pediatr Nurs 2002; 28:487–490.
21. Barnes VA, Davis HC, Murzynowski JB, Treiber FA. Impact of meditation on resting and ambulatory blood pressure and heart rate in youth. Psychosom Med 2004;66:909–914.

22. Astin JA, Harkness E, Ernst E. The efficacy of "distant healing": a systematic review of randomized trials. Ann Intern Med 2000;132:903–910.

23. Starn JR. Energy healing with women and children. 1998.

24. Pasero CL. Pain control: Is laughter the best medicine? Am J Nurs 1998;98:12–14.

25. Sarrell EM, Cohen HA, Kahan E. Naturopathic treatment for ear pain in children. Pediatrics 2003;111: e574–579.

26. Tsao JCI, Meldrum M, Kim SC, Jacob MC, Zeltzer LK. Treatment preferences for CAM in children with chronic pain. Evid Based Complement Alternat Med 2006;November:1–8.

27. Tsao JC, Meldrum M, Bursch B, Jacob MC, Kim SC, Zeltzer LK. Treatment expectations for CAM interventions in pediatric chronic pain patients and their parents. Evid Based Complement Alternat Med 2005; 2:521–527.

Part IV
Common Recurrent and Chronic Pain Problems in Primary Care

17
Functional Abdominal Pain

Lisa Scharff and Laura E. Simons

Abstract: Functional abdominal pain (FAP) is a frequent complaint seen in the pediatric primary care setting. Current diagnostic criteria for functional gastrointestinal disorders (FGIDs) are defined in the Rome III criteria, which outline a positive symptom profile for diagnosis. In addition, clinicians should be aware of specific "red flag" rule-out symptoms that may suggest organic disease rather than FAP. Although an organic etiology for functional abdominal pain is unclear, substantive research supports the role of "visceral hyperalgesia" and biopsychosocial determinants in the maintenance of FAP. Prognostic factors for this condition suggest that individuals reluctant to adopt a biopsychosocial model of pain are more likely to experience continued symptoms and impairment into adulthood. Assessment of FAP generally involves a thorough history and minimal laboratory tests. For treatment, several promising biobehavioral strategies have received empirical support for successfully addressing FAP symptoms. This chapter will review our current understanding of FAP, how to adequately assess for this condition, and promising treatment strategies for children with living with painful FGIDs.

Key words: Abdominal pain, chronic pain, biopsychosocial, pediatric, functional pain.

Introduction

Functional abdominal pain (FAP) is a frequent complaint in childhood and accounts for 2 to 4 percent of pediatrician visits per year [1]. Depending on background, context, and associated symptoms the complaint of frequent abdominal pain could either signal an important organic disease process or a relatively benign, but persistent pain problem. While this chapter will discuss some of the "red flags" that indicate a need for further workup of abdominal pain, our primary focus will be on guidelines for diagnosis and treatment of FAP in children and adolescents.

1. Definition of FAP

FAP itself is actually a diagnostic category within a broader scope of functional gastrointestinal disorders (FGIDs) and was designed to be a more accurate diagnostic guide than the early concept of "recurrent abdominal pain," (RAP) [2]. RAP was initially defined as at least three episodes of pain, occurring within three months, in the area of the umbilicus, that are severe enough to affect the child's activities. The Rome III criteria for pediatric FGIDs (generated through an international collaboration of gastroenterologists, to which *Gastroenterology* 130, 2006 is devoted) defines a broad pain-related FGIDs category which includes: functional dyspepsia, irritable bowel syndrome, functional abdominal pain syndrome (see Table 17-1), and abdominal migraine [3]. These diagnostic entities supply positive symptom lists that allow health care professionals to identify functional disorders in a manner that avoids the traditional "trash basket" approach of simply ruling out more potentially dangerous disease processes [4]. The Rome III criteria for functional abdominal pain

G.A. Walco and K.R. Goldschneider (eds.), *Pain in Children: A Practical Guide for Primary Care.*
© Humana Press, a part of Springer Science + Business Media, 2008

(FAP) represent several changes from the Rome II criteria set out in 1999 [5]. A major thrust behind the changes is to empower the primary care physician to make the diagnosis and reduce the need for referrals to gastroenterologists. The changes include shortening the duration criteria of abdominal pain from 3 months to 2 months, allowing for episodic or intermittent pain versus requiring continuous pain, allowing for the presence of physiological events below threshold for diagnosing irritable bowel syndrome (IBS), no longer requiring the physician to determine that the pain was not "feigned," and, lastly, eliminating the requirement of some loss of daily function so that motivated children and adaptive parental response are no longer penalized behaviors. For those who experience loss of daily function and/or associated somatic symptoms, this group is now referred to as having Functional Abdominal Pain Syndrome (FAPS; see Table 17-1 to clarify the distinction between functional abdominal pain and functional abdominal pain syndrome). Nonetheless, because these diagnostic categories are relatively new, most of the research that has been conducted with children with FGIDs/FAP reviewed in this chapter has used the older "RAP" definition in recruiting study participants.

TABLE 17-1. Rome III diagnostic criteria for childhood functional abdominal pain.

Functional abdominal pain*

Must include *all* of the following:

1) Episodic or continuous abdominal pain
2) Insufficient criteria for other FGIDs
3) No evidence of an inflammatory, anatomic, metabolic or neoplastic process that explains the patient's symptoms

Functional abdominal pain syndrome*

Must include childhood functional abdominal pain at least 25% of the time and one or more of the following:

1) Some loss of daily functioning
2) Additional somatic symptoms such as headache, limb pain or difficulty sleeping

*Criteria fulfilled at least once per week for at least two months before diagnosis.
Note: For diagnostic criteria for other FGIDs (functional dyspepsia, irritable bowel syndrome, abdominal migraine) see ref. [3].

FAP can be distinguished from other FGIDs according to attributes of the pain, as well as accompanying symptoms. Abdominal migraine, for example, is defined as episodic pain that lasts for one hour or more, with weeks to months between episodes. The pain must interfere with activities and be associated with two of the following: anorexia, nausea, vomiting, headache, photophobia, or pallor. Functional dyspepsia is pain or discomfort centered in the upper abdomen, above the umbilicus, with no associated bowel form or frequency change and no pain relief with defecation.

2. Prevalence

Between 4 and 25 percent of school-age children complain of abdominal pain severe enough to interfere with daily activities [2, 6, 7]. Prevalence varies by age and gender, with an increase in prevalence in ages 4 to 6, and again in early adolescence [8, 9]. FAP also tends to be more common in females, particularly after age 12, and is frequently associated with other types of pain (e.g., headache, back, limb pain), most commonly, headache [10]. There is also a higher prevalence of FAP in living situations with more social stressors [6, 11], indicating a strong psychosocial component. The majority of children with broadly defined "RAP" are likely better classified as having irritable bowel syndrome, and many children with abdominal pain without the hallmark symptom of altered bowel habits may develop this over time.

3. Etiology

Approximately 10 percent of children with FAP are diagnosed with organic pain. Warning signs or "red flags" that need to be investigated are listed in Table 17-2. The most common red flag is simply an atypical description of the pain. Abdominal pain that does not occur around the umbilicus is more likely to have an organic cause. This has been termed "Apley's law."

Common suspects for organic contributions to pain include lactose malabsorption, helicobacter pylori, chronic abdominal wall pain, and slipping rib syndrome. Barr [12] identified a 40 to 50 percent incidence of lactose malabsorption in

TABLE 17-2. Red flags.

Persistent right upper or right lower quadrant pain	Family history of inflammatory bowel disease, celiac disease, or peptic ulcer disease
Unexplained fever	Arthritis
Involuntary weight loss	Perirectal disease
Deceleration of linear growth	Delayed puberty
Gastrointestinal blood loss	Pain awakening the child at night
Significant vomiting	Nocturnal diarrhea
Dysuria	Dysphagia

children with recurrent abdominal pain. When these children were placed on a lactose-free diet, 25 percent of them reported a more than 50 percent reduction in pain [12, 13]. These findings have not been successfully reproduced, however. Other investigators have reported a lower incidence of lactose intolerance in children with RAP and a placebo effect of dietary restriction [14]. In general, lactose intolerance probably accounts for pain in only a small subset of FGID patients, but it should be especially considered in children of susceptible ethnic backgrounds.

Helicobacter pylori is a gram-negative spiral shaped bacteria that is able to colonize the gastric mucosa in humans and cause gastritis. It tends to be prevalent in crowded households in poorer areas of the world. *H. pylori* is not common in the United States, with a rate of incidence of 1 percent per year. There is an association between duodenal ulcers and infection with *H. pylori*, and eradication of the organism prevents recurrence of the ulcer. However, the role of *H. pylori* in causing recurrent abdominal pain in children is also controversial. The weight of evidence suggests that *H. pylori* infection is very unlikely to be the cause of FAP as there is no strong evidence that it causes pain in the absence of peptic ulceration [15]. Therefore, screening for *H. pylori* infection is not recommended for these patients.

Chronic abdominal wall pain is often caused by nerve entrapment and can be distinguished from FAP by a thorough physical examination [16] that identifies tender points on the abdomen. Often the most intense tender points, which can also be associated with allodynia, will be very specific and focused at a site as small as a fingertip. If the pain is unrelated to movement of the spine, associated with a surgical scar, or localized to the abdomen then the abdominal wall is implicated [17]. Treatment with a trigger point anesthetic injection is usually associated with immediate and significant pain relief.

The slipping rib syndrome can be related to referred abdominal pain in some patients, and there are positive signs that can be identified upon physical examination to determine this diagnosis as well. The pain is often focused on one side, although the pain can also be referred throughout the abdomen. Certain types of movement usually aggravate the pain, such as those associated with deep breathing or movement of the upper extremities. Pain caused by slipping rib can be reproduced by the "hooking maneuver," when the examiner hooks his or her fingers under the costal margin and pulls gently both superiorly and anteriorly (this will sublux the loosened rib cartilage) [18]. Intercostal nerve blocks often relieve the pain at least temporarily, and resection of the involved rib and cartilage are associated with complete and lasting pain relief [19].

FAP has often been associated with anxiety and depression [20, 21]; however, the presence of abdominal pain, regardless of etiology, is associated with increased levels of distress [22]. Stressful life events, lowered quality of life, and a lack of coping skills are symptom triggers in both IBS and inflammatory bowel disease (IBD) [23, 24]. It is tempting to conclude that psychological distress or stressful life events are responsible for the development of FAP symptoms, but the evidence does not support this conclusion. On the other hand, adult patients who develop IBS following bacterial colitis have a higher incidence of anxiety than those who do not [25, 26]. Psychological issues do need to be assessed in children with FGIDs, even though it is no longer acceptable to conclude there is a direct causal relationship. Treatment seeking behavior is clearly dependent on the functional status of the child and parental psychological distress. Children with FAP who have psychologically distressed mothers and those that are missing a great deal of school are those that tend to seek treatment for pain [27, 28].

4. Biopsychosocial Model

The biopsychosocial model is the current framework for understanding FAP. Within this model physiologic and psychosocial processes interact and manifest in abdominal pain that is termed the "brain-gut axis" [29]. Thus, psychological stress heightens visceral sensation. DiLorenzo and colleagues found that children with FAP had lower thresholds of visceral perception in the rectum and stomach, compared to control patients, with 45 percent of the FAP group patients having elevated anxiety scores [30]. The biopsychosocial model is not only important for the medical provider's conceptualization and subsequent treatment of FAP, as parents who adopt this framework are more likely to have children whose symptoms resolve over time [31]. Parents need to understand that an underlying physiological process is what "sets the stage" for their child's symptoms, that this is not a disease, and that symptoms can be managed by determining the pain's triggers and teaching the child coping techniques to use when symptoms are triggered.

5. Prognosis

Thirty to 60 percent of children with FAP will experience a remission of pain [32, 33]. Long-term follow-up studies have noted, however, that these children are also more likely to report abdominal pain several years after evaluation in comparison to healthy controls [34]. FAP symptoms are much less likely to remit in children with elevated psychological distress [35] or whose family members have irritable bowel syndrome [36]. Poor outcomes are found in families who are resistant to adopting a biopsychosocial model of illness and refuse to engage with psychological services, characterized by high levels of health care utilization, persistent abdominal pain in the child, and the child's failure to return to normal functioning [31, 37]. There is also evidence that children with FAP are at greater risk for developing psychiatric disorders, particularly anxiety disorders [38, 39].

Importantly, not all patients with abdominal pain will have clinically elevated anxiety or depressive symptoms, but those who do are at the greatest risk for persistent disability. There is sufficient evidence that FAP is a risk factor for the subsequent development of psychological disorders later in life, and so it should not be dismissed as a transient reaction to adverse stress.

6. Assessment of FAP

The essential components of a sound workup for abdominal pain are a complete history and physical exam. In gathering history, ask detailed questions about the pain, including but not exclusive to, pain descriptors, location of pain, patterns of the pain (intermittent versus constant), intensity, associated symptoms, pain triggers, disability secondary to the pain, and current pain management strategies. "Red flags" that should be attended to are outlined in Table 17-2. It is also vital to be attuned to the biopsychosocial framework of abdominal pain. Triggering factors that may interact with a biological predisposition include: family conflict, problems with peers or school, anxiety symptoms, depressive symptoms, and potential sources of secondary gain, such as school or activity avoidance, history of physical or sexual abuse, and other stressful life events. After conducting a thorough physical exam, a limited and reasonable screening includes a complete blood cell count, erythrocyte sedimentation rate or C-reactive protein measurement, urinalysis and urine culture [3]. More extensive tests are often not indicated and do not provide a significant yield unless the physical examination or history suggest a potential organic cause [40].

7. Treatment

A biopsychosocial approach to treatment is essential for children with FGIDs. The pain itself needs to be validated while providing the family with support and reassurance that no organic pathology exists. As parents are often looking for the specific cause of the abdominal pain, take time to discuss the inseparability of physical and psychological triggers of symptoms, and explain the possible mechanism involving the brain–gut interaction. Other options are available, including some evidence that pharmacological, psychological, and dietary treatment in the form of peppermint oil supplements may be useful for these patients.

7.1. Pharmacological Therapy

Many pharmacological interventions have been used clinically to treat FAP, with antidepressants quite possibly being the most popular [41]. A

Cochrane review concluded that there was little evidence to support the use of pharmacology in FAP outside of clinical trials [42]. More recently, Campo and colleagues [43] reported promising outcomes in an open-label trial of citalopram in 25 children with FAP and comorbid anxiety (72 % of sample) and depression (44 % of sample). Twenty-one patients (84%) noted significant improvements in pain, anxiety, depressive symptoms, other somatic symptoms, and functional impairments at the end of a 12-week flexible dose medication trial. This study is the only investigation known to the authors to examine the effectiveness of SSRIs in children with FAP.

Other medication trials have demonstrated positive results in children with FGIDs. See et al. [44] conducted a double-blind placebo-controlled crossover trial of famotidine in 25 children with dyspepsia and concluded that the active medication was associated with significant improvement in the dyspeptic symptoms, but no improvement in pain ratings. Symon and Russel [45] conducted a double-blind crossover placebo-controlled trial of pizotifen syrup in 14 children with abdominal migraine. The medication was associated with decreased pain frequency and severity compared to placebo. Thus, specific medications do show some promise in the treatment of FGIDs. Overall, there is a paucity of empirical support for these methods, compared to the frequency of their use.

7.2. Dietary Management

Clinically, children and parents often associate their FAP symptoms with eating in general and specific foods in particular. As reviewed above, lactose intolerance can be a potential contributor to FAP and is worth investigating in children with a predisposition; however, a positive test result and elimination of lactose from the diet is not necessarily associated with pain relief, as these two presentations appear to be separate entities [46]. Sorbital malabsorption has similarly been cited as a potential cause of chronic abdominal pain [47].

Food diaries are easy and economical to maintain and may be helpful in investigating the relationship between specific foods, mealtimes, and pain. Many families will initiate dietary restrictions on their own. It is not uncommon to find at least a clinical relationship between greasy foods, large meals, and altered bowel habits. If constipation is a part of the clinical presentation, fiber supplements have proven to be an effective treatment [48].

Unfortunately, very little evidence exists to support the role of most dietary treatments in FAP [49]. Despite the clinical associations made between specific foods and FAP, there are few investigations regarding dietary restrictions in FAP patients, and there is often a strong placebo response in controlled studies of dietary change. One exception is some evidence that supports treating IBS with peppermint oil [50]. Seventy-six percent of IBS patients who received peppermint oil supplements for 2 weeks reported decreases in the severity of symptoms, compared with only 19 percent who received placebo. Dosing is one capsule about 20 minutes prior to meals. Peppermint oil can cause gastroesophageal reflux, so should be used cautiously in patients with a history of reflux.

7.3. Psychological Interventions

The majority of research in the treatment of FAP has emphasized cognitive behavioral therapeutic (CBT) interventions that are designed to teach the child coping skills and relaxation strategies, as well as to teach the parents how to reinforce healthy, functional behavior (see Chapter 15). These treatments emphasize a rehabilitative approach wherein the child returns to daily activities and responsibilities (e.g., school) prior to definitive symptomatic relief. Shifting the focus from trying to find a "cure" to finding a way to cope with and overcome a distressing, persistent physical symptom is essential for the child's recovery. Within this framework the child is the active agent of change empowered to overcome a difficult, but manageable problem with a new set of skills and tools on which to rely. Such treatments generally report good results.

Sanders and colleagues [51] conducted a controlled study of CBT treatment in 16 children with recurrent abdominal, and reported that 75 percent of the treated group became pain free, compared to 25 percent of the controls. In a second study Sanders et al. [52] randomized 44 children with RAP into CBT or "reassurance" treatment. Over half the patients receiving CBT reported being pain free at post-treatment, compared to 23.8 percent of controls. Improvement was maintained at a 12-month follow-up. Robins et al. [53] conducted a similar randomized study with 69 children with RAP using CBT and standard medical follow-up groups. Significantly less pain and school absences were found in the CBT group, compared to controls, and improvement was maintained one year later.

Although continued research is necessary, evidence for the use of psychological therapies to treat FAP is mounting [40]. The key elements of the above treatments for painful FGIDs include supplying the children with skills to cope with both the triggers of pain and the pain itself, such as relaxation training and stress management, as well as parent training to help encourage normal, healthy functioning and reduce disability. Other psychology-based treatment elements described in the research literature show promise, but have not been investigated as thoroughly. These include self-hypnosis training [54] and biofeedback [55].

Not all mental health providers are experienced in treating children with chronic pain and it is important to find a practitioner with expertise in both behavioral medicine and pediatrics who has a cognitive-behavioral approach to treatment. Referrals are appropriate in cases where children are missing an excessive amount of school, clearly have anxiety issues, or even cases where stress management training may be useful. In general, with uncomplicated cases, children can be successfully treated in less than 12 sessions.

7.4. Other Treatment Options

Several other treatment options are available for the child with FAP, but little is known about their efficacy. Acupuncture has been increasingly utilized, but a Cochrane review of acupuncture in adults with irritable bowel syndrome [56] was inconclusive. Acupuncture practitioners have emphasized that this type of treatment is a general approach that is not limited to needle insertion and manipulation, and that it is difficult to research the effect of Chinese medicine as a whole. Reflexology massage, also investigated in adult IBS patients, has demonstrated no clear benefit [57]. Mechanical treatment via transcutaneous electrical nerve stimulation is used [58], but has not been researched in a controlled manner.

8. Conclusion

In recent years a great deal of research has been conducted with children who suffer from FAP. Unfortunately, there are only a few well-researched options for treatment. The most progress has been made in the development of diagnostic criteria to establish subtypes of FGIDs that are defined by specific symptoms. Pharmacological research has been inadequate at this point in time and dietary treatments, while having a certain amount of face validity, also remain questionable. Psychological interventions have the most promise for treating persistent cases of FGID; however, families who are "stuck" on medical models and organic etiology for pain may have a difficult time accepting these types of interventions. Making time to explain the biopsychosocial model to families and getting them to buy into this approach for symptom management will likely be the most influential piece to their symptom improvement.

Take-Home Points

- 2 to 4 percent of children present in the primary care setting with functional abdominal pain (FAP).
- FAP is a subset of abdominal pain-related functional gastrointestinal disorders (FGIDs). These include functional dyspepsia, irritable bowel syndrome, abdominal migraine, and functional abdominal pain syndrome.
- FAP is most commonly found in children 4 to 6 years, in adolescence, in female children (particularly adolescents), and is often associated with other types of pain (most commonly headache).
- Approximately only 10 percent of children with abdominal pain have an organic cause that can often be detected by paying attention to the "red flags" (see Table 17-2).
- Stress and psychological distress have a reciprocal relationship with FAP, termed the "brain–gut" axis.
- The biopsychosocial model is the current framework for understanding FAP.
- The two key ingredients for successful assessment of FAP are a complete history and thorough physical exam. Limit medical screening and tests.
- For treatment, reassurance may be enough for some. For others, psychologically based treatment shows the most efficacy. Pharmacologic

treatments, including peppermint oil, antidepressants, and anti-migraine medications have roles, although research data are sparse.

References

1. Starfield B, Hoekelman RA, McCormick M, et al. Who provides health care to children and adolescents in the United States? Pediatrics 1984;74:991–997.
2. Apley J, Naish N. Recurrent abdominal pains: A field study of 1,000 schoolchildren. Arch Dis Child 1958;33:165–170.
3. Rasquin A, Di Lorenzo C, Forbes D, et al. Childhood functional gastrointestinal disorders: child/adolescent. Gastroenterology 2006;130:1527–1537.
4. Subcommittee on Chronic Abdominal Pain. Chronic abdominal pain in children. Pediatrics 2005;115: 212–815.
5. Rasquin-Weber A, Hyman PE, Cucchiara S, et al. Childhood functional gastrointestinal disorders. Gut 1999;45 (Suppl 2):II60–68.
6. Faull C, Nicol AR. Abdominal pain in six-year-olds: an epidemiological study in a new town. J Child Psychol Psychiatry 1986;27(2):251–60.
7. Malaty HM, Abudayyeh S, O'Malley KJ, et al. Development of a multidimensional measure for recurrent abdominal pain in children: Population-based studies in three settings. Pediatrics 2005;115: e210–215.
8. Chitkara DK, Rawat DJ, Talley NJ. The epidemiology of childhood recurrent abdominal pain in Western countries: a systematic review. Am J Gastroenterol 2005;100:1868–1875.
9. Ramchandani PG, Hotopf M, Sandhu B, Stein A. The epidemiology of recurrent abdominal pain from 2 to 6 years of age: Results of a large, population-based study. Pediatrics 2005;116:46–50.
10. Perquin CW, Hazebroek-Kampschreur AA, Hunfeld JA, et al. Pain in children and adolescents: A common experience. Pain 2000;87:51–58.
11. Alfven G. The covariation of common psychosomatic symptoms among children from socio-economically differing residential areas: An epidemiological study. Acta Paediatr 1993;82:484–487.
12. Barr RG, Levine MD, Watkins JB. Recurrent abdominal pain of childhood due to lactose intolerance. N Engl J Med 1979;300:1449–1452.
13. Barr R, Francoeur TE, Westwood M, Walsh S. Recurrent abdominal pain due to lactose intolerance revisited. Amer J Dis Child 1986;140:302.
14. Ceriani R, Zuccato E, Fontana M, et al. Lactose malabsorption and recurrent pain in Italian children. J Pediatr Gastroenterol Nutr 1988;7:852–857.
15. O'Donohoe JM, Sullivan PB, Scott R, Rogers T, Brueton MJ, Barltrop D. Recurrent abdominal pain and Helicobacter pylori in a community-based sample of London children. Acta Paediatr 1996;85: 961–964.
16. Srinivasan R, Greenbaum DS. Chronic abdominal wall pain: A frequently overlooked problem. Am J Gastroenterol 2002;97:824–830.
17. Gallegos NC, Hobsley M. Abdominal wall pain: an alternative diagnosis. Br J Surg 1990;77: 1167–1170.
18. Heinz GJ, Zavala DC. Slipping rib syndrome. J Am Med Assoc 1977;237:794–795.
19. Saltzman DA, Schmitz ML, Smith SD, Wagner CW, Jackson RJ, Harp S. The slipping rib syndrome in children. Pediatr Anesth 2001;11:740–743.
20. Hodges K, Kline JJ, Barbero G, Woodruff C. Anxiety in children with recurrent abdominal pain and their parents. Psychosomatics 1985;26:859–866.
21. Campo JV, Bridge J, Ehmann M, et al. Recurrent abdominal pain, anxiety, and depression in primary care. Pediatrics 2004;113:817–824.
22. Walker LS, Greene JW. Children with recurrent abdominal pain and their parents: more somatic complaints, anxiety, and depression than other patient families? J Pediatr Psychol 1989;14:231–243.
23. Varni JW, Lane MM, Burwinkle TM, et al. Health-related quality of life in pediatric patients with irritable bowel syndrome: a comparative analysis. J Dev Behav Pediatr 2006;27:451–458.
24. Jones MP, Wessinger S, Crowell MD. Coping strategies and interpersonal support in patients with irritable bowel syndrome and inflammatory bowel disease. Clin Gastroenterol Hepatol 2006;4:474–481.
25. Thabane M, Kottachchi DT, Marshall JK. Systematic review and meta-analysis: the incidence and prognosis of post-infectious irritable bowel syndrome. Aliment Pharmacol Thera 2007;26:535–544.
26. Ruigomez A, Garcia Rodriguez LA, Panes J. Risk of irritable bowel syndrome after an episode of bacterial gastroenteritis in general practice: Influence of comorbidities. Clin Gastroenterol Hepatol 2007;5:465–469.
27. Levy RL, Langer SL, Walker LS, Feld LD, Whitehead WE. Relationship between the decision to take a child to the clinic for abdominal pain and maternal psychological distress. Arch Pediatr Adolesc Med 2006;160:961–965.
28. Venepalli NK, Van Tilburg MA, Whitehead WE. Recurrent abdominal pain: what determines medical consulting behavior? Dig Dis Sci 2006;51: 192–201.
29. Drossman DA, Creed FH, Olden KW, Svedlund J, Toner BB, Whitehead WE. Psychosocial aspects of

the functional gastrointestinal disorders. Gut 1999;45 (Suppl 2):II25–30.

30. Di Lorenzo C, Youssef NN, Sigurdsson L, Scharff L, Griffiths J, Wald A. Visceral hyperalgesia in children with functional abdominal pain. J Pediat 2001;139: 838–843.

31. Crushell E, Rowland M, Doherty M, et al. Importance of parental conceptual model of illness in severe recurrent abdominal pain. Pediatrics 2003;112: 1368–1372.

32. Stickler GB, Murphy DB. Recurrent abdominal pain. Am J Dis Child 1979;133:486–489.

33. Bury RG. A study of 111 children with recurrent abdominal pain. Aust Paediatr J 1987;24:117–119.

34. Walker LS, Garber J, Van Slyke DA, Greene JW. Long-term health outcomes in patients with recurrent abdominal pain. Special Issue: Pediatric chronic conditions. J Pediatr Psychol 1995;20:233–245.

35. Mulvaney S, Lambert EW, Garber J, Walker LS. Trajectories of symptoms and impairment for pediatric patients with functional abdominal pain: a 5-year longitudinal study. J Am Acad Child Adol Psych 2006;45:737–744.

36. Pace F, Zuin G, Di Giacomo S, et al. Family history of irritable bowel syndrome is the major determinant of persistent abdominal complaints in young adults with a history of pediatric recurrent abdominal pain. World J Gastroenterol 2006;12: 3874–3877.

37. Lindley KJ, Glaser D, Milla PJ. Consumerism in health care can be detrimental to child health: lessons from children with functional abdominal pain. Arch Dis Child 2005;90:335–337.

38. Campo JV, Di Lorenzo C, Chiappetta L, et al. Adult outcomes of pediatric recurrent abdominal pain: Do they just grow out of it? Pediatrics 2001;108:E1.

39. Hotopf M, Carr S, Mayou R, Wadsworth M, Wessely S. Why do children have chronic abdominal pain, and what happens to them when they grow up? Population based cohort study. BMJ (Clinical research ed) 1998;316: 1196–1200.

40. Chronic abdominal pain in children. Pediatrics 2005;115:e370–381.

41. Olden KW. The use of antidepressants in functional gastrointestinal disorders: new uses for old drugs. CNS Spectr 2005;10:891–896.

42. Huertas-Ceballos A, Macarthur C, Logan S. Pharmacological interventions for recurrent abdominal pain (RAP) in childhood. Cochrane Database Syst Rev 2002:CD003017.

43. Campo JV, Perel J, Lucas A, et al. Citalopram treatment of pediatric recurrent abdominal pain and comorbid internalizing disorders: an exploratory study. J Am Acad Child Adolesc Psychiatry 2004;43:1234–1242.

44. See MC, Birnbaum AH, Schechter CB, Goldenberg MM, Benkov KJ. Double-blind, placebo-controlled trial of famotidine in children with abdominal pain and dyspepsia: global and quantitative assessment. Dig Dis Sci 2001;46:985–992.

45. Symon DN, Russell G. Double blind placebo controlled trial of pizotifen syrup in the treatment of abdominal migraine. Arch Dis Child 1995;72:48–50.

46. Lebenthal E, Rossi TM, Nord KS, Branski D. Recurrent abdominal pain and lactose absorption in children. Pediatrics 1981;67:828–832.

47. Hyams JS. Sorbitol intolerance: an unappreciated cause of functional gastrointestinal complaints. Gastroenterology 1983;84:30–33.

48. Feldman W, McGrath P, Hodgson C, Ritter H, Shipman RT. The use of dietary fiber in the management of simple, childhood, idiopathic, recurrent, abdominal pain. Results in a prospective, double-blind, randomized, controlled trial. Am J Dis Child 1985;139:1216–1218.

49. Huertas-Ceballos A, Macarthur C, Logan S. Dietary interventions for recurrent abdominal pain (RAP) in childhood. Cochrane Database Syst Rev 2002: CD003019.

50. Kline RM, Kline JJ, Di Palma J, Barbero GJ. Enteric-coated, pH-dependent peppermint oil capsules for the treatment of irritable bowel syndrome in children. J Pediat 2001;138:125–128.

51. Sanders MR, Rebgetz M, Morrison M, Bor W, et al. Cognitive-behavioral treatment of recurrent nonspecific abdominal pain in children: An analysis of generalization, maintenance, and side effects. J Consult Clin Psychol 1989;57:294–300.

52. Sanders MR, Shepherd RW, Cleghorn G, Woolford H. The treatment of recurrent abdominal pain in children: a controlled comparison of cognitive-behavioral family intervention and standard pediatric care. J Consult Clin Psychol 1994;62:306–314.

53. Robins PM, Smith SM, Glutting JJ, Bishop CT. A randomized controlled trial of a cognitive-behavioral family intervention for pediatric recurrent abdominal pain. J Pediatr Psychol 2005;30:397–408. Epub 2005 Feb 23.

54. Anbar RD. Self-hypnosis for the treatment of functional abdominal pain in childhood. Clin Pediatr 2001;40:447–451.

55. Humphreys PA, Gevirtz RN. Treatment of recurrent abdominal pain: components analysis of four treatment protocols. J Pediatr Gastroenterol Nutr 2000;31:47–51.

56. Lim B, Manheimer E, Lao L, et al. Acupuncture for treatment of irritable bowel syndrome. Cochrane Database Syst Rev 2006;18:CD005111.

57. Tovey P. A single-blind trial of reflexology for irritable bowel syndrome. Br J Gen Pract 2002;52:19–23.

58. Sylvester K, Kendall GP, Lennard-Jones JE. Treatment of functional abdominal pain by transcutaneous electrical nerve stimulation. Br Med J (Clin Res Ed) 1986;293:481–482.

18
Headaches

Navil F. Sethna and Alyssa A. Lebel

Abstract: Recurrent headaches are important clinical problems in school-aged children that may cause significant suffering and functional disability, especially regarding school attendance and physical activity. Applying early, aggressive, individualized pharmacological and nonpharmacological therapies for recurrent and chronic daily headaches is crucial to diminish discomfort, improve quality of life, and limit persistence of symptoms into adulthood. The objective of this chapter is to summarize the revised diagnostic criteria of childhood headaches and evidence-based treatment guidelines.

Key words: International Classification of Headache Disorders, children, adolescents, migraine, chronic daily headache, disability, multidisciplinary treatment.

Introduction

Recurrent headaches, particularly migraines and tension-type headaches, are frequently present in otherwise healthy children and adolescents in primary care. In a recent survey of 622 school children, headache is the most prevalent (60%) pain complaint present from more than three months [1]. Prevalence increases with age and varies with case definition, ranging from 37 to 51 percent in children under 7 years of age, to 57 to 82 percent by 15 years of age. Headaches are also more common in pre-pubertal boys and in peri- and post-pubertal females [2]. Poorly treated headaches may limit school attendance, socialization, sleep, and overall quality of life for young sufferers and their families [3].

Effective management of headaches requires specific assessment of subtypes of patients' headache(s); some patients may experience more than one type of headache. The classification of headache disorders has been recently revised by the International Classification of Headache Disorders (ICHD-2) to include new information about some headache disorders, recognition of new disorders, and modification of criteria for children age 15 years and younger to improve the validity of diagnostic criteria [4]. As per the previous 1988 International Headache Society guidelines, headache disorders are grouped into primary and secondary disorders. The diagnosis of primary headaches is established by consensus-based criteria and requires exclusion of secondary headache due to an underlying cause (Table 18-1). Primary headache is further defined by specific historical features and clinical "pattern recognition." Definition guides effective management and outcome assessment. Routine laboratory studies (CBC, ESR, electrolytes LFT, urine analysis), lumbar puncture, EEG, and neuroimaging studies (e.g., CT, MRI) are of little value in diagnosing primary headaches in children when the clinical history is not associated with risk factors, and if physical and neurologic examinations are normal [2].

G.A. Walco and K.R. Goldschneider (eds.), *Pain in Children: A Practical Guide for Primary Care.*
© Humana Press, a part of Springer Science + Business Media, 2008

TABLE 18-1. Classification of pediatric migraine with and without aura.

Migraine without aura*	Migraine with aura**
A. At least five attacks fulfilling criteria B through D	A. At least two attacks fulfilling criteria B to D
B. Headache attacks lasting 1 to 48 hours	B. Aura consisting of at least one of the following, but no motor weakness:
C. Headache has at least two of the following:	1. Fully reversible visual symptoms including positive features (e.g., flickering lights, spots, or lines) and/or negative features (e.g., loss of vision)
1. Unilateral location	2. Fully reversible sensory symptoms including positive features (e.g., pins and needles) and/or negative features (e.g., numbness)
2. Pulsating quality	3. Fully reversible dysphasic speech disturbance
3. Moderate or severe pain intensity	C. At least two of the following:
4. Aggravation by or causing avoidance of routine physical activity (e.g., walking or climbing stairs)	1. Homonymous visual symptoms and/or unilateral sensory symptoms
D. During headache at least one of the following:	2. At least one aura symptom develops gradually over ≥ 5 and ≤ 60 minutes
1. Nausea, vomiting, or both	D. Headache fulfilling criteria B to D for migraine without aura begins during the aura or follows aura within 60 minutes
2. Photophobia and phonophobia	E. Not attributed to another disorder
E. Not attributed to another disorder	

*Previously known as common migraines
**Previously known as classic migraines
Table adapted from ref. [4].

1. Migraine

1.1. Migraine without Aura

The revised pediatric criteria (Table 18-1) are less restrictive, as a migraine episode may last one to 48 hours in children younger than 15 years, compared to four to 72 hours in patients older than 15 years of age. They also improve specificity, but remain of low sensitivity and present a diagnostic challenge in the primary care setting. The criterion of five or more episodes may delay diagnosis and treatment for months. The presence of unilateral migraine headache has high diagnostic specificity, but bilateral headache is common in children. This criterion is now offset by choice of an alternative feature in subtype C of the definition (Table 18-1). Certain criteria have reasonable specificity, but could be difficult to elicit per history, such as a pulsatile quality of pain or photophobia. Accurate information could be ascertained by using an alternative descriptor that the child could relate to such as "throbbing, vibrating, pounding, beating, or hammering," inferring from the child's behavior (closes an eye or prefers dark room to avoid sensitivity to light), or by eliciting one of the alternative subtype features [5, 6].

1.2. Migraine with Aura

An important change in classifying migraine with aura does not alter the basic definition of typical aura, but organizes this phenomenon into understandable clinical features (Table 18-1). The updated classification describes subcategories of typical aura that may occur with non-migrainous headache, or that may occur independent of headache pain. The diagnostic criteria for hemiplegic migraine, which is characterized by variable duration (up to 24 hours) and degree of motor weakness (hemiparesis), are now distinctly divided into familial hemiplegic migraine, the dominantly inherited type of migraine, and sporadic (no family history of such headaches) hemiplegic migraines. The features of these two types of migraines are distinguished from basilar migraine, which is now termed basilar-type migraine and involves symptoms related to posterior fossa dysfunction (intense dizziness, vertigo, visual disturbances, ataxia, and diplopia). Such features may also be appreciated during hemiplegic migraine, but basilar-type migraine is not associated with motor weakness.

1.3. Complications of Migraine

1. Chronic migraine is considered when migraine headache persists for two weeks per month or longer, and last three months or longer, in the absence of medication overuse (use of anti-migraine drug and/or opioids for 10 days per month or longer, or other analgesics for two weeks per month or longer). The diagnosis of chronic migraine due to analgesic rebound is confirmed when improvement occurs within two months of discontinuing overused medications.

2. Status migrainosus is defined as a severe and disabling migraine episode that persists for 72 hours or longer.

3. Persistent aura without infarct refers to otherwise typical past attacks of migraine with aura that last longer than a week in the absence of infarct on brain imaging.

4. Migrainous infarct is a rare condition that may present with an otherwise typical aura that persists longer than one hour and neuroimaging reveals ischemic infarct. Patients with migraine using tobacco, oral contraceptive agents, or other potential vasoconstrictors are at greatest risk for this complication.

5. Migraine-triggered seizures are uncommon, but may occur during or within an hour of migraine attack.

6. Probable migraine is diagnosed when headache features do not fulfill all criteria of migraine and its subtypes. This type of migraine is common and can be equally severe and debilitating as other types of migraines.

1.4. Other Features Characteristic of Juvenile Migraines

1. Alice in Wonderland syndrome is an unusual form of aura involving visual-spatial distortions of objects appearing smaller (micropsia), larger (macropsia), far away (teleopsia), or distorted (metamorphopsia). It is also reported after viral infections, occipital seizures, and intake of hallucinogenic drugs [7, 8].

2. Acute confusional migraines may present with an acute confusional state that mimics the presentations of hemiplegic and basilar migraines, and may include agitation, disorientation, hemiparesis, blindness, aphasia, paresthesias, or amnesia. The differential diagnosis includes infectious encephalopathies, drug intoxication, cerebrovascular disease, and seizures. It may eventually evolve to typical migraine. This syndrome often affects boys, triggered by head trauma, and is associated with a strong family history of migraine [9, 10].

2. Childhood Periodic Syndromes

Variants of migraine in childhood are now included under the heading of childhood periodic syndromes, and are often precursors of migraine with and without aura.

1. Cyclical vomiting syndrome is a relatively rare disorder which occurs in 2.5 percent of school children [11]. It is characterized by repeated episodes of nausea and vomiting that last for hours to days, separated by symptom-free periods of variable length [12]. Vomiting occurs in the absence of signs of gastrointestinal disease in young children and typically stops spontaneously at puberty, although some adolescents are affected.

2. Abdominal migraine occurs in up to 12 percent of school children [13]. It presents with recurrent episodes of abdominal pain, ranging from dull to severe, and usually in the peri-umbilical area or poorly localized. Abdominal pain is associated with at least two additional features that may include anorexia, nausea, vomiting, and pallor.

3. Benign paroxysmal vertigo of childhood (BPV) is common in toddlers (median age 18 months), but may present between the ages of 1 to 4 years. The suggested prevalence among school children is 2.6 percent [14]. Episode frequency ranges from twice a week to once every few months, declining over time, and resolving in most children by age 10 years, although in a small proportion of children BPV may progress to migraine. Onset of symptoms is sudden and characterized by anxiety and fear of falling due to unsteadiness, with patients often attempting to grasp onto nearby objects to remain immobile. Vertigo may be associated with pallor, sweating, nausea, vomiting, photo- and phonophobia, and nystagmus. BPV

TABLE 18-2. Tension-type headache (TTH).

A. Type
    Infrequent ETTH: At least 10 episodes of < 1 day per month on average (< 12 days per year) and fulfilling B-D.
    Frequent ETTH: At least 10 episodes on 1 to 15 days per month for ≥ 3 months (12 to 180 days per year)
       and fulfilling B-D.
    CTTH: Headache occurring on ≥ 15 days per month for > 3 months (≥ 180 days per year and fulfilling B-D).
B. Duration
    Infrequent TTH: lasting 30 minutes to 7 days
    Frequent TTH: lasting 30 minutes to 7 days
    CTTH: lasting for hours or may be continuous
C. Headache has at least two of the following characteristics:
    1. bilateral location
    2. pressing/tightening (non-pulsating) quality
    3. mild or moderate intensity
    4. not aggravated by routine physical activity such as walking or climbing stairs
D. Both of the following:
    1. no nausea or vomiting (anorexia may occur)
    2. no more than one of photophobia or phonophobia
E. Not attributed to another disorder

Note: ETTH = episodic tension-type headache; CTTH = chronic tension-type headache.
Table adapted from ref. [4].

may be followed by somnolence, but is not associated with loss of consciousness. There is often a strong family history of migraine and motion sickness. The underlying etiology is unknown, neurological examination is normal, and investigation, including EEG, ophthalmologic exam, and otolaryngologic evaluation, is unrevealing [15].

4. Retinal migraine, a very rare condition in children, is characterized by recurrent and brief (< 60 minutes) episodes of unilateral visual disturbance, including scintillations, scotomata, or blindness, which precede, follow, or occur during migraine headache. The cause is unknown; an animal model suggests a local neurogenic inflammatory process [16]. The diagnosis is considered after excluding other causes of unilateral visual loss such as transient ischemic attack, retinal detachment, or optic neuropathy.

3. Tension-Type Headache (TTH)

Tension-type headache is as common a cause of headache in children and adolescents as migraine and has an overall 1-year prevalence of 9.8 percent among school children ages 7 to 15 years. The prevalence rate of both types

of headache increase with age, and at a greater preponderance among teenage females [17]. TTH is classified as episodic (ETTH) or chronic (CTTH), and the diagnostic criteria are outlined in Table 18-2.

Like chronic migraine headache, chronic TTH evolves from episodic TTH in most instances and cannot be diagnosed in patients overusing acute medication unless the headache persists after withdrawal of medication. A diagnosis of probable TTH is considered if one criterion of TTH definition is absent.

The etiology of TTH is unknown, and the earlier hypothesis of persistent muscle contraction causing ischemia is no longer accepted. Current data suggest that the pathophysiology of TTH is similar to migraine, but with less intense pain and sometimes of shorter duration [18]. Many experts believe that TTH and migraine form a continuum within a spectrum of the headache disorders and often are not readily discernible.

4. New Daily Persistent Headache (NDPH)

This type of headache fulfills the criteria of CTTH (Table 18-2), but it is not preceded by episodic headache or medication overuse, occurs daily and

TABLE 18-3. Reasons for referral to secondary and tertiary care specialists.

- Inability to rule out serious disease: brain tumor, congenital anomalies (hydrocephalus, obstructive Arnold-Chiari malformation, vascular anomalies, venous sinus thrombosis), subacute infections (viral, fungal, Lyme), intracranial hypertension and pseudo-tumor cerebri (with and without papilledema), spontaneous or posttraumatic CSF leak
- Inaccessibility to neuroimaging tests
- Patient and family factors: illness behavior, noncompliance with therapy, perceived seriousness of the symptom, severity of symptoms, degree of disability (e.g., school absenteeism, insomnia), patient and family health beliefs, mood disturbance and psychosocial stress
- Inaccessibility to psychological counseling or an interdisciplinary care model of headache clinic

within 3 days of onset, and is clearly recalled by the patients. The previous inclusive diagnosis of chronic daily headache (CDH) that included transformed migraine (TM), NDPH, CTTH and hemicrania continua is incorporated in the ICHD-revised. CDH represents a small proportion (3%) of children presenting to neurology ambulatory practice [19]. It predominantly affects females in mid-teen years and evolves from TM often complicated by medication overuse. The etiology of CDH is unclear and probably results from diverse determinants, including an inherited predisposition, environmental stressors, and psychological factors.

5. Referral to Secondary/Tertiary Care

A minority of children with headaches seen in the primary care setting are referred to specialists such as neurologists, pain medicine physicians, and interdisciplinary headache clinics (see Table 18.3). Fortunately, most childhood headaches are benign, not associated with serious neurological or medical conditions. Most secondary headaches are generally eliminated by a thorough medical and family history, followed by a physical and a complete neurological examination. However, the "red flags" outlined in Table 18-4, should also prompt referral to a pediatric neurologist or emergency department.

6. Management

Generally, management of headaches and, in particular, migraine and tension-type headaches, in children follows the same general principles

TABLE 18-4. Warning signs of possible serious conditions.

- Age < 5 years without a family history of migraine
- Sudden and severe onset of a new headache
- Mental status changes during headache course
- Recent infection or fever
- Pain began during vigorous exercise or head/neck trauma
- Pain radiation to posterior thorax (meningeal involvement)
- History of toxic exposure and/or substance use
- History of cancer or HIV
- Pregnancy

as for adults, including patient education (reassurance of absence of serious organic disease, explanation of the nature of the migraine and tension-type headache disorders, realistic expectation from management approach in the absence of cure, limit reliance on pain medication), life-style modification, pharmacological, and psychological approaches. The selected strategies should be tailored to the individual child's headache severity, frequency and duration, and impact on quality of life.

Before initiating drug therapy for migraine or tension-type headaches, behavioral modification and eliminating triggers is a necessary first step to improve responsiveness of the acute episodes to other therapies; e.g., eliminating certain foods, odors, excessive caffeine (which may affect mood or disturb sleep) alcohol, avoid skipping meals, inadequate or excessive sleep poor hydration, medication overuse (frequent and daily medications intake), and stressors at school, home and interpersonal relationships. While all children and adolescents with migraine and tension-type headaches may benefit from psychological counseling as an adjunct to pharmacological therapy, early intervention is advisable in cases of severe headaches that restrict school attendance, social and play activities, or overly stressed adolescents that are driven to excel at academics and in extracurricular activities, and those with interpersonal difficulties or who have preexisting psychological states that may trigger or aggravate headaches [20, 21].

6.1. Management of Acute Migraine

The goals of management are to control symptoms of acute episodes and prevent further episodes through pharmacological, behavioral, or a combination of approaches. The first line of treatment is simple rest and nonspecific analgesics. The most useful immediate action for the child is to rest in a quiet, dark room, and sleep, which often completely relieves the headache. The initial and most effective medications with the highest proven efficacy are acetaminophen and ibuprofen (Table 18-5) [22, 23].

1. If severe migraine episodes persist despite the above therapy, a combination of medications may be prescribed—Fiorinal® (butalbital, aspirin and caffeine), Fiorecet® (butalbital, acetaminophen and caffeine), and Midrin® (isometheptene, acetaminophen, dichloralphenazone)—that may be effective in some children over the age of 12 years in doses of one to two capsules as an additional rescue therapy. Butalbital is a barbiturate drug that causes sedation, tolerance, and potential withdrawal, and rebound headache can occur upon abrupt discontinuation. Other options include mild opioids (e.g., oxycodone, codeine), but, like barbiturates, may cause psychological dependence and should be used occasionally if the patient is intolerant or unresponsive to various migraine medications. Both combination medications and opioids should be used with the caveat that there is no evidence-based data on their efficacy, and they are not indicated by the FDA for management of headaches in children and adolescents.

2. In the presence of severe vomiting, intravenous or intramuscular ketorolac tromethamine (an NSAID) is an effective rescue drug for many patients with an acute episode of migraine, but there are no controlled data available on its efficacy in children. Antiemetics should be prescribed for nausea and emesis, such as promethazine 0.25 to 0.5 mg/kg/dose (maximum 25 mg) via IV, IM, or orally every 4 to 6 hours as needed in children over the age of 2 years. Prochlorperazine is indicated in children over the age of 2 years, or body weight of 10 kg, taken orally at a dose of 0.4 mg/kg/day divided over 6 or 8 hours as needed. If emesis is severe, it can be administered intramuscularly at doses of 0.1 to 0.15 mg/kg/dose every 6 to 8 hours. Metoclopramide can be given 1 to 2 mg/kg/dose orally or by IV every 2 to 6 hours as needed for intense emesis. All these drugs have the potential for producing extrapyramidal side effects (e.g., acute dystonia) [24]. Ondansetron

TABLE 18-5. Acute treatment analgesics for migraines.

Analgesics	Dosage	Evidence based recommendation
Mild-to-Moderate Migraine		
Ibuprofen (4–16 y)	10 mg/kg	Level A
Acetaminophen (4–16 y)	10–15 mg/kg	Level B
Moderate-to-Severe Migraine		
Sumatriptan nasal spray (6–14 y)	5–20 mg	Level A
Oral triptans		Level U
Sumatriptan (8–16 y)	50, 100 mg	
Rizatriptan (12–17 y)	5 mg	
Zolmitriptan (12–17 y)	2.5, 5 mg	
Subcutaneous sumatriptan (6–16 y)	3 mg, 6 mg or 0.06 mg/kg	Level U

Level A rating denotes established effectiveness; level B rating denotes probably effectiveness; level U rating denotes data inadequate or conflicting.

is also used in doses of 0.15 mg via IV every 4 hours up to 3 doses per day for severe vomiting, or orally 2 to 4 mg every 8 hours as needed.

3. Migraine-specific agents (triptans and dihydroergotamine [DHE]) are indicated for moderate to severe headaches that respond poorly to the above first-line regimen. While these drug categories are not yet FDA-approved for use in children, several controlled blinded and open-label trials in children over the age 12 years have shown safety and efficacy relative to placebo, but there are no comparative efficacy studies among the various triptans (Table 18-6). The goal of triptan therapy is to alleviate the headache within two hours of onset; if unsuccessful the same triptan agent may be repeated [25–31]. A recent systematic review of efficacy of triptan agents found no differences in effectiveness between oral triptans and placebo, and concluded that high quality studies are needed in large sample sizes of children and adolescents to confirm triptan agents' efficacy [32].

Nasal spray (20 mg) or subcutaneous sumatriptan is selected when severe vomiting is present in children over the age of 12 years; adverse effects are more frequent with the subcutaneous route. The most common adverse effect with the nasal spray is taste disturbance, which occured in 25 percent of adolescents receiving sumatriptan. Alternatively, zolmitriptan nasal spray (5 mg) and oral disintegrating tablet (2.5 to 5 mg) or oral-dissolving wafers of rizatriptan (5 to 10 mg) can be used (Table 18-6) [25, 28, 29, 33, 34].

6.2. Management of Chronic Migraines

For children who respond poorly to acute therapy, progress to have frequent and more intense recurrence of headaches, and are unable to carry out normal activities, psychological counseling is recommended to assess comorbidities, such as anxiety and depression, and daily preventive medications are considered. As with the rescue medications stated above, the data on efficacy and safety of various preventive medications in children is even more limited and a host of medications of diverse pharmacological actions are used. The use of these medications is based on data extrapolated from adult clinical experience and is based on the individual patient's response using trial and error to determine efficacy or intolerance; therefore, this requires frequent monitoring (Table 18-7). In general, these medications are recommended for short-term use (weeks to months) and are gradually withdrawn after symptom frequency diminishes, or their use is limited to the school year calendar. These medications should be prescribed in low doses and gradually raised to the lowest effective dose [35].

6.3. Managing Chronic Daily Headaches

Chronic daily headache is most difficult to manage. Most headache specialty clinics advocate using an interdisciplinary care team that cares for the patient rather than using isolated pharmacological interventions to manage primary chronic headache. This approach allows more comprehensive and holistic care to address individual psychosocial factors that usually complicate chronic headache and includes education about the nature of the headache, avoidance of

TABLE 18-6. Acute migraine therapies with triptans

Generic name (trade name)	Dosage	Recommended dose
Sumatriptan (Imitrex®)	25, 50, 100 mg oral tablets	Repeated in 2 hours; maximum 200 mg/day
	5, 20 mg nasal spray	Repeated in 2 hours; maximum 40 mg/day
	4–6 mg subcutaneous injection	Repeated after 1 hour; maximum 12 mg/24 hours
Rizatriptan (Maxalt®)	5, 10 mg oral tablets	Repeat after 2 hours; maximum 30 mg/24 hours
(Maxalt ODT®)	5, 10 mg oral disintegrating tablets	
Zolmitriptan (Zomig®)	2.5, 5 mg oral tablets	Repeat every 2 hours; maximum 10 mg/24 hours
(Zomig ZMT®)	2.5, 5 mg oral disintegrating tablets	
Zolmitriptan nasal spray	5 mg	
Naratriptan (Amerge®)	1, 2.5 mg oral tablets	Repeat every 4 hours; maximum 5 mg/ 24 hours

Note: Trade names are used for example only, and do not imply brand preference.
(It is recommended to limit the analgesics to 2 to 3 times per week to avoid medication overuse).

TABLE 18-7. Preventive agents for childhood migraine.

Medication	Dose options	Available forms	Side effects
Cyproheptadine	0.25–1.5 mg/kg	2 mg/tsp syrup; 4 mg tablets	Sedation, weight gain
BETA BLOCKERS*			
Propranolol	2–4 mg/kg/day	10, 20, 40, 60, or 80 mg tablets 60, 80, 120, or 160 mg long-acting capsules	Hypotension, sleep disorder, decreased stamina, depression
Metoprolol	2–6 mg/kg/day	50 or 100 mg tablets	Hypotension, sleep disorder, decreased stamina, depression
Nadolol	0.5–2.5 mg/kg/day	20, 40, or 80 mg tablets	Hypotension, sleep disorder, decreased stamina, depression
ANTICONVULSANTS			
Topiramate	1–10 mg/kg/day	15 or 25 mg sprinkles 25 or 100 mg tablets	Sedation, paresthesias, weight loss, glaucoma, kidney stones
Divalproex	20–40 mg/kg/day (usually 250 mg twice per day)	250 mg/tsp syrup 125 mg sprinkles 250 or 500 mg tablets	Weight gain, bruising, hair loss, heptotoxicity, ovarian cysts
Gabapentin	10–40 mg/kg/day	250 mg /tsp syrup 600 or 800 mg tablets 100, 300, 400 mg capsules	Fatigue, ataxia, tinnitus
ANTIDEPRESSANTS			
Amitriptyline	10–25 mg every night at bedtime	10, 25, or 50 mg tablets	Sedation
Nortriptyline	10–75 mg every night at bedtime	10, 25, 50 or 75 mg tablets	Weight gain
Fluoxetine	10–40 mg every morning	10 or 20 mg capsules	Insomnia, anxiety, weight gain
NONSTEROIDAL ANTI-INFLAMMATORY AGENTS			
Naproxen sodium	250–500 mg twice per day	220, 250, 375, or 500 mg tablets	Gastric upset
CALCIUM CHANNEL BLOCKERS			
Verapamil	4–10 mg/kg/day given three times per day	40, 80, or 120 mg tablets 120, 180, 240 mg sustained-release tablets	Hypotension, nausea, atrio-ventricular block, weight gain

Reprinted with permission from SLACK Incorporated [35].

medication-overuse, stress management, biofeedback, relaxation, cognitive-behavioral therapy, sleep regulation and regular aerobic exercise.

Only a few prospective randomized-controlled trials (RCT) in children with chronic daily headache are available to guide practitioners on safety and efficacy of the various currently used medications, and their use is extrapolated from adults experience [36, 37].

6.4. Biobehavioral Treatment

Severe headaches can result in considerable pain, distress (e.g., anger, frustration, anxiety), and functional impairment (e.g., missing school

and social activities). Psychological states (e.g., anxiety, depression) may precede or follow the onset of headaches, particularly in children with chronic daily headache [38]. Therefore, addressing the psychological factors is an integral part of effectively managing migraines, tension-type, and chronic daily headaches. Psychological interventions for headaches have shown good evidence of efficacy and include biofeedback, relaxation training, and cognitive-behavioral modification to a more positive lifestyle outlook. For some children, family counseling is essential to coach their children and positively reinforce a child's healthy behavior while discouraging the pain and illness behaviors. In general, children over the age of 7 years are most suitable for these interventions, although preschool-aged children may also benefit from developmentally appropriate adjustment of some of these biobehavioral interventions [21]. A recent meta-analysis of RCTs demonstrated consistent efficacy of psychological treatments in reducing pediatric headache symptoms by 50 percent or greater, based on evidence level 1 that was maintained up to 1 year follow-up. However, the sample size was relatively small to determine the effect of psychological interventions on various types of headache [39]. Prospective RCTs are needed to compare psychological interventions to various pharmacological treatments for long-term efficacy, as well as impact on the quality of life of pediatric patients with headache.

6.5. Dietary Modifications and Supplements

Recommendations to avoid certain food and food additives have been based on patient self-reporting or observational studies. For an instance, reviews found no correlation between vasoactive amines (present in cheese, red wine, and chocolate) and migraine headaches. [40, 41] Although the evidence is conflicting for dietary triggers and usefulness of dietary supplements, individual triggers do exist. The benefit of dietary supplements such as magnesium, riboflavin, a healthy low fat diet that contains omega-3-fatty acids or olive oil are supported by small trials and could be beneficial to some patients [42]. Coenzyme Q10 supplementation may play a role in headache management. Hershey et al. found a large percentage of pediatric migraine patients to be deficient in CoQ10. Treatment with CoQ10 produced a significant reduction in headaches and improvement in quality of life [43].

6.6. Physical Therapy

Physical therapy is indicated particularly for TTHs to correct poor posture, reduce muscular tension by stretching and strengthening, and improve cervical range of movements. Teaching the patient to do home exercises can provide long-standing benefits. Simple means of massage, warm or cold applications, ultrasound therapy and stretching can alleviate tension of the neck and upper shoulder muscles [44].

6.7. Acupressure and Acupuncture

In the United States, acupressure and acupuncture has become increasingly practiced during the past two decades, despite its lack of evidence as an effective pain reliever. The analgesic effect of acupuncture techniques, whether based on Chinese medicine principles, trigger point stimulation, with or without electrical stimulation or pharmacological adjunct offer modest relief at best [45]. Because properly practiced acupuncture is associated with low risk and cost, acupuncture therapy is generally an acceptable adjunct or alternative to a conventional treatment when the latter treatment is ineffectual or equally effective. A recent, adequately powered, multicenter RCT in adults with migraine compared semi-standardized traditional Chinese acupuncture to semi-standardized sham acupuncture and standard prophylactic migraine treatments of beta-blockers, flunarizine, and valproic acid as the first, second, and third choice, respectively [46]. The results showed no difference in treatment outcomes between patients treated with Chinese acupuncture, sham acupuncture, or standard migraine therapies. More rigorous study designs and methodologies are needed to conclusively determine the therapeutic value of acupuncture.

Take-Home Points

- The first step in any treatment strategy primarily involves the development of a therapeutic alliance and rapport with the patient and family.
- Recurrent primary headaches are common in children and are identified largely by history and physical examination. Proper diagnosis of subtypes is the best guide to optimal administration of specific treatments and education of the patient and family about the headache disorder.
- Migraine and TTH are the most common headaches. Prompt, safe, and effective treatment of initial symptoms is the key to successful control of pain and suffering. Failure to treat recurrent headaches effectively may lead to poor quality of life and progression to persistent headaches. Prophylactic agents may reduce pain intensity

and frequency for some patients with chronic headache.

- Individualized lifestyle adjustment interventions are indispensable components, complimenting pharmacological therapies of coordinated management for all types of headaches. These include regular conditioning exercise, dietary trigger avoidance, sleep hygiene, self-management, and psychological counseling to reduce life stresses and manage comorbid affective disorders.

- Clinical evidence supporting the efficacy and safety of acute treatment of migraine in children and adolescents is most striking for ibuprofen, acetaminophen, and nasal spray of sumatriptan and zolmitriptan. Preventive (prophylactic) medications have not been rigorously investigated except for flunarezine (not available in the United States), and their daily use is limited for sufficiently severe or frequent headache episodes that interfere with daily activities.

Recommended Reading

Lewis DW, Winner P: The pharmacological treatment options for pediatric migraine: an evidence-based appraisal. Neurorx: The Journal of The American Society For Experimental Neurotherapeutics 2006; 3: 181–191

Lipton RB, Bigal ME, Steiner TJ, Silberstein SD, Olesen J: Classification of primary headaches. Neurology 2004; 63: 427–435

References

1. Roth-Isigkeit A, Thyen U, Stoven H, Schwarzenberger J, Schmucker P. Pain among children and adolescents: Restrictions in daily living and triggering factors. Pediatrics 2005;115:e152–162.

2. Lewis DW, Ashwal S, Dahl G, et al. Practice parameter: Evaluation of children and adolescents with recurrent headaches: report of the Quality Standards Subcommittee of the American Academy of Neurology and the Practice Committee of the Child Neurology Society. Neurology 2002;59:490–498.

3. Hunfeld JA, Perquin CW, Duivenvoorden HJ, et al. Chronic pain and its impact on quality of life in adolescents and their families. J Pediatr Psychol 2001;26:145–153.

4. The International Classification of Headache Disorders, 2nd ed. Cephalalgia 2004;24 (Suppl 1):9–160.

5. Maytal J, Young M, Shechter A, Lipton RB. Pediatric migraine and the International Headache Society (IHS) criteria. Neurology 1997;48:602–607.

6. Winner P, Hershey AD. Diagnosing migraine in the pediatric population. Current Pain and Headache Reports 2006;10:363–369.

7. Golden GS. The Alice in Wonderland syndrome in juvenile migraine. Pediatrics 1979;63:517–519.

8. Cinbis M, Aysun S. Alice in Wonderland syndrome as an initial manifestation of Epstein-Barr virus infection. Br J Ophthalmol 1992;76:316.

9. Ehyai A, Fenichel GM. The natural history of acute confusional migraine. Arch Neurol 1978;35:368–369.

10. Ferrera PC, Reicho PR. Acute confusional migraine and trauma-triggered migraine. Am J Emerg Med 1996;14:276–278.

11. Lipton RB, Bigal ME, Steiner TJ, Silberstein SD, Olesen J. Classification of primary headaches. Neurology 2004;63:427–435.

12. Fleisher DR, Matar M. The cyclic vomiting syndrome: a report of 71 cases and literature review. J Pediatr Gastroenterol Nutr 1993;17:361–369.

13. Al-Twaijri WA, Shevell MI. Pediatric migraine equivalents: occurrence and clinical features in practice. Pediatr Neurol 2002;26:365–368.

14. Russell G, Abu-Arafeh I. Paroxysmal vertigo in children–an epidemiological study. Int J Pediatr Otorhinolaryngol 1999;49 Suppl 1:S105–107.

15. Drigo P, Carli G, Laverda AM. Benign paroxysmal vertigo of childhood. Brain Dev 2001;23:38–41.

16. May A, Shepheard SL, Knorr M, et al. Retinal plasma extravasation in animals but not in humans: implications for the pathophysiology of migraine. Brain 1998;121 :1231–1237.

17. Laurell K, Larsson B, Eeg-Olofsson O. Prevalence of headache in Swedish school children, with a focus on tension-type headache. Cephalalgia 2004;24:380–388.

18. Gobel H, Weigle L, Kropp P, Soyka D. Pain sensitivity and pain reactivity of pericranial muscles in migraine and tension-type headache. Cephalalgia 1992;12:142–151.

19. Moore AJ, Shevell M. Chronic daily headaches in pediatric neurology practice. J Child Neurol 2004;19: 925–929.

20. Pakalnis A, Gibson J, Colvin A. Comorbidity of psychiatric and behavioral disorders in pediatric migraine. Headache 2005;45:590–596.

21. Powers SW, Andrasik F. Biobehavioral treatment, disability, and psychological effects of pediatric headache. Pediatr Ann 2005;34:461–465.

22. Hamalainen ML, Hoppu K, Valkeila E, Santavuori P. Ibuprofen or acetaminophen for the acute treatment of migraine in children: a double-blind, randomized, placebo-controlled, crossover study. Neurology 1997;48:103–107.

23. Lewis DW, Kellstein D, Dahl G, et al. Children's ibuprofen suspension for the acute treatment of pediatric migraine. Headache 2002;42:780–786.

24. Lewis DW, Diamond S, Scott D, Jones V. Prophylactic treatment of pediatric migraine. Headache 2004;44:230–237.

25. Ahonen K, Hamalainen ML, Rantala H, Hoppu K. Nasal sumatriptan is effective in treatment of migraine attacks in children: A randomized trial. Neurology 2004;62:883–887.

26. Tepper SJ, Cady R, Dodick D, et al. Oral sumatriptan for the acute treatment of probable migraine: first randomized, controlled study. Headache 2006;46:115–124.

27. Visser WH, Winner P, Strohmaier K, et al. Rizatriptan 5 mg for the acute treatment of migraine in adolescents: results from a double-blind, single-attack study and two open-label, multiple-attack studies. Headache 2004;44:891–899.

28. Winner P, Lewis D, Visser WH, Jiang K, Ahrens S, Evans JK. Rizatriptan 5 mg for the acute treatment of migraine in adolescents: A randomized, double-blind, placebo-controlled study. Headache 2002;42:49–55.

29. Winner P, Rothner AD, Wooten JD, Webster C, Ames M. Sumatriptan nasal spray in adolescent migraineurs: a randomized, double-blind, placebo-controlled, acute study. Headache 2006;46:212–222.

30. Elkind AH, Wade A, Ishkanian G. Pharmacokinetics of frovatriptan in adolescent migraineurs. J Clin Pharmacol 2004;44:1158–1165.

31. Hershey AD, Powers SW, LeCates S, Bentti AL. Effectiveness of nasal sumatriptan in 5- to 12-year old children. Headache 2001;41:693–697.

32. Damen L, Bruijn JK, Verhagen AP, Berger MY, Passchier J, Koes BW. Symptomatic treatment of migraine in children: a systematic review of medication trials. Pediatrics 2005;116:e295–302.

33. Linder SL. Subcutaneous sumatriptan in the clinical setting: The first 50 consecutive patients with acute migraine in a pediatric neurology office practice. Headache 1996;36:419–422.

34. Lewis DW, Winner P, Hershey AD, Wasiewski WW. Efficacy of zolmitriptan nasal spray in adolescent migraine. Pediatrics 2007;120:390–396.

35. Lewis DW, Yonker M, Winner P, Sowell M. The treatment of pediatric migraine. Pediatr Ann 2005;34:448–460.

36. Gladstein J, Mack KJ. Chronic daily headache in adolescents. Pediatr Ann 2005;34(6):472–9.

37. Lewis DW, Winner P. The pharmacological treatment options for pediatric migraine: an evidence-based appraisal. Neurorx: The Journal of the American Society For Experimental Neurotherapeutics 2006;3:181–191.

38. Galli F, Patron L, Russo PM, Bruni O, Ferini-Strambi L, Guidetti V. Chronic daily headache in childhood and adolescence: clinical aspects and a 4-year follow-up. Cephalalgia 2004;24:850–858.

39. Trautmann E, Lackschewitz H, Kroner-Herwig B. Psychological treatment of recurrent headache in children and adolescents–a meta-analysis. Cephalalgia 2006;26:1411–1426.

40. Jansen SC, van Dusseldorp M, Bottema KC, Dubois AE. Intolerance to dietary biogenic amines: a review. Ann Allergy Asthma Immunol 2003;91:233–240.

41. Salfield SA, Wardley BL, Houlsby WT, et al. Controlled study of exclusion of dietary vasoactive amines in migraine. Arch Dis Child 1987;62:458–460.

42. Crawford P, Simmons M, Hoock J. Clinical inquiries. What dietary modifications are indicated for migraines? J Fam Pract 2006;55:62–3, 6.

43. Hershey AD, Powers SW, Vockell AL, et al. Coenzyme Q10 deficiency and response to supplementation in pediatric and adolescent migraine. Headache 2007;47:73–80.

44. Hammill JM, Cook TM, Rosecrance JC. Effectiveness of a physical therapy regimen in the treatment of tension-type headache. Headache 1996;36:149–153.

45. Butler S, Chapman C. Richard. Bonica's Management of Pain, 3rd ed. Philadelphia: Lippincott, Williams & Wilkins; 2001.

46. Diener HC, Kronfeld K, Boewing G, et al. Efficacy of acupuncture for the prophylaxis of migraine: a multicentre randomized controlled clinical trial. Lancet Neurol 2006;5:310–316.

19
Evaluating and Managing Pediatric Musculoskeletal Pain in Primary Care

Mark A. Connelly and Laura E. Schanberg

Abstract: Musculoskeletal pain is common in pediatric populations, reported in up to half of children from community samples, and is a frequent presenting complaint in pediatric primary care. Evaluating pediatric musculoskeletal pain is complicated by the extensive differential diagnosis. Some of the diagnoses require immediate treatment decisions at the primary care level to prevent future problems and disability. In this chapter we review general evaluation and treatment approaches to pediatric patients who present to primary care providers with musculoskeletal pain complaints. We begin by providing guidelines for evaluating these children, including the history, physical exam, and appropriate use of imaging and laboratory data, emphasizing that some causes of musculoskeletal pain in children are diagnosed entirely on the basis of the history and physical. Subsequently we briefly discuss two relatively uncommon musculoskeletal pain conditions in children (back pain and complex regional pain syndrome), where prompt and accurate diagnosis by the primary care physician improves outcome. Finally, we suggest guidelines for referral to pediatric subspecialists.

Key words: Arthritis, back pain, musculoskeletal pain, chronic pain, limb pain, complex regional pain syndrome.

Introduction

Pediatric primary care physicians regularly see children and adolescents complaining of musculoskeletal pain. National surveys indicate that musculoskeletal pain as a primary complaint comprises approximately 7 percent of all pediatric visits [1]. The most common musculoskeletal pain complaints in children seen in primary care clinics include arthralgias of the knee (33%) and other joints (e.g., ankles, wrists, elbows; 28%), followed by soft tissue pain (18%), heel pain (8%), hip pain (6%), and back pain (6%) [2]. Nearly all of these complaints are benign in nature and attributable to trauma, overuse, or developmental variants [2]. In fact, musculoskeletal pain is a normal part of the developmental experience of youngsters, with estimates of prevalence typically falling between 25 to 50 percent in community samples of children [3–6].

Given the pervasiveness of musculoskeletal pain in healthy children and the extensive differential diagnosis, the challenge for primary care physicians is recognizing pain indicative of a serious underlying health problem that requires timely additional testing and specialized care. Although there is substantial disagreement on how to make this determination [7], the importance of the primary care assessment of musculoskeletal pain is undeniable. In this chapter, we present a rational approach to deciphering the meaning of pediatric musculoskeletal pain for the primary care physician, including important issues to bear in mind when taking a history, conducting the physical exam, and considering laboratory tests and radiological studies. Improved early diagnosis and treatment of children presenting with musculoskeletal complaints by primary care physicians prevents excessive use of health care resources, unnecessary and often invasive medical tests, and increasing functional disability. In fact, the over-medicalization of benign persistent musculoskeletal pain makes successful treatment and resolution more difficult. In the vast majority of cases, it is in the primary care setting that benign persistent pain is most effectively diagnosed and managed.

1. Diagnostic Issues in Pediatric Musculoskeletal Pain

1.1. Overview

The vast majority of musculoskeletal complaints in children presenting to primary care providers are not life-threatening in nature. Trauma or sports-related injuries are most common [2], but malignancies and rheumatologic conditions also often present with musculoskeletal pain as the primary symptom [8–12]. Furthermore, "benign" or idiopathic pain can result in the development of persistent musculoskeletal pain syndromes with significant morbidity and functional disability, particularly in the adolescent years [13, 14]. The overarching goal in evaluating children presenting with musculoskeletal pain is to identify when intervention (other than reassurance and follow-up) is necessary, using the minimum amount of testing to make the appropriate diagnosis. Subspecialty referral is rarely indicated.

Before considering other possibilities, the primary care physician must rule out conditions that require immediate attention, such as pyarthrosis, trauma, and malignancy. A delay in diagnosing these conditions may severely compromise long-term outcome. Fortunately, the distinction between children having a relatively benign cause for their musculoskeletal pain complaints and those with more serious disease is generally evident from a complete history and physical exam. For example, an infected joint typically presents with fever, severe localized pain, and decreased range of motion or tenderness of the affected area on exam. Systemic lupus erythematosus may have weight loss, fatigue, fever, joint pain and/or swelling, rash, and laboratory abnormalities. Table 19-1 provides additional variables that may be helpful in distinguishing benign and serious causes of musculoskeletal pain, although there are always exceptions. As noted in the table, most systemic disease will

TABLE 19-1. Potential indicators of benign versus serious causes of musculoskeletal pain

Clinical finding	Benign cause of musculoskeletal pain	Serious cause of musculoskeletal pain
Effects of rest versus activity on pain	Relieved by rest and worsened by activity	Relieved by activity and present at rest
Time of day pain occurs	End of the day	Morning
Objective joint swelling	No	Yes
Joint characteristics	Hypermobile or normal	Stiffness, limited range of motion
Bony tenderness	No	Yes
Muscle strength	Normal	Muscle weakness
Growth	Normal growth pattern or weight gain	Poor growth and/or weight loss
Constitutional symptoms (e.g., fever, malaise)	Fatigue without other constitutional symptoms	Yes
Lab findings	Normal CBC, ESR, CRP	Abnormal CBC, raised ESR and CRP
Radiographic findings	Normal	Effusion, osteopenia, radiolucent metaphyseal lines, joint space loss, bony destruction

Source: "Rheumatology: 16. Diagnosing musculoskeletal pain in children"—Adapted from: CMAJ, 24-Jul-01; 165(2), 183–188, by permission of the publisher.

present with objective abnormalities as well as subjective complaints.

A useful protocol for assessing the child presenting with musculoskeletal pain has recently been published [15]. First, a thorough history and complete physical exam should be conducted to look for obvious etiology (such as sprains, strains, or fractures), characteristics of the pain (localized or diffuse), and evidence of systemic involvement [10]. Table 19-2 lists possible diagnoses classified solely on the basis of pain localization and signs of systemic involvement. If the etiology remains unclear after the history and physical, but the physical exam is normal and the child's activity level and functioning have not been significantly affected, reassurance (and follow-up if concerns persist) is generally

TABLE 19-2. Diagnoses to consider as a function of pain localization and evidence of systemic involvement.

Localized Pain	
Child is well	Child is systematically unwell
Growing pains	Infectious and post-infectious
Mechanical knee pains	arthritis
Strains and sprains	Osteomyelitis
Bone tumors	Malignancy
Pauciarticular chronic inflammatory arthritis	
Complex Regional Pain Syndrome	

Diffuse Pain	
Child is well	Child is systematically unwell
Benign Hypermobility Syndrome	Leukemia
	Neuroblastoma
Diffuse idiopathic pain syndrome (e.g., juvenile primary fibromyalgia)	Systemic-onset JRA
	Chronic inflammatory arthritis
	Systemic lupus erythematosus
	Inflammatory bowel disease
Chronic inflammatory arthritis	Infectious and post-infectious arthritis

Source: "Rheumatology: 16. Diagnosing musculoskeletal pain in children"—Adapted from: CMAJ, 24-Jul-01; 165(2), 183–188, by permission of the publisher.

appropriate. However, if the etiology is unclear and the child's activity level has changed or the physical exam is abnormal, judicious laboratory tests (e.g., CBC, ESR, CRP, thyroid function tests) and plain radiographs of the affected area should be ordered. Though often omitted, a brief screen of emotional and social functioning (e.g., depression or anxiety symptoms, school performance and absences, sleep quality, and relating to peers) and family history is also important in cases of idiopathic musculoskeletal pain lasting for several months to gauge level of disability and guide possible referral.

1.2. Important Considerations when Taking a History

Many diseases that present with musculoskeletal complaints can be diagnosed without the aid of laboratory tests (e.g., all types of chronic inflammatory arthritis, fibromyalgia, and transient synovitis of the hip). Thus, a comprehensive history is critical for narrowing the differential diagnosis of musculoskeletal pain in children. The history may provide clues to the presence of systemic disease or psychosocial factors impacting pain complaints. For example, the presence of current or recent fever can be indicative of an inflammatory or neoplastic process, particularly in the context of worsening symptoms and/or weight loss. Growth failure points to the presence of chronic illness. School issues, abuse, mood disorders, family trauma, and parental enmeshment may contribute to sustaining pain complaints and enhancing pain perception.

Soliciting detailed information about pain characteristics can also be helpful in ruling out traumatic causes as well as a variety of other possible conditions. Specifically, one should obtain information on pain onset, location, duration, intensity, alleviating and aggravating factors, progression, and radiation. Whether pain came on suddenly or developed over several days or weeks may suggest trauma, sepsis, or malignancy (if pain onset was rapid), or an inflammatory process (if pain onset was gradual). Pain that begins shortly after an illness is often suggestive of post-infectious etiology, whereas onset of pain shortly after the initiation of new athletic activity would be suggestive of a possible overuse syndrome. However, musculoskeletal pain in any location that lacks focal signs or symptoms is more likely to be "functional."

A child's chronological age narrows the likely diagnoses for musculoskeletal pain. For example, although trauma can occur at all ages, sprains and strains rarely occur in very young children, while child abuse is of increased concern in this age group. Similarly, infections can occur across the age spectrum, but the offending organisms vary (e.g., an adolescent with a septic knee may have a gonococcal infection). Neoplasms also occur at all ages, but specific malignancies are characteristically present in certain age groups (e.g., acute lymphoblastic leukemia and neuroblastoma are more frequent in children less than 4 years old, whereas osteogenic sarcoma and Ewing's sarcoma tend to occur in older children). Other conditions such as Legg-Calve-Perthes Disease (LCP) and growing pains are typically seen in younger children (ages 4 to 10), whereas slipped capital femoral epiphysis (SCFE) is usually seen in children older than 10 years of age. Inflammatory processes such as juvenile rheumatoid arthritis (JRA) and reactive arthritis can present in all age groups, but it would be unusual to have a young child present with systemic lupus erythematosus (SLE).

Obtaining a comprehensive family history may also help focus a diagnosis. In particular, certain inflammatory or autoimmune disorders have a well-known genetic component. For example, spondyloarthropathy or psoriasis may be associated with the genetic marker HLA-B27 and run in families. Data also suggest that gathering information from parents about their own pain histories may help health care providers identify children at risk for developing maladaptive pain coping strategies and higher levels of disability [16].

1.3. Physical Exam

A complete physical exam is essential and can help exclude infectious, traumatic, and oncologic etiologies. In fact, the diagnosis of inflammatory arthritis is made by physical exam alone; laboratory studies are not necessarily helpful in determining whether or not arthritis is present [10]. A careful neurologic exam, including testing for muscle strength, also is important. The musculoskeletal portion of the physical exam should include determination of leg lengths, range of motion of all joints, gait, and assessment of spinal curvature. In particular, the important distinction between arthralgia (pain in a joint) and arthritis (synovitis in a joint) is made based on a complete joint examination, including the spine, temporomandibular joints, and entheses (site of tendon insertion into bone). The joint exam should give careful attention to symptoms that may indicate inflammation, including warmth, effusion or synovial thickening, erythema, tenderness or pain with motion, and decreased or loss of range of motion. It is important to bear in mind that joint pain in young children may be referred from another area. Consequently, the joints above and below the symptomatic joint must be examined carefully. In addition, it is useful to remember that arthritis must be present in the same joint on physical exam for 6 weeks to meet diagnostic criteria for juvenile rheumatoid arthritis. Table 19-3 lists additional considerations on the physical exam (and other components of the initial evaluation) for distinguishing potential etiologies of musculoskeletal pain.

1.4. Laboratory Tests

In most cases, diagnosis and management of musculoskeletal pain in children is appropriately based on the history and physical alone. Reliance on a "rheumatoid panel" to screen for rheumatic disease is not recommended because it can lead to unnecessary expense, in addition to patient and parent worry from false positives [10]. For example, a positive ANA can be found in 5 to 15 percent of the general population [17] and in up to 30 percent of children in whom it is ordered [18], making a positive test almost meaningless in the absence of other abnormal tests and physical findings. In addition, the rheumatoid factor is only present in 10 percent of children with arthritis [19] and 30 percent of children with SLE, rendering it also useless as a screening test in children [20].

Appropriate decisions regarding which laboratory tests to obtain at the first visit depend on the nature of the presenting complaints. For example, a classic presentation of "benign nocturnal limb pain of childhood" or "growing pains" (e.g., pain without a limp in an otherwise well school-aged child with frequent night wakening due to acute onset of pain which resolves spontaneously by morning) rarely warrants laboratory testing. The most commonly ordered tests for further evaluation of musculoskeletal pain in a primary care setting include a complete blood count (CBC) with differential, erythrocyte sedimentation rate (ESR), and C-reactive protein (CRP). The CBC is used to detect inflammation (suggested by leukocytosis or thrombocytosis) or cytopenias (present in malignancy, viral syndrome and SLE). The ESR is often, but not reliably, elevated with infection, malignancy, and inflammatory disease (e.g., SLE, some types of arthritis, and vasculitis). Serious underlying disease is estimated to be seven times more likely in patients with musculoskeletal pain if the ESR is greater than 50 mm/hr, as compared to patients with an ESR of less than 20 mm/hr. Three-quarters (78%), but not all, patients with an ESR greater than 100 have been found to have "significant diagnoses" [21]. A complete blood count and ESR are unlikely to be normal in a child with a bone or joint infection, SLE, or a malignancy; however, repeat testing may be indicated to detect evolving disease. The presence of hematuria and/or

TABLE 19-3. Considerations for differential diagnosis and management of musculoskeletal pain in children.

Differential diagnosis	Things to consider in history and physical	Suggested lab studies, radiographs and initial treatment
Traumatic ■ Fractures ■ Soft tissue injury ■ Child abuse ■ Foreign body ■ Overuse injuries	■ Pattern of repetitive physical activity or repetitive relatively minor trauma ■ Child immediately stopped whatever activity he/she was engaged in following a trauma ■ Delay in bringing the child to medical attention following the "accident," bruises of varying ages, and/or torn frenulum of the lips and retinal hemorrhages are "red flags" for child abuse	■ Plain films as an initial study or a bone scan to detect subtle fractures ■ Repeat imaging if pain persists for greater than 2 weeks ■ Treat pain with NSAIDs and acetaminophen and consider immobilization of the affected area
Orthopedic/Mechanical ■ Legg-Calve-Perthes ■ Slipped capital femoral epiphysis (SCFE) ■ Congenital hip dysplasia ■ Osgood-Schlatter ■ Hypermobility	■ Pain is likely to have insidious onset, involve point tenderness, and be worse at the end of the day or with increased activity ■ Often presents with a limp in younger children ■ Hypermobility syndrome will typically be evident from the physical exam	■ Obtain plain films, including frog-leg lateral view to assess SCFE ■ Obtain MRI if Legg-Calve-Perthes disease is suspected and plain films are negative (or consider bone scan to assess for avascular necrosis) ■ Consult with or refer to orthopedist as soon as possible ■ Child should avoid extended weight bearing until orthopedic consultation is obtained
Infectious ■ Osteomyelitis ■ Septic arthritis ■ Diskitis ■ Soft tissue infections/ myositis ■ Lyme disease ■ Iliopsoas abscess	■ Should be suspected any time the child's symptoms have been acutely present (one to two days) and the child is unwell, febrile, and/or has a very tender bone or the inability to move a joint ■ Erythema overlying the tender area ■ Chief complaint for infectious pain etiology is often refusal to walk or significantly decreased use of extremity	■ Obtain blood culture, CBC with differential, ESR, and CRP for suspected infectious cause ■ Joint aspiration should be performed immediately and the child administered IV antibiotics while awaiting the culture results ■ 99 mTc bone scan should be considered if osteomyelitis is suspected and a bone scan with SPECT should be considered if diskitis is suspected ■ Therapy is directed at the causative organism (e.g., *Staphylococcus aureus,* coagulase negative staphylococci, *Pseudomonas aeruginosa, Streptococcus pyogenes, Streptococcus pneumoniae,* and *Salmonella* species are the most common organisms in an otherwise healthy child)
Inflammatory ■ JRA ■ Spondyloarthropathy ■ Post-infectious arthritis ■ Acute rheumatic fever ■ Dermatomyositis ■ Systemic lupus erythematosus ■ Mixed connective tissue disease ■ Transient synovitis of the hip ■ Henoch-Schonlein purpura ■ Inflammatory bowel disease ■ Psoriatic arthritis ■ Vasculitides	■ Morning stiffness or gel with pain worse in the mornings or after naps or sitting for extended period, and pain better with use/activity ■ Physical exam suggestive of inflammation (e.g., warmth, effusion or synovial thickening, erythema, tenderness or pain with motion, and decreased or loss of range of motion) ■ Constitutional symptoms (fever, weight loss, fatigue) may be present ■ Walk refusal in the absence of fever, decreased range of motion, a flexed, abducted, and externally rotated hip, and a previous history of an upper respiratory infection is often elicited in cases of transient hip synovitis	■ Obtain CBC and ESR (decreased hemoglobin, elevated ESR, and increased acute phase proteins and cytokines correlate with clinical symptoms of disease activity in JRA) ■ Ultrasound can demonstrate fluid in the hip with 95% accuracy ■ Refer to rheumatology clinic for disease management. Typically treated with NSAIDs (e.g., naproxen) and remittive agents (e.g., methotrexate) or biologic agents (e.g., etanercept) ■ Refer to pediatric rheumatology and/or obtain a bone marrow before starting steroid treatment in children with fever, rash, anemia and arthritis

(continued)

TABLE 19-3. (continued)

Differential diagnosis	Things to consider in history and physical	Suggested lab studies, radiographs and initial treatment
Neoplastic ■ Leukemia ■ Lymphoma ■ Neuroblastoma ■ Ewing's sarcoma ■ Osteoid osteoma ■ Osteogenic sarcoma ■ Chondrosarcoma ■ Histiocytosis X	■ Concerning features for neoplasm include severe back pain, night sweats, and nonarticular bone pain ■ Unremitting fever and weight loss are additional red flags ■ Acute leukemia in particular can present as a limping child ■ Osteoid osteomas are associated with night pain often relieved dramatically by small doses of NSAIDs ■ Bony tenderness (which extends beyond the joint capsule) is suggestive of leukemia	■ CBC with peripheral smear, ESR, uric acid and LDH are appropriate initial laboratory screening tests ■ Imaging studies are dictated by the type of complaint (i.e., plain films may be appropriate for localized bony symptoms, whereas MRI could be considered for soft tissue findings, and a bone scan for more generalized pain) ■ Referral to a pediatric hematologist/oncologist is necessary in cases of suspected malignancy. Obtaining bone marrow aspirations and extensive imaging studies before referral is costly and may delay diagnosis and treatment
Idiopathic Pain Syndromes ■ Growing pains ■ Juvenile primary fibromyalgia syndrome ■ Complex regional pain syndrome ■ Localized pain syndrome ■ Low back pain	■ Growing pains present with "classic" complaints of symmetrical lower limb pain of short duration that awakens the child from sleep approximately three to four nights each month and resolves by morning ■ Idiopathic pain syndromes typically present with longstanding symptoms. Onset is often preceded by trauma (injury, illness, significant psychological stressors) or there is a history of mood, family, and/or behavior problems ■ Physical exam may reveal tender points in the absence of arthritis, which may suggest juvenile fibromyalgia ■ Children may show few pain behaviors and move around with no apparent difficulty during examination though will often use unique descriptors for pain such as "miserable," "intense," or "unbearable," and report high pain intensity levels	■ Laboratory tests including CBC, ESR, CRP, and TFTs are recommended to exclude other etiologies of persistent pain ■ Multimodal treatment (e.g., medication, aerobic exercise, pain coping skills training, stress management, family therapy) should be initiated in cases with functional disability. Referral to a pediatric pain clinic is recommended when available. If not available, this can be initiated by primary care physician using local resources ■ Growing pains can be treated without referral. Reassurance, massage, and analgesic therapy (typically NSAIDs) are generally sufficient

proteinuria on urinalysis suggests SLE or vasculitis and a need for subspecialty referral.

If an infectious etiology is strongly considered based on history and physical exam, cultures of both the blood and affected joint(s) should be obtained for cell count and gram stain immediately. Aspiration of joint fluid may be both therapeutic and diagnostic. Since the hip joint is a closed space, moderate to large effusions of the hip may require aspiration to improve comfort and prevent sequelae, even if a septic joint is not suspected. Joint fluid can also help differentiate infection from trauma and inflammatory disease.

1.5. Radiographs

A worrisome history of localized pain, atypical or systemic symptoms, or abnormal physical findings in a child with musculoskeletal pain is an indication for use of radiologic studies. Radiographs are usually quite sensitive for bone tumors or fracture. However, a normal radiograph does not necessarily rule out cancer as a possible cause; several cancers that may present with musculoskeletal pain, such as leukemia or lymphoma, may not have radiologic abnormalities. Similarly, normal radiographic findings do not exclude the diagnosis of chronic inflammatory arthritis or early osteomyelitis.

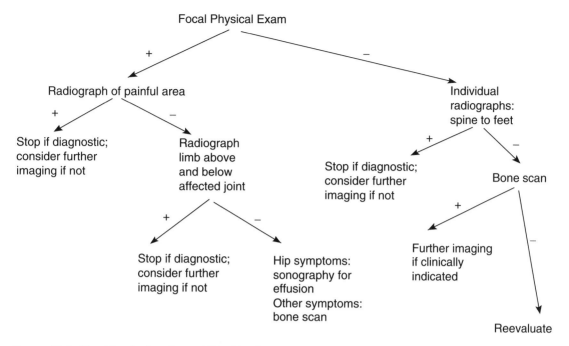

FIGURE 19-1. Algorithm for imaging a child with a limp (*Source*: "Pediatric imaging perspective: acute limp." Used with permission from: Journal of Pediatrics; 132:906–908 by permission of the publisher).

In the presence of a focal exam, the affected area should be radiographed first (see Fig. 19-1 for a sample algorithm of imaging the child presenting with a limp [22]). If the diagnosis remains unclear, the limb both above and below the involved area should be radiographed. If the latter films are negative, then an ultrasound of the hip (if hip symptoms are present) or a bone scan (for non-hip symptoms) may be necessary. Although plain films are rarely useful in the initial evaluation of children who present with arthritis, these films should always be ordered before arranging for more expensive scans. Magnetic resonance imaging has the greatest sensitivity for inflammatory processes, but at the expense of time- and cost-efficiency; thus, MRI should be used judiciously [15]. Nonetheless, computed tomography or an MRI can be particularly helpful to characterize anatomy when the location of the affected joint makes physical examination difficult (e.g., in the hip, back, or temporomandibular joint).

2. Specific Musculoskeletal Pain Problems

Although space limitations preclude a comprehensive review of the presentation and approach of each condition presenting with musculoskeletal pain, we have chosen to highlight two pain problems, back pain and complex regional pain syndrome (CRPS).

2.1. Back Pain

Back pain is less prevalent as a presenting condition in children than adults and warrants special consideration, given several possible serious etiologies which, if unrecognized, may have severe consequences and lead to increasing disability [23]. The differential diagnosis for back pain in children is extensive and there are informative reviews available [24–26]. Table 19-4 includes some of the main conditions presenting as back pain in

TABLE 19-4. Differential diagnosis of common reasons for pediatric back pain.

Diagnosis	Indications
Tumors of the spine	◆ Non-mechanical unremitting pain (not relieved by activity cessation or recumbency), highly localized with consistent tenderness on exam ◆ Progressive disability ◆ Back held stiffly on exam, and jumping is painful or refused ◆ Confirmed by abnormal lab studies and radiographs, or SPECT bone scan with CT or MRI follow-up if SPECT is positive
Infections of the spine (diskitis, sacroiliitis)	◆ Severe pain with insidious onset over days to weeks with localized tenderness ◆ Progressively increasing disability ◆ Constipation (reluctant to perform Valsalva's maneuver for normal stooling) ◆ Reluctance, stiffness with movement ◆ Radiograph shows disk space narrowing (diskitis) ◆ Marked limp or refusal to walk (sacroiliitis) ◆ Pathology readily located by bone scan
Spondylolysis	◆ Presents as mechanical back pain localized lateral to the midline, discomfort worse with extension and rotation of the spine while standing ◆ Most common in adolescents, rarely seen in children younger than three ◆ History suggestive of repeated subclinical injury involving low back rotation and extension (e.g., gymnastics, football, diving) ◆ Tenderness to palpation across the involved level ◆ Radiographs show "collar around the Scotty dog"
Spondylolisthesis	◆ Mechanical low back pain often presenting with abnormal gait and tight hamstrings ◆ Forward subluxation of one vertebral body on the level below; seen on plain radiographs
Herniated nucleus pulposis	◆ Mechanical low back pain with radicular radiation emanating from back and extending down to the ankle or foot ◆ Worse with coughing or sneezing ◆ Child may list to one side or be uncomfortable sitting on the buttock of one side ◆ Passive straight leg maneuver will elicit nerve root irritation ◆ Diagnosis confirmed with MRI
Ring apophysis fracture	◆ Acute onset of pain with a lifting activity, typically occurring in an adolescent ◆ Evident on plain radiograph, or if not, MRI
Lumbar Scheurmann's	◆ Mechanical pain with upper lumbar tenderness and occasional radiation to the thigh ◆ History of cumulative subclinical trauma ◆ Plain radiograph diagnostic (disc space narrowing at involved level and evidence of erosion of anterior lip of vertebral body)
Musculo-ligamentous back pain	◆ Represents the majority of pediatric patients with back pain ◆ Insidious onset of mechanical pain with poor, vague, or variable localization and poorly localized and broad tenderness on physical exam ◆ Often associated with trigger points and tight musculature ◆ Requires exclusion of the above disorders ◆ No neurologic findings and normal radiographs

children and their indicators, based on a recent review article [25]. Similar to other musculoskeletal pain presentations in children, back pain may require several follow-up visits to ensure adequate diagnosis of the underlying etiology.

Back pain from minor strains and repetitive microtrauma is common in children and should be fairly obvious from history. These minor injuries typically result in mild to moderate pain that resolves on its own in a few weeks without requiring further follow-up other than perhaps education on injury prevention; brief follow-up either in clinic or by telephone for the few weeks following the initial evaluation will help ensure the pain was indeed self-limited. Vertebral defects (e.g., spondylolysis and spondylolisthesis) are very rare in young children, but commonly occur in young adolescents who are active in sports (e.g., contact sports, gymnastics, diving) [24, 25]. Plain radiographs of the lumbosacral spine, or technetium bone scans and CT scans in the case of questionable radiographic findings, typically are adequate for localizing the problem and confirming the diagnosis. Recently, 18F-fluoride PET-CT also has been shown to detect spinal lesions such as spondylolysis with high diagnostic accuracy in adolescents with back pain [27]. Congenital spinal deformities, such as scoliosis, in adolescents typically do not manifest as significant back pain. However, in cases of scoliosis with back pain, radiographs are required to rule out concerning pain etiologies (e.g., osteoid osteoma or infection). Referral for an orthopedic evaluation is important when scoliosis is initially detected.

Diskitis should be suspected in young children (typically under age 10) who refuse to walk or sit; have pain in the back, hip, or abdomen; have localized back tenderness and who complain of back pain with straight leg-raising [25, 28]. Often MRI or a bone scan with single-photon emission CT is recommended when diskitis is suspected since early radiographic findings may be negative [28]. Primary vertebral tumors in children (e.g., osteoid osteoma, benign osteoblastoma, Ewing's sarcoma) and primary skeletal lymphoma of the spine are quite uncommon, but often present with back pain as a primary complaint [12]. Suggestive indicators of such neoplastic etiologies are mentioned in Table 19-4. Similarly, intervertebral disc herniation in children is relatively rare, but may suddenly occur in athletes after exertion and may be associated with neurologic signs. CT scans are superior to plain radiographs for demonstrating such herniations. However, plain radiographs are typically sufficient for identifying Scheuermann's disease by demonstrating vertebral body wedging, narrowing of intervertebral disk space and Schmorl's nodes [24]. Note that herniated discs are not rare in the adolescent population, and may or may not explain low back pain in a particular patient. Disc encroachment upon a neuroforamina, coupled with radicular symptoms in the appropriate dermatome, more strongly indicate the disc as the pain generator.

The significance of strain from heavy backpacks and computer use in pediatric presentations of back pain is actively debated, with some researchers going as far as making specific "safe weight" guidelines for backpacks (e.g., ≤ 10% of child's body weight) [29–32]. In our practice the use of backpacks is a frequent cause of thoracic back pain, particularly in adolescent girls. The extent to which emotional and social variables are significant in the initiation and maintenance of back pain in children is unclear [33–35], but should be considered in patients. However, heavy backpacks or highly distraught families should not lead the provider to a premature conclusion about the etiology of back pain. Unlike in adults, back pain presentations in children are more often related to serious underlying causes with immediate treatment needs.

After "red flags" have been ruled out, nonspecific and myofascial back pain can be addressed without invasive or complex treatment plans. A biopsychosocial approach is appropriate (see Fig. 25-1 in Chapter 25). NSAIDs and perhaps a muscle relaxant are the pharmacologic staples. Biofeedback-guided muscle relaxation can promote body awareness, as well as reduce muscle tension and stress (see Chapter 15 for details). Stretching and attention to core strength comprise the basics of the physical therapy treatment scheme. A transcutaneous electrical nerve stimulator (TENS) unit can be helpful on the low back or lower neck areas, when the pain is fairly localized. Trigger point injections can be helpful when discrete trigger points are found, as part of a diagnosis of myofascial pain. For patients who have an unusually difficult time becoming more active, aquatic therapy, or at least spending time moving about in a warm pool, can be helpful.

2.2. Complex Regional Pain Syndrome

The diagnosis and treatment of complex regional pain syndrome (CRPS) continue to generate significant controversy [36], but general diagnostic and treatment guidelines have been established (albeit, not specific for children) [37]. CRPS, previously referred to as reflex sympathetic dystrophy (RSD), typically presents in children and adolescents as ongoing burning lower limb pain following an initiating noxious event or immobilization, and has key features of pain disproportionate to the inciting event, persisting allodynia (a heightened pain response to normally non-noxious stimuli), hyperalgesia (exaggerated pain reactivity to noxious stimuli), and indicators of autonomic nervous system dysfunction (e.g., edema in the affected area, cyanosis, mottling, and hyperhydrosis) [37–39]. Although most pediatric patients with CRPS present between the ages of 9 to 15 with a history of minor trauma or repeated stress injury (e.g., caused by competitive sports), many are unable to identify a precipitating event [40]. Girls outnumber boys by as much as 6:1 and unlike the adult form, lower extremities are most commonly affected [39]. The incidence of CRPS in children is unknown, in large part because it is often undiagnosed or diagnosed late, with the diagnosis frequently delayed by nearly a year [41–44]. A missed early diagnosis of CRPS increases the difficulty of treatment, at least in adults, and can have severe consequences including bone demineralization, muscle wasting, and joint contractures. Although a bone scan may show increased uptake in the involved limb if performed early enough in the process, there are no laboratory findings that help make the diagnosis of CRPS. When the above signs and symptoms are noted in a child, the diagnosis of CRPS is made based on a thorough history and physical exam to exclude infection, stress fracture, or neoplasm. The role of bone scans, MRI, and laboratory testing is to rule out other potential diagnoses, not to make the diagnosis of CRPS.

Treatment for childhood CRPS, as for other pain syndromes, seeks to improve function as well as relieve pain. Families and providers need to work together to clearly outline the goals by which to measure treatment successes. Recommended treatment modalities include aggressive physical and occupational therapy, cognitive-behavioral interventions, medications, and sympathetic nerve blocks. Identifying CRPS should prompt immediate referral for physical therapy, which is the cornerstone of therapy. Physical therapy, including desensitization, graduated weight bearing, range of motion, and remobilization, may be required as frequently as four times per week. Children may need analgesic pre-medication in order to tolerate physical therapy at the onset of treatment.

If possible, timely referral to a pediatric chronic pain clinic can be instrumental in reducing further disability in cases of CRPS. Treatment at these clinics involves a multidisciplinary approach including therapies that facilitate intensive physical therapy and promote restoration of functioning (e.g., medication management and cognitive-behavioral therapy). In a minority of children and adolescents with

CRPS, sympathetic blockade, intravenous regional blockade, or continuous epidural block may be required to facilitate aggressive physical therapy. Nerve blocks are not recommended as initial therapy and should be undertaken only after other therapies have failed and only under the auspices of pediatric pain specialists. Multiple studies have shown noninvasive treatments, particularly cognitive behavioral therapy and physical therapy, are at least as efficacious as nerve blocks in children [40, 41, 45–47].

3. Follow-Up and Referral

3.1. When to Refer to a Pediatric Rheumatologist

The American College of Rheumatology issued a position statement to inform primary care physicians of the indications for referral to a pediatric rheumatologist [48]. Other referral guidelines also are available (see reference [49]). These indications include patients with an unclear diagnosis and functional impairment (e.g., regression in physical skills and inability to attend school), normal laboratory findings but local or generalized pain and/or swelling, unexplained physical findings or complaints not consistent with lab findings and physical exam, and suspected rheumatologic or autoimmune explanation for pain. However, indications for referral to pediatric rheumatologists appear to remain unclear based on data showing up to 20 physicians are consulted and up to 10 years elapse between the onset of symptoms and the first consultation with a pediatric rheumatologist for children eventually diagnosed with juvenile idiopathic arthritis [50].

Len and colleagues recently sought to develop a screening tool to be used in primary care settings to assist the physician with determining appropriate referrals to a pediatric rheumatologist [51]. The final version of the questionnaire consists of 12 items, takes less than five minutes to complete, and has been shown to have good inter-observer reliability ($r = 933$). Items are shown in Table 19-5. The authors recommend that children scoring higher than 5 are candidates for referral to a pediatric rheumatologist. This cut-off score was derived empirically and shown to differentiate children

TABLE 19-5. Screening questionnaire for referral to a rheumatologist.

Question #	Question	Response
1	Have you noticed swollen joints or articulations in your child for the last 7 days?	☐ Yes ☐ No ☐ Don't Know
2	Has your child complained of pain in the joints, muscles or bones for the last 7 days (not related to trauma)?	☐ Yes ☐ No ☐ Don't Know
3	Has your child ever presented any swelling on the joints or articulations that lasted more than 30 days?	☐ Yes ☐ No ☐ Don't Know
4	Has your child ever presented pain in the joints or articulations that lasted more than 30 days (not related to trauma)?	☐ Yes ☐ No ☐ Don't Know
5	Has your child ever presented difficulties in closing the hands, folding the wrists, knees or ankles?	☐ Yes ☐ No ☐ Don't Know
6	Has your child limped or walked in a different way in the last month?	☐ Yes ☐ No ☐ Don't Know
7	Is there anything that your child cannot do, like playing or running, because he/she has presented any problems in the joints or articulations?	☐ Yes ☐ No ☐ Don't Know
8	Has your child ever awakened complaining of his/her joints or articulations?	☐ Yes ☐ No ☐ Don't Know
9	Has your child ever had to cancel any everyday activity, like going to school or playing, because of pain in the joints or articulations?	☐ Yes ☐ No ☐ Don't Know
10	Does your child present any deformity in any joint or articulation?	☐ Yes ☐ No ☐ Don't Know
11	Has your child ever had fever for more than 30 days without any apparent cause, followed by swelling or pain in the joints or articulations?	☐ Yes ☐ No ☐ Don't Know
12	Has your child ever presented any redness in the body followed by swelling or pain in the joints or articulations?	☐ Yes ☐ No ☐ Don't Know

Note: "Yes" is scored as 1, and "no" and "I don't know" are scored as 0. Final score = sum of all 12 questions (range = 0–12). Children with a score >=5 should be referred to a rheumatologist. Adapted with permission from [51].

with rheumatic conditions from both children with idiopathic generalized musculoskeletal pain and healthy controls.

Although the screening tool for referral to a pediatric rheumatologist has the potential to benefit many busy primary care physicians evaluating children with musculoskeletal pain, it is important to note that many rheumatic entities develop over weeks or months. Thus, in cases where a rheumatic cause is suspected, but there is no clear indication for referral at the initial evaluation, close follow-up with the primary care physician is necessary. Subsequent resolution of symptoms and absence of worrisome features can reassure the child and family that a malignancy or chronic inflammatory disease is not present and the development of additional signs and symptoms can direct further evaluation or referral.

In general, nonsteroidal anti-inflammatory agents are the primary pharmacological agent used for the treatment of musculoskeletal pain and, most often, additional medications are not needed. NSAIDs and other analgesics including acetaminophen, tramadol, and rarely, opioids can be safely used in children and adolescents to alleviate pain while awaiting referral to pediatric rheumatology. Recently, the COX-2 inhibitor, celecoxib, was approved by the FDA to treat JRA in children and is useful when gastrointestinal side effects limit the use of traditional NSAIDs. See Table 19-6 for dosing guidelines.

Steroids should not be used to treat musculoskeletal pain prior to consultation with a pediatric rheumatologist to prevent masking malignancy or rheumatic disease. If arthritis is present, controlling the underlying disease is the first step in pain management. This may include methotrexate, anti-tumor necrosis factor and other biologic agents, in addition to NSAIDs. Additional symptomatic relief is provided by acetaminophen, heat or cold, splints, adaptive devices, physical therapy, and rarely, opioids. Opioids, when used properly, can safely and efficaciously treat the pain often associated with arthritis [52].

As in adults, adjuvant medications are often useful for managing chronic pain in children. These medications most commonly include tricyclic antidepressants for generalized chronic pain associated with sleep disturbance. The tricyclic antidepressants (e.g., amitriptyline) are used in low doses given at night (see Table 19-6).

3.2. When to Refer to a Pediatric Pain Clinic

Early referral to dedicated pediatric pain clinics is primarily indicated in the case of suspected "benign" pain syndromes, as the interdisciplinary team approach typical of these clinics can help reduce further functional disability and family frustration. Adult pain clinics have variable clinical experience working with these children and often rely too heavily on procedural interventions, ignoring the psychosocial aspects of pain common in children and adolescents. Early use of blocks and overly sedating medications may actually complicate rather than facilitate treatment. Dedicated pediatric pain clinics are thus best able to address the complex needs of children with chronic pain and their families.

However, since dedicated pediatric pain clinics are few and far between, treatment should be initiated by the primary care physician. Indications for referral to a pediatric pain clinic include a history of musculoskeletal pain persisting for at least three months with no evidence of medical "red flags" and accompanied by ongoing limitations in physical, academic, social, or emotional functioning despite initiation of treatment with improved sleep hygiene, education, graduated aerobic exercise, and medication (see Chapter 13). As stated by Konijnenberg and colleagues [7], the momentum to discuss a broader conceptualization of pain (including psychosocial contributions) is best created in the first

TABLE 19-6. Pediatric dosing guidelines for selected medications used to treat musculoskeletal pain.

Medication	Total daily dose	Frequency	Daily maximum
NSAIDs			
Ibuprofen	30–40 mg/kg	3 times/day	2400 mg
Naproxen	10–20 mg	2 times/day	1000 mg
Nabumetone	30 mg/kg	Daily	2000 mg
Meloxicam	0.125 mg/kg	Daily	7.5 mg
Celecoxib	100 mg (≤25 kg)	2 times/day	200 mg
	200 mg (>25 kg)		
Other analgesics			
Acetaminophen	10–15 mg/kg/dose	Every 4 hours	Lesser of 90 mg/kg or 4 g
Hydrocodone	0.15 mg/kg	Every 4 hours	Limited by side effects
Oxycodone	0.05–0.2 mg/kg	Every 3–6 hours	Limited by side effects
Tramadol	25–100 mg	Every 4–6 hours	300 mg
Amitriptyline	10–30 mg	At bedtime	75 mg at bedtime

contacts with families and should be initiated in primary care. Chapter 13 provides recommendations for speaking to families about an array of pain syndromes.

3.3. Other Referrals

The need to refer to other subspecialties may be apparent based on findings from the initial evaluation or become apparent over time. For example, evidence from the initial evaluation of a traumatic or mechanical etiology that may benefit from surgical correction or assistive devices should be referred to a pediatric orthopedics clinic or pediatric physical therapist. Congenital disorders of the spine and vertebral defects should also be referred for orthopedic evaluation. A pediatric oncology referral should be prompted when the initial evaluation indicates a possible neoplastic etiology. Even in cases where referral is indicated, however, it is essential that the primary care physician remain involved in the child's care to facilitate appropriate follow-up and provide support.

Take-Home Points

- Benign musculoskeletal pain is surprisingly common in childhood and adolescence.
- Acute assessment of the child with musculoskeletal pain by history, physical, and laboratory testing should focus on ruling out a diagnosis of trauma, infection, and malignancy.
- Chronic causes of musculoskeletal pain, such as rheumatic disease and pain syndromes (e.g., fibromyalgia and complex regional pain syndrome) may take several visits to identify. In fact, arthritis must be present for six weeks before the diagnosis of chronic inflammatory arthritis is made.
- There are no laboratory tests, including the ANA, that indicate arthritis is present. The diagnosis of arthritis is based entirely on the physical exam.
- Management of pain syndromes is best done in the primary care setting with close follow-up and local resources.
- Subspecialty referral is indicated when the diagnosis is unclear after several visits, joint swelling is present for over 30 days, there is evidence of systemic illness, or functional disability is present

and worsening. Referral should be accomplished prior to the use of steroids to prevent masking malignancy or rheumatic disease.

References

1. Schappert S, Nelson C. National ambulatory medical care survey: 1995–1996 summary. Vital Health Stat 13 1996;142:1–122.
2. De Inocencio J. Musculoskeletal pain in primary pediatric care: Analysis of 1,000 consecutive 661 general pediatric clinic visits. Pediatrics 1998;102: e63–67.
3. El-Metwally A, Salminen J, Auvinen A, Kautiainen H, Mikkelsson M. Prognosis of non-specific musculoskeletal pain in preadolescents: A prospective 4-year follow-up study till adolescence. Pain 2004;110:550–559.
4. Mikkelsson M, Salminen J, Kautiainen H. Non-specific musculoskeletal pain in preadolescents. Prevalence and 1-year persistence. Pain 1997;73:29–35.
5. Passo M. Aches and limb pain. Pediatr Clin North Am 1982;29:209–219.
6. Perquin C, Hazebroek-Kampschreur A, Hunfeld J, et al. Pain in children and adolescents: a common experience. Pain 2000;87:51–58.
7. Konijnenberg A, De Graeff-Meeder E, Kimpen J, et al. Children with unexplained chronic pain: do pediatricians agree regarding the diagnostic approach and presumed primary cause? Pediatrics 2004;114: 1220–1226.
8. Beresford M, Cleary A. Evaluation of a limping child. Current Paediatrics 2005;15:15–22.
9. Cabral D, Tucker L. Malignancies in children who initially present with rheumatic complaints. J Pediatr 1999;134:53–57.
10. Malleson P, Beauchamp R. Rheumatology: Diagnosing musculoskeletal pain in children. Can Med Assoc J 2001;165:183–188.
11. Trapani S, Grisolia F, Simonini G, Calabri G, Falcini F. Incidence of occult cancer in children presenting with musculoskeletal symptoms: A 10-year survey in a pediatric rheumatology unit. Semin Arthritis Rheum 2000;29:348–359.
12. Wilne S, Collier J, Kennedy C, Koller K, Grundy R, Walker D. Presentation of childhood CNS tumors: a systematic review and meta-analysis. Lancet Oncol 2007;8:685–695.
13. Connelly M, Schanberg L. Latest developments in the assessment and management of chronic musculoskeletal pain syndromes in children. Curr Opin Rheumatol 2006;18:496–502.
14. Malleson P, Clinch J. Pain syndromes in children. Curr Opin Rheumatol 2003;15:572–580.

15. Junnila J, Cartwright V. Chronic musculoskeletal pain in children: part I. Initial evaluation. Am Fam Physician 2006;74:115–122.

16. Schanberg L, Anthony K, Gil K, Lefebvre J, Kredich D, Macharoni L. Family pain history predicts child health status in children with chronic rheumatic disease. Pediatrics 2001;108:E47–E53.

17. Illei G, Klippel J. Why is the ANA result positive? Bull Rheum Dis 1999;48:1–4.

18. Malleson P, Sailer M, Mackinnon M. Usefulness of antinuclear antibody testing to screen for rheumatic diseases. Arch Dis Child 1997;77:299–304.

19. Eichenfield A, Arthrey B, Doughty R, Cebul R. Utility of rheumatoid factor in the diagnosis of juvenile rheumatoid arthritis. Pediatrics 1986;78:480–484.

20. Brewer E, Bass J, Baum J. Current proposed revision of JRA criteria. Arthritis Rheum 1977;20:195–199.

21. Huttenlocher A, Newman T. Evaluation of the erythrocyte sedimentation rate in children presenting with limp, fever, or abdominal pain. Clin Pediatr 1997;36:339–344.

22. Fordham L, Auringer S, Frush D. Pediatric imaging perspective: acute limp. J Pediatr 1998;132:906–908.

23. Matullo K, Samdani A, Betz R. Low-back pain and unrecognized Cobb syndrome in a child resulting in paraplegia. Orthopedics 2007;30:237–238.

24. Afshani E, Kuhn J. Common causes of low back pain in children. Radiographics 1991;11:269–291.

25. Glancy G. The diagnosis and treatment of back pain in children and adolescents: an update. Adv Pediatr 2006;53:227–240.

26. Khoury N, Hourani M, Arabi M, Abi-Fakher F, Haddad M. Imaging of back pain in children and adolescents. Curr Probl Diagn Radiol 2006;35:224–244.

27. Ovadia D, Metser U, Lievshitz G, Yaniv M, Wientroub S, Even-Sapir E. Back pain in adolescents: assessment with integrated 18F-fluoride positron-emission tomography-computed tomography. J Pediatr Orthop 2007;27:90–93.

28. Kulas D, Schanberg L. Musculoskeletal pain in children. In: Schechter N, Berde C, Yaster M, editors. Pain in Infants, Children, and Adolescents, 2nd ed. Philadelphia: Lippincott, Williams, & Wilkins; 2003:578–98.

29. Bejia I, Abid N, Salem K, et al. Low back pain in a cohort of 622 Tunisian school children and adolescents: an epidemiological study. Eur Spine J 2005;14:331–336.

30. Diepenmaat A, Van der Wal M, De Vet H, Hirasing R. Neck/shoulder, low back, and arm pain in relation to computer use, physical activity, stress, and depression among Dutch adolescents. Pediatrics 2006;117:412–416.

31. Moore M, White G, Moore D. Association of relative backpack weight with reported pain, pain sites, medical utilization, and lost school time in children and adolescents. J Sch Health 2007;77:232–239.

32. Negrini S, Negrini A. Postural effects of symmetrical and asymmetrical loads on the spines of school children. Scoliosis 2007;2:8.

33. Currie S, Wang J. More data on major depression as an antecedent risk factor for first onset of chronic back pain. Psychol Med 2005;35:1275–1282.

34. Jones G, Macfarlane G. Epidemiology of low back pain in children and adolescents. Arch Dis Child 2005;90:312–316.

35. Kopek J, Sayre E. Stressful experiences in childhood and chronic back pain in the general population. Clin J Pain 2005;21:478–483.

36. Berde C, Lebel A. Complex regional pain syndromes in children and adolescents. Anesthesiology 2005;102:252–255.

37. Reflex Sympathetic Dystrophy Syndrome Association. Complex regional pain syndrome: Treatment guidelines. Milford: Reflex Sympathetic Dystrophy Syndrome Association; 2006.

38. Merskey H, Bogduk N. Classification of Chronic Pain: Descriptions of Chronic Pain Syndromes and Definitions of Pain Terms. Seattle: IASP Press, 1994.

39. Low A, Ward K, Wines A. Pediatric complex regional pain syndrome. J Pediatr Orthop 2007;27:567–572.

40. Dangel T. Chronic pain management in children. Part II: reflex sympathetic dystrophy. Paediatr Anaesth 1998;8:105–112.

41. Bernstein B, Singsen B, Kent J, et al. Reflex neurovascular dystrophy in childhood. J Pediatr 1978;93:211–215.

42. Maillard S, Davies K, Khubchandani R, Woo P, Murray K. Reflex sympathetic dystrophy: A multidisciplinary approach. Arthritis Rheum 2004;51:284–290.

43. Stanton R, Malcolm J, Wesdock K, Singsen B, Name O. Reflex sympathetic dystrophy in children: an orthopedic perspective. Orthopedics 1993;16:773–779.

44. Veldman P, Reynen H, Arntz I, Goris R. Signs and symptoms of reflex sympathetic dystrophy: prospective study of 829 patients. Lancet 1993;342:1012–1016.

45. Lee B, Scharff L, Sethna N, et al. Physical therapy and cognitive-behavioral treatment for complex regional pain syndromes. J Pediatr 2002;141:135–140.

46. Sherry D, Wallace C, Kelley C, Kidder M, Sapp L. Short- and long-term outcomes of children with complex regional pain syndrome type 1 treated with exercise therapy. Clin J Pain 1999;15:218–223.

47. Wilder R, Berde C, Wolohan M, Vieyra M, Masek BJ, Micheli LJ. Reflex sympathetic dystrophy in children: Clinical characteristics and follow-up of seventy patients. J Bone Joint Surg Am 1992;74:910–919.

48. Guidelines for referral of children and adolescents to pediatric rheumatologists. American College of Rheumatology, 1997. (Accessed January 5th, 2007, at *http://www.rheumatology.org/publications/position/pediatricreferrals.asp?aud=mem.*)

49. Foster H, Khawajab K. When to request a paediatric rheumatology opinion. Current Paediatrics 2005;15:1–8.

50. Len C, Liphaus B, Machado C, et al. Juvenile rheumatoid arthritis: delay in the diagnosis and referral to the specialist. Rev Paul Pediatr 2002;20:280–292.

51. Len C, Terreri M, Puccini R, et al. Development of a tool for early referral of children and adolescents with signs and symptoms suggestive of chronic arthropathy to pediatric rheumatology centers. Arthritis Rheum 2006;55:373–377.

52. Connelly M, Schanberg L. Opioid therapy for the treatment of refractory pain in children with juvenile rheumatoid arthritis. Nat Clin Prac Rheumat 2006;2:636–637.

20
Pain in Sickle Cell Disease

Carlton Dampier

Abstract: Vaso-occlusive pain from sickle cell disease is one of the most challenging pain syndromes in pediatrics. Pain symptoms can occur in patients of all ages, from young infants to young adults. Pain can represent a very rare event for some individuals, but can be a daily occurrence for others. Pain symptoms in younger children are usually relatively mild and of short duration, and management strategies need to focus on the use of rapidly acting, short-duration analgesics, and comforting nonpharmacologic strategies. Symptoms become more frequent and of longer duration in older children and adolescents, requiring a more complex management strategy. Long-acting analgesics may provide more optimal relief for those with persistent pain, and short-acting analgesics may be needed for breakthrough pain. Selected patients may benefit from adjuvant analgesics such as antidepressants or anxiolytics. If available, training in the use of cognitive-behavioral techniques may improve self-esteem and perceived control over pain symptoms. As pain symptoms are just one of many symptoms of this complex disorder, the family and the health care provider must work as a team, together with sickle cell disease specialists, so that optimal disease management can go hand-in-hand with optimal pain management. Ongoing clinical research is likely to lead to more effective disease management in the future, which may lessen the burden of pain for patients and families affected by this disorder.

Key words: Sickle cell disease, vaso-occlusive episode, pain crisis, pediatric pain.

Introduction

Pain, the most common manifestation of sickle cell disease, begins early in the first year of life in highly symptomatic individuals. Almost all children, even those with milder forms of this disorder, will ultimately experience pain as they progress through childhood into adolescence and then young adulthood. A small minority of individuals will transition, often in their preteen or early adolescent years, from sporadic episodic acute pain to frequently recurrent acute pain. These individuals represent the majority of patients hospitalized for the management of acute pain. Persistent or chronic pain may also develop, presumably from bone, joint, or nerve damage from repeated vascular occlusion.

These pain symptoms occur in the context of an inherited disorder largely affecting African-American or Hispanic minority populations, many of whom live in medically underserved areas in the nation's inner city or in rural southern communities and face numerous economic and social challenges. The impact of these pain symptoms and other disease-related complications go beyond the substantial use of health care resources, with adverse effects on the child's physical functioning, school attendance and academic performance, and social roles [1]. Parents and other caregivers face similar difficulties with job attendance and performance. As with many other pediatric disorders, most patients and their families show remarkable resilience in the face of the many challenges of living with this disorder. However, some children and their families show poor psychosocial adaptation and experience

G.A. Walco and K.R. Goldschneider (eds.), *Pain in Children: A Practical Guide for Primary Care.*
© Humana Press, a part of Springer Science + Business Media, 2008

substantial mental health comorbidities, and often experience exacerbation of pain symptoms and utilize excessive health care resources [2].

Primary care providers are in a unique position to assist with the management of pain from this disorder because providing ongoing longitudinal care facilitates the development of a trusting relationship between health care providers and the patient and family. This therapeutic alliance facilitates introducing interventions and adherence to therapy over time. The success or failure of interventions for episodic pain recommended by specialists is also best evaluated in this longitudinal primary care context. Primary care providers' knowledge of the family's interests, beliefs, and values can also support the family's adherence to the mixture of pharmacologic and nonpharmacologic techniques often required for optimal symptom management.

1. Disease Pathophysiology

Acute vascular occlusion with subsequent tissue ischemia leading to activation of peripheral nociceptors is the presumed etiology for the episodic pain syndrome typically referred to as a "sickle crisis," vaso-occlusive episode, or sickle painful episode. Deoxygenation of sickle hemoglobin leads to the formation of a nucleus containing a small number of hemoglobin molecules that subsequently polymerize quickly into long fibers. These fibers organize in helical twisted rope-like structures with remarkable physical strength that physically deform red blood cells into stiff elongated "sickle" shapes. The initial theories of vaso-occlusion suggested that these stiff red cells become mechanically lodged in small blood vessels, thus disrupting blood flow and causing subsequent tissue ischemia, the so-called vicious cycle of sickling. Current proposals for the pathophysiology of vaso-occlusion suggest a much more complex process with critical involvement of the vascular endothelium and plasma components, in addition to multiple red blood cell changes beyond those of sickle hemoglobin polymer formation [3].

The endothelial cell, which lines blood vessels, ordinarily provides a smooth relatively inert surface that prevents interaction with cellular components of the blood to reduce the risk of thrombogenesis and other harmful vascular events, but has

a mechanism which allows interaction with various white blood cells, particularly in the context of an inflammatory response. Red blood cells in individuals with sickling disorders have acquired membrane changes that allow them to strongly adhere to vascular endothelial cells using receptor mediated mechanisms, as do white blood cells. A variety of plasma factors are also thought to be important in the pathophysiology of sickle vaso-occlusion. Plasma proteins such as fibrinogen, fibronectin, and von Willebrand factor may act as bridging molecules between receptors on the endothelial cells and those on the sickled red blood cells. These molecules are acute phase reactants whose levels increase as part of the inflammatory response. Thus, acute inflammatory changes from fever or infection may be a common initiating event to vascular occlusion from sickled red blood cell-endothelial cell interactions [4].

An important physiologic system that coordinates the interaction between the plasma compartment and the vascular endothelium involves the generation and destruction of nitric oxide, a major endogenous vasodilator that regulates vascular tone in many different vascular beds. Sickle cell disease is now thought to be a disorder associated with a significant nitric oxide deficiency, as hemoglobin released into the circulation during red blood cell hemolysis rapidly scavenges nitric oxide and converts it into an inactive form. A number of other similar changes reduce the available precursors of nitric oxide formation, and impair the ability of its enzymatic production. These changes may cause a significant endothelial dysfunction, not unlike that seen in diabetes or atherosclerosis, that may contribute to the initiation or perpetuation of vascular occlusion by sickle erythrocytes [5, 6].

Bone marrow or stem cell transplant leading to endogenous production of non-sickling erythrocytes is the only curative therapy for sickling disorders, but has limited utility because of current constraints for highly human leukocyte antigen-matched donors and the occurrence of considerable peri-and post-transplant complications [7]. Hydroxyurea, a chemotherapeutic agent that increases fetal hemoglobin production in susceptible individuals, is FDA-approved for adult individuals with sickling disorders who experience frequent hospitalizations for pain or pulmonary vaso-occlusive complications [8, 9]. Its off-label use in older children and adolescents with frequent pain has become relatively widespread, and ongoing clinical trials are exploring its potential benefit in young children prior to the onset of organ damage. Alternatives to hydroxyurea that may have a broader spectrum of efficacy on preventing sickling-related vaso-occlusion are also being developed. A decision to start hydroxyurea therapy in children for frequent pain should be a collaborative decision between the sickle cell specialist, primary care provider, and the patient and their family, based on a careful assessment of individual risks and benefits. Similarly, a careful plan for monitoring hematologic toxicity and other adverse effects needs to be established and adherence to dosing recommendations must be reinforced.

Other clinical trials for acute vaso-occlusive pain are exploring a variety of approaches to modulate nitric oxide metabolism or production, or to reduce hemolysis to decreased nitric oxide consumption [6]. Various anti-inflammatory therapies are also being tested, particularly for pulmonary vaso-occlusive complications. However, until these agents provide effective control of vaso-occlusion, management of its associated pain will remain the primary therapeutic modality.

2. Clinical Characteristics of Vaso-Occlusive Pain

Vaso-occlusive pain represents a continuum of frequency and intensity, but variation is larger between patients than between episodes within individual patients. Many patients experience a prodromal phase heralding the onset of pain, while others experience sudden onset of pain that can wake them from sleep [10]. With experience, most patients and families become relatively adept at assessing and managing their typical vaso-occlusive pain and only seek acute care services when the characteristic of the episode is unusual or is too severe to manage at home. Due to lack of training, family resources, or past experiences, some families are unable to manage even relatively uncomplicated painful episodes at home and instead seek acute health care services at hospital emergency departments. A consistent, trusted health care provider can be instrumental in providing medical supervision to patients and families for the home management of pain during most vaso-occlusive episodes, and consistent acute care management in a local emergency department.

Dactylitis, a painful swelling of the dorsum of the hands or feet often with associated swelling of the proximal portions of the fingers and toes, is the common initial presentation of vaso-occlusive pain in infants and young children [11]. Current ongoing observational studies suggest that children with the SS genotype have a significantly shorter median age to first dactylitis episode than those with SC genotype (1.9 versus 3.9 years). These first sickle pain episodes can range in length from less than 12 hours to over 8 days, with a median duration of 2 days. Some children, mostly with the SS genotype, continue to have episodes of recurrent vaso-occlusive pain throughout early childhood, which are usually of 1 to 2 days duration and are manageable with oral analgesics in the home setting, unless there is coexistent fever or respiratory symptoms that require hospital management. On average, pain is experienced on about 2 percent of days in preschool age children, while school-age children and young adolescents report vaso-occlusive pain that occurs on 5 to 10 percent of days [12]. For children who are old enough to self-report pain, the vaso-occlusive pain experienced during these episodes is generally of mild to moderate intensity, but severe pain can occur on 10 to 15 percent of pain days. As compared to adolescents, school-age children tend to have less intense pain, and girls tend to report a higher number of painful sites than boys.

In terms of episodes rather than days, 40 to 50 percent of school-age children experience one pain episode per month, while about 10 percent experience more than two episodes a month [13]. About half of these episodes are relatively brief, lasting 1 day or less. However, about 5 percent of episodes in older children last longer than 2 weeks. Adolescents, females, and individuals with the SS genotype tend to have vaso-occlusive episodes of longer durations.

Identifying prospective patients at increased risk of more severe or frequent pain has been frustrating and largely unsuccessful. Higher levels of fetal hemoglobin, either naturally occurring or acquired from the use of hydroxyurea, reduce the frequency of vaso-occlusive pain. Surprisingly, more severe anemia from lower levels of hemoglobin also reduces the frequency of vaso-occlusive pain, but the precise physiology of this reduction is unclear [13]. However, current clinical research is suggesting that these very anemic individuals are at increased risk for other vascular events such as stroke, pulmonary hypertension, priapism, and leg ulcers. Thus, sickle cell disease may represent a complex disorder of two overlapping phenotypes, a vaso-occlusive phenotype and a vasculopathy phenotype [14].

3. Other Pain Syndromes

While episodic extremity pain is the prototypical pain experienced during vaso-occlusive episodes, many other pain symptoms or syndromes are possible and can represent a significant diagnostic challenge for medical providers and family caregivers alike.

3.1. Chest Pain

Chest pain localized to the sternum or lateral lower rib cage can occur as an isolated site of vaso-occlusive pain or more commonly in combination with extremity pain. The rib pain, as is the extremity bone pain, is secondary to infarction of bone marrow, cortical bone, or periosteum. It is frequently pleuritic in nature and can be associated with an underlying pleural effusion and, because of associated splinting, may be a risk factor for developing an acute chest syndrome. A chest X-ray is appropriate in those patients with fever or respiratory symptoms to determine if there is underlying pulmonary pathology. Diffuse abdominal pain with an associated ileus, sometimes mimicking an acute abdomen, can be a presenting symptom of a vaso-occlusive episode particularly in younger children. Inflammatory markers are usually elevated, and radiographic studies are usually nonspecific. Given the very low frequency of etiologies leading to an acute abdomen and the increased risk of surgery in these patients, surgical intervention is very rarely warranted. Close observation by sickle cell specialists and judicious fluid and analgesic management is the treatment of choice in the absence of other signs and symptoms suggestive of more severe pathology.

3.2. Headache

Headache pain may also complicate otherwise typical vaso-occlusive episodes. These headaches are typically frontal in location and can sometimes have features similar to migraine headaches with nausea, photophobia, and throbbing characteristics. Whether these symptoms are secondary to vaso-occlusion in bones of the face or skull, or from more typical headache pathophysiology, is uncertain. Metoclopramide is sometimes helpful in addition to analgesics.

As an isolated pain syndrome, headache is relatively common, but has been poorly characterized [15]. Some may have features characteristic of migraine headaches, while others may be more typical of tension-type headaches. A small number of individuals satisfy current diagnostic criteria for chronic daily headache. Headaches may be somewhat more frequent in children with a history of sickle cell-related cerebrovascular events such as stroke, making these yet another pain syndrome that will require careful subspecialty evaluation. As in children without sickle cell disease, referral to a neurologist with experience in headache management is appropriate for frequent or prolonged headaches. Since many of the medications typically used for acute migraine headache management, such as the tryptan-class of medications, are likely contraindicated in sickle cell patients, therapeutic approaches using anticonvulsant or antidepressant medications for headache prophylaxis may be more practical.

3.3. Abdominal Pain

Other pain syndromes which are likely distinct from these types of vaso-occlusive episodes are also common. Young children with acute splenic sequestration can experience significant left upper quadrant visceral pain from rapid enlargement of the splenic capsule. These physical findings are often appropriately identified by well-trained family caregivers who can bring their children in for prompt emergency evaluation and potentially life-saving transfusion therapy. Subsequent transfusion therapy and splenectomy are indicated for children with recurrent episodes. Older children can experience episodic right upper quadrant colicky abdominal pain and jaundice from cholelithiasis, which is best documented by ultrasonography. Surgical evaluation with subsequent elective cholecystectomy is the typical therapeutic approach.

3.4. Avascular Necrosis

Bone infarction leading to avascular necrosis in the vertebral column, shoulder, or hip, can be a cause of acute and chronic pain in adolescent and young adult patients. Persistent or recurrent joint pain symptoms require diagnostic imaging and referral to an orthopedic specialist experienced with managing these patients. Physical therapy is often helpful for initial symptom management, but some patients will have progressive joint changes, particularly in the hips, that will ultimately require joint replacement for relief of chronic pain or to improve physical functioning.

4. Pain Treatment in the Home Setting

Most families prefer to manage vaso-occlusive pain at home. The home setting is likely to be more comfortable for children and less disruptive to the family. Successful management depends on the presence of a caregiver relatively skilled in pain assessment with access to adequate analgesic medication, and some extended family support as these episodes may last for several days and require around-the-clock medication for adequate management. Home management and proper emergency department utilization is facilitated by telephone access to a trusted medical professional with experience in sickle cell disease, who can address additional management concerns or questions.

Low potency analgesics, such as acetaminophen or ibuprofen, are typically chosen as initial therapy by most families and are often adequate for mild pain, particularly in younger children. These analgesics are often chosen out of concern for the adverse consequences of the more potent opioid analgesics. Older children, particularly those with more intense pain, are more likely to choose opioid analgesics. The combination of opioids and ibuprofen provides the most pain relief [16]. Families need to be reminded to provide these medications on an appropriate time-contingent basis as most studies and anecdotal experience suggest that families administer these medications less frequently than recommended [16].

In addition to pharmacologic interventions, families naturally provide a variety of nonpharmacologic interventions that can be effective pain relieving strategies [17, 18]. Relatively passive distraction-based strategies such as rest, watching TV, talking with friends, and playing video games are commonly used. Also relatively common are the use of physical modalities such as the application of heat or of gentle massage. Guided imagery and self-hypnosis are among a group of cognitive behavioral techniques that have been shown to be helpful in the home management of vaso-occlusive pain [19]. Unfortunately, few patients and families can take advantage of these latter techniques, as they do not have access to the mental health professionals experienced in teaching their use. Primary providers can take a proactive role in treatment by referring patients to community resources between acute painful events. Cognitive-behavioral techniques are better learned and practiced when the patient is not in the midst of a vaso-occlusive episode.

Optimum pain management for adolescents with sickle cell disease can be challenging for health care providers. This can be a time of increasing pain intensity and duration when some adolescents may have difficulty communicating to their parents, and some parents may have difficulty relinquishing health care control to their children. This may be particularly problematic for families with a heightened concerned for potential adverse consequences of frequent opioid use. Meetings between family members and the health care team may be very helpful in this setting to deal with concerns and issues, and to agree on strategies that can be effectively implemented.

5. Pain Treatment in the ED

An urgent visit to the emergency department truly represents a "crisis" for many families who may be distraught by their inability to successfully manage the pain at home, or may be concerned by the unusual severity of the pain or its associated symptoms. At the same time, the emergency department staff is often struggling to provide health care to increasing numbers of medically underserved individuals, and is often frustrated by the symptoms of sickle cell pain which have few objective physical or laboratory signs that can guide management or response to therapy. Cultural and economic disparities and a lack of consistent staffing can also be a source of mistrust and frustration. Primary care providers can play a critically important role in the management of vaso-occlusive pain in the emergency department setting by providing a consistent management strategy and by acting as a resource for both the family and emergency department staff, sharing details of medical history and previous successful therapies.

6. Pain Treatment in the Hospital Setting

For those patients who require hospitalization, vaso-occlusive pain is uniformly intense and may be complicated by infection or other sickle-related complications. These patients are best managed by health care providers with extensive knowledge of sickle cell disease and its complications, who are comfortable with the usage of opioid analgesics, usually delivered via patient-controlled analgesia devices. Whether because of pain intensity or because of metabolic changes related to sickle cell disease, patients frequently require opioid analgesic dosages that are several fold higher than that required for typical postoperative pain management. A variety of adjuvant analgesics, including NSAIDs, are used, as are medications to control sedation, pruritus, nausea, and constipation. Epidurals and other interventional treatments may have a role in vaso-occlusive episode management in selected situations.

Patients and families are often wary of new or different treatments, especially those offered by people they do not know or trust. Hearing about treatment options ahead of time (e.g., pre-hospital or during well-child checks) can facilitate the process of treatment, when the stress of the pain and admission can be overwhelming. Also, helping the family to understand what will happen upon admission, and how to advocate for themselves, can be extremely valuable to both patients and the health care team.

Most admissions for uncomplicated vaso-occlusive pain require the administration of analgesics for 4 to 7 days [20]. High doses are used at the beginning to control pain, and then are gradually weaned as the pain intensity subsides. Younger children, whose pain is often of short duration, can be transitioned to short-acting oral analgesics prior to discharge. Adolescents with more persistent pain and longer hospitalization may benefit from a long-acting oral analgesics started mid-way through their hospital stay. Starting long-acting opioids can facilitate weaning from parenteral opioids, lessen the likelihood of subsequent opioid withdrawal symptoms, and provide more effective analgesia for any persistent pain after discharge. The family's usual outpatient health care provider must be part of the discharge planning process, particularly for adolescent patients, to assist with the management of persistent or rebound pain that may otherwise lead to subsequent readmission to the hospital.

7. Closing Thoughts

Large urban hospitals or academic medical centers in metropolitan areas with large minority populations have specialized comprehensive sickle cell clinics and dedicated acute care units for sickle cell patients. However, most individuals with sickle cell disease, much like individuals with other chronic diseases, are cared for by a combination of physicians, often in multiple practice locations for both health maintenance and acute care issues. Given their unique knowledge of local and family resources, the pediatrician is often in the best position to facilitate successful pain relief by coordinating home care and acute care management of sickle pain. Given their long-term relationship with each family, they are also best positioned to support and reinforce education efforts by specialists, and to advocate for changes in management strategies as the disease process changes over time.

Take-Home Points

- As with any chronic condition, sickle cell disease patients benefit from ongoing health maintenance care, including education regarding the natural history of the disease and its potential treatment options, and for the management of acute complications.
- Many cognitive-behavioral strategies are naturally used by families for pain relief and should be supported and encouraged. More complex therapies such as self-hypnosis require expert guidance and are best introduced and learned ahead of time, rather than in times of crisis.

- Analgesics should be tailored to the intensity and duration of pain. Moderate to severe pain is best managed with a combination of NSAIDs and opioids of varying potency.
- Trust and rapport can often be lacking in the acute care setting, and the primary physician can play a valuable role in being the liaison between the family and acute care team, particularly for new or different therapies or when unusual complications have occurred.

References

1. Panepinto JA, O'Mahar KM, DeBaun MR, Loberiza FR, Scott JP. Health-related quality of life in children with sickle cell disease: child and parent perception. Brit J Haematol 2005;130:437–444.
2. Barakat LP, Lash LA, Lutz MJ, Nicolaou DC. Psychosocial Adaptation of Children and Adolescents with Sickle Cell Disease. New York, NY: Oxford University Press, 2006.
3. Frenette PS. Sickle cell vaso-occlusion: multistep and multicellular paradigm Curr Opin Hematol 2002;9:101–106.
4. Hebbel RP, Osarogiagbon R, Kaul D. Endothelial biology of sickle cell disease: inflammation and a chronic vasculopathy. Microcirculation 2004;11:129–151.
5. Rother RP, Bell L, Hillmen P, et al. The clinical sequelae of intravascular hemolysis and extracellular plasma hemoglobin. JAMA 2005;293:1653–1662.
6. Macka AK, Kato GJ. Sickle cell disease and nitric oxide: a paradigm shift? Internat J Biochem Cell Biol 2006;38:1237–1243.
7. Krishnamurti L. Hematopoietic cell transplantation for sickle cell disease: state of the art. Expert Opin Biol Ther 2007;7:161–172.
8. Charache S, Terrin ML, Moore RD, et al. Effect of hydroxyurea on the frequency of painful crises in sickle cell anemia. N Engl J Med 1995;332:1317–1322.
9. Steinberg MH, Barton F, Castro O, et al. Effect of hydroxyurea on mortality and morbidity in adult sickle cell anemia. JAMA 2003;289:1645–1651.
10. Jacob E, Beyer JE, Miaskowski C, Savedra M, Treadwell M, Styles L. Are there phases to the vaso-occlusive painful episode in sickle cell disease? J Pain Sympt Manage 2005;29:392–400.
11. Ely B, Dampier C, Gilday M, O'Neal P, Brodecki D. Caregiver report of pain in infants and toddlers with sickle cell disease: reliability and validity of a daily diary. J Pain 2002;3:50–57.
12. Dampier C, Ely E, Brodecki D, et al. Characteristics of pain managed at home in children and adolescents with sickle cell disease by using diary self-reports. J Pain 2002;3:461–470.
13. Dampier C, Setty BNY, Eggleston B, Brodecki D, O'Neal P, Stuart M. Vaso-occlusion in children with sickle cell disease clinical characteristics and biologic correlates J Pediatr Hematol Oncol 2004;26:785–790.
14. Kato GJ, Gladwin MT, Steinberg H. Deconstructing sickle cell disease: reappraisal of the role of hemolysis in the development of clinical subphenotypes. Blood Rev 2007;21:37–47.
15. Niebanck AE, Pollock AN, Smith-Whitley K, Raffini LJ, Zimmerman RA, Ohene-Frempong K, Kwiatkowski JL. Headache in children with sickle cell disease: prevalence and associated factors J Pediatr 2007;151:67–72.
16. Dampier C, Ely E, Brodecki D, et al. Home management of sickle cell pain: a daily diary study in children and adolescents. J Pediatr Hematol Oncol 2002;24:643–647.
17. Dampier C, Ely E, Eggleston B, Brodecki D, O'Neal P, Dampier C, et al. Physical and cognitive-behavioral activities used in the home management of sickle pain: a daily diary study in children and adolescents. Pediatr Blood Cancer 2004;43:674–678.
18. Yoon SL, Black S. Comprehensive, integrative, management of pain for patients with sickle cell disease. J Alternat Complement Med 2006;12:995–1001.
19. Chen E, Cole SW, Kato PM. A review of empirically supported psychosocial interventions for pain and adherence outcomes in sickle cell disease. J Pediatr Psychol 2004;29:197–209.
20. Panepinto JA, Brousseau DC, Hillery CA, Scott JP. Variation in hospitalizations and hospital length of stay in children with vaso-occlusive crises in sickle cell disease Pediatr Blood Cancer 2005;44:182–186.

21
Chronic Pelvic Pain

Christine D. Greco

Abstract: Pelvic pain is a common but clinically challenging problem seen among adolescents. Dysmenorrhea and endometriosis are frequent gynecologic causes of pelvic pain; however, gastrointestinal, urologic, and musculokeletal conditions can mimic pain of gynecologic origin. Initial therapy is aimed at treating the underlying condition. Nonsteroidal medications, antidepressants and anticonvulsants are sometimes used in the treatment of pelvic pain. Patients who continue to experience pain may benefit from a multidisciplinary treatment approach consisting of medication trials, cognitive-behavioral therapy, physical therapy, and complementary and alternative therapies.

Key words: Pelvic pain, endometriosis, chronic pain, adolescence, irritable bowel syndrome, dysmenorrhea, interstitial cystitis.

Introduction

Pelvic pain is a common condition among adolescents and can result in significant disability and suffering. According to a survey of 2,700 adolescent girls, almost 60 percent experienced dysmenorrhea and 15 percent reported school absences because of pelvic pain [1]. Chronic pelvic pain accounts for approximately 10 percent of all referrals to gynecologists and 40 percent of all gynecologic diagnostic laparoscopies [2, 3]. Steege and Jamieson reported a 39 percent prevalence of pelvic pain among women presenting to primary care offices [3]. The treatment of chronic pelvic pain poses a considerable challenge to health care providers.

Common gynecologic conditions that cause pelvic pain in adolescents include dysmenorrhea and endometriosis. However, other conditions can be associated with pelvic pain such as irritable bowel syndrome, chronic constipation, interstitial cystitis, musculoskeletal conditions, and psychosocial conditions.

1. Evaluation

1.1. History

A thorough history and physical exam can help determine gynecologic and non-gynecologic causes of pain, and can help identify coexisting factors that exacerbate pain. Questions should focus on location, character and duration of pain, timing to menstrual cycle, and association with stress, activity, gastrointestinal symptoms, or urologic symptoms. The history should address issues of physical and sexual abuse, sleep hygiene, depression, and anxiety. Patients should be questioned about associated symptoms such as headaches and back pain.

1.2. Physical Exam

The abdomen should be examined for masses, allodynia, and location of pain. A thorough musculoskeletal exam can help identify areas of myofascial pain or other musculoskeletal causes. For instance, examining the abdominal musculature may reveal small, discreet bundles of muscle

G.A. Walco and K.R. Goldschneider (eds.), *Pain in Children: A Practical Guide for Primary Care.*
© Humana Press, a part of Springer Science + Business Media, 2008

that, when compressed, are not only tender, but also radiate pain in nondermatomally appropriate directions. Such trigger points are easily missed, unless the abdominal wall is considered as a potential site of pain. Hip flexion against resistance can identify a psoas muscle abscess in patients where fever and pain on walking are part of the clinical picture.

A pelvic exam should be performed; however, a rectal-abdominal exam may be better tolerated in adolescents who are not sexually active [4]. Presence of masses and areas of tenderness should be noted; tenderness in the cul-de-sac can often be a sign of endometriosis [4]. An examination of the lower reproductive tract can help rule out a congenital anomaly or imperforate hymen, which can be associated with endometriosis [5].

1.3. Testing

The history and findings on physical exam should be used as a guide for laboratory and diagnostic testing. Baseline recommended laboratory testing includes a CBC and CRP to help determine inflammatory processes, a pregnancy test, and a urinalysis and urine culture to help identify urologic causes of pain. A rectal exam with stool guaiac should be performed to help identify gastrointestinal causes of pain. A pelvic ultrasound may be indicated in some cases to determine the presence of masses, ovarian cysts, or congenital anomalies. Pelvic ultrasound may also be indicated when an adolescent declines a pelvic exam. Operative laparoscopy may help to establish a diagnosis, particularly when a patient fails conservative therapy.

2. Primary Dysmenorrhea

Primary dysmenorrhea refers to cramping in the lower abdomen during the menstrual cycle in females who have no underlying pelvic abnormalities. Other related symptoms can also occur such as headaches, nausea, and diarrhea. Pain can also radiate to the back and upper thighs. Dysmenorrhea is a common complaint among adolescents and is a frequent cause of school and work absences. The prevalence of dysmenorrhea in one study of 586 adolescents was 72 percent, with 38 percent of patients reporting moderate to severe symptoms

[6]. Harlow and Park found that 42 percent of college females missed some activity and 25 percent missed school due to menstrual pain [7]. One study showed that 90 percent of women presenting to primary care offices reported some degree of dysmenorrhea [3].

Symptoms of dysmenorrhea result from inflammation mediated by prostaglandins and leukotrienes which are produced by the endometrium in the uterus [8]. The cascade of prostaglandins and leukotrienes results in vasoconstriction and myometrial contractions, leading to ischemia and pain.

Nonsteroidal anti-inflammatory drugs (NSAIDs) inhibit cyclo-oxygenase and are frequently used for the treatment of primary dysmenorrhea see (Table 21-1). A systematic review showed that NSAIDs were significantly more effective in treating menstrual-related pain when compared to placebo [9]. A number of randomized-controlled trials have shown efficacy of a variety of NSAID preparations for the treatment of primary dysmenorrhea, indicating that proper dosing may be more efficacious than the choice of NSAID preparation [9–12]. For patients who consistently experience moderate to severe pain during menstrual flow, scheduled dosing of NSAIDs may provide more consistent pain relief than prescribing them to be taken "as needed." Since NSAIDs inhibit prostaglandin production, but not leukotriene or other inflammatory mediator production, some adolescents may continue to experience pain despite adequate NSAID dosing. Oral contraceptive pills (OCPs) suppress ovulation and reduce prostaglandin and leukotriene production. There is robust evidence to support the use of OCPs in reducing pain and other symptoms of dysmenorrhea, particularly when used in conjunction with NSAIDs [13, 14]. Patients who continue to experience significant pain should be further evaluated for causes of pain, such as endometriosis or structural anomalies.

3. Endometriosis

Endometriosis is a condition where endometrial implants are located outside of the uterine cavity. The ectopic endometrial implants respond to hormonal influences similarly to endometrial tissue within the uterus and are involved in the inflammatory response mediated by prostaglandin and leuko-

TABLE 21-1. Commonly used non-opioid analgesics.

Drug	Dose (mg/kg) (<60 kg)	Dose (mg) (>60 kg)	Interval (hr)	Daily maximal dose (mg/kg) <60 kg	Daily maximal dose (mg/kg) >60 kg
Acetaminophen (po)	10–15	650–1,000	4	90[a]	4000
Naproxen[b] (po)	5–6	250–375	12	24	1000
Ibuprofen[b] (po)	6–10	400–600	6	40	2400
Ketorolac (IV)	0.5	30	6		

[a]Maximal daily doses for acetaminophen should be reduced for infants and preterm neonates.
[b]Dosing guidelines for infants and neonates have not been established.
Note: For larger weight patients, daily maximum dose should not exceed recommended maximum dosing for adults.

triene cascades. Common sites of endometrial implants include ovaries, cul-de-sac, peritoneum, appendix, and cervix.

Studies by Vercellini and others have reported a prevalence of 25 to 38 percent among adolescents with chronic pelvic pain [15, 16]. It is estimated that as many as 70 to 90 percent of adult women with chronic pelvic pain have endometriosis [16]. Laufer et al. showed that almost 70 percent of adolescents who did not respond to conventional therapy of NSAIDs and OCPs were found to have endometriosis at the time of laparoscopy, indicating that adolescents who continue to experience chronic pelvic pain despite conventional therapy should be referred to a pediatric gynecologist for more definitive diagnosis and treatment [17]. Endometriosis can result in severe pelvic pain and should be suspected when empiric therapy fails to relieve pain. Data suggest that the severity of pain does not necessarily correlate with the extent of disease found on laparoscopy [18].

Endometriosis in adolescent women often presents differently than in adult women. Adult women with endometriosis typically experience chronic pain which is cyclic in nature. Other signs and symptoms in adult women include dyspareunia, endometriomas, and infertility. In contrast, adolescents with endometriosis can present with cyclic or acyclic pain [4]. In a study by Laufer et al., 62 percent of adolescents with endometriosis experience cyclic and acyclic pain, 34 percent experience gastrointestinal symptoms, and 12 percent experience urinary symptoms [17]. Endometriomas are rarely found in adolescent women.

Combinations of NSAIDs and OCPs are most commonly used for initial treatment of suspected endometriosis. For patients who do not experience effective relief of symptoms, operative laparo-scopy may be needed for a definitive diagnosis and removal of endometriosis. Data from randomized-controlled

trials among adult women show that medical treatment following surgical therapy was more effective for relieving pain than surgical therapy alone, presumably due to residual microscopic disease [19, 20]. Gonadotropin-releasing hormone (GnRH) agonists, such as leuprolide acetate, significantly reduce estradiole production and subsequent hormonal stimulation of endometriosis [21]. Because of concerns of bone density loss, GnRH agonists are typically used for adolescents following surgery with documented endometriosis who are over the age of 16 years [17]. Continuous OCPs are also used following surgery to suppress endometriosis, particularly in younger adolescents.

Procedures aimed at interrupting nerve transmission have been used in the treatment of chronic pelvic pain. Laparoscopic uterosacral nerve ablation (LUNA) disrupts efferent nerve fibers in the uterosacral ligament. Presacral neurectomy (PSN) disrupts sympathetic efferents from the uterus. The limited data from randomized-controlled trials do not support effectiveness of neuroablative treatment for either short-term or long-term pain relief [22], so referral to specialists for these interventional treatments is not warranted.

4. Irritable Bowel Syndrome

Irritable bowel syndrome is a functional gastrointestinal disorder that can present with a variety of symptoms and can be a non-gynecologic factor in the etiology of chronic pelvic pain (see Chapter 17 for details). Approximately 12.4 percent of adolescents with endometriosis have gastrointestinal symptoms [17]. In a study of 987 patients presenting to a pelvic pain clinic, 35 percent met criteria for IBS [23]. Diagnostic criteria include abdominal pain or discomfort that is associated with altered bowel function, such as a change in frequency or appearance of stool or pain which is improved with defecation [24]. Endometriosis can produce pain on defection (or urination), but a change in stool characteristics is not typical.

Patients should have no underlying pathology to explain the symptoms and should have a normal physical exam. Associated symptoms include bloating or abdominal distention and passage of mucous. Signs such as fever, poor growth, weight loss, or guaiac positive stools may indicate a more serious systemic illness. In the absence of concerning findings on history or physical exam, routine screening tests should include CBC, sedimentation rate, and stool culture. Routine extensive diagnostic testing is not indicated without warnings signs of systemic disease and may heighten patient anxiety.

Visceral hypersensitivity has been proposed as a possible underlying mechanism in IBS. VanGinkel et al., studied rectal sensation and rectal contractile response following a test meal in children with IBS [25]. When compared to healthy volunteers, children with IBS had a lowered threshold for pain and a disturbed contractile response to a meal, indicating that sensory and motor abnormalities may have a causative role in children with IBS.

The management of IBS should be directed at individual symptoms and the degree of disability. In general, therapy should consist of education and reassurance about their condition, dietary changes, psychologic counseling, and possible medication trials. Regular school attendance and participation in normal activities should be emphasized. Studies report that 50 to 90 percent of patients with IBS who seek medical care have anxiety, depression, social phobia, and other psychiatric diagnoses [26]. Since psychological factors appear to play an important role in IBS, ongoing cognitive-behavioral therapy, including relaxation techniques and self-hypnosis, are very helpful for many patients with IBS. A subgroup of patients may require psychopharmacologic evaluation. There are limited data on the efficacy of anticholinergics in the treatment of IBS in adolescents. Amitriptyline can be useful, particularly in patients who have predominance of diarrhea or for those with poor sleep. Kline et al. showed good results with peppermint oil capsules in relieving abdominal pain associated with IBS [27]. Fiber supplementation may provide relief in patients with a predominance of constipation, although some may experience an increase in pain due to abdominal distension.

5. Musculoskeletal Pain

There is some evidence to support that pain from pelvic musculoskeletal structures can be a contributing factor in chronic pelvic pain. In a study by Hertweck et al., 66 percent of patients aged nine to 23 years with unexplained pelvic pain were found to have musculoskeletal etiologies of pelvic pain [28]. On physical exam, 10 percent of patients were found to have trigger points. Ninety-five percent of patients had resolution of their symptoms after completing a physical therapy program.

In a study of 987 women with chronic pelvic pain, Steege et al. found that 22 percent of patients had tenderness of the levator ani muscles, and 14 percent had tenderness of the piriformis muscle, indicating musculoskeletal factors may play a significant role in chronic pelvic pain [29]. Patients with levator ani and piriformis tenderness had higher Beck Depression Inventory scores, higher McGill Pain Inventory scores, and had pain that was worsened with bowel movements. There is very little consensus on diagnostic criteria for musculoskeletal causes of pelvic pain and a lack of evidenced-based data on treatment. It may be worthwhile to refer patients with musculoskeletal pain to physical therapists who specialize in pelvic floor therapies.

6. Interstitial Cystitis

Interstitial cystitis (IC) is a condition characterized by pain (94%), urinary frequency (91.7%) and urgency (89.3%) [30]. The prevalence of IC varies according to criteria used to establish a diagnosis. When female third-year medical students were surveyed, 30.6 percent were identified as having probable IC-based on symptoms [31]. Parsons and colleagues reported a prevalence of IC in approximately 22 percent of women attending health care lectures [32].

The diagnosis of IC is typically made on the basis of history, physical exam, and negative diagnostic tests, including urinalysis, urine culture, urine cytology, and cystoscopy in select patients. Pain originating in the bladder can be localized to the suprapubic, vaginal, and perineal area, or may be perceived as diffuse pelvic pain [33]. Thirty-eight percent of women with IC report abdominal cramping [34]. In a study by Driscoll and Teichman, 33 percent of patients with IC presented with pelvic pain alone, without urinary symptoms, and there is evidence that some women experience exacerbations of IC symptoms during their menstrual cycle [30]. Depressed mood is a common feature among patients with IC; reports indicate that as many as 55 to 67 percent of patients present with depression at the time of diagnosis [30]. Physical examination may be normal; however, 30 to 50 percent of patients have suprapubic tenderness and 37 percent have levator ani tenderness [33].

The referred nature of bladder pain to the pelvis, often in the absence of other urinary symptoms, combined with an association of pain with menstrual cycles leads to difficulties in distinguishing pain of bladder origin from gynecologic sources. Myers et al. reported that 38 percent of women scheduled to undergo laparoscopy for chronic pelvic pain were found to have IC, based on the presence of symptoms and positive cystoscopy results [35]. In a prospective study by Feng et al., 69 percent of women with chronic pelvic pain had testing indicative of IC; laparoscopic findings revealed endometriosis in 28 percent of patients [36]. Data suggest that there is a high prevalence (96%) of IC among women with chronic pelvic pain and endometriosis [37].

Treatment of IC generally includes medication trials, often combined with cognitive-behavioral therapy, biofeedback, and physical therapy. Patient education is helpful in establishing realistic treatment goals. Pentosan sodium polysulfate is an approved medication for IC, typically used in adult patients. Data showing efficacy has been mixed, although some controlled studies have reported good response rates [38]. Tricyclic antidepressants and antihistamines such as hydroxyzine are also used in treatment of IC; however, there is a lack of evidence showing efficacy. Anecdotal evidence supports the use of gabapentin, but clinical trials are lacking. Since a significant portion of patients with IC may have depressed mood, cognitive-behavioral therapy may be indicated for many patients, in addition to other treatment modalities. Physical therapy aimed at strengthening and conditioning pelvic floor muscles may be beneficial

in select patients, particularly those with urgency and frequency; however, there are limited data on effectiveness [39].

7. Pediatric Pain Center: A Multidisciplinary Approach

Chronic pelvic pain may be due to a number of contributing factors such as endometriosis, irritable bowel symptoms, interstitial cystitis, and musculoskeletal causes. Patients may have a number of factors that coexist and contribute to overall pain. Many patients with chronic pelvic pain maintain normal activities; however, patients referred to pediatric pain centers represent a subgroup of patients who continue to experience severe pain and varying degrees of disability despite aggressive medical, and sometimes surgical, management [40]. There is evidence that use of a multidisciplinary approach for patients with chronic pelvic pain, that focuses on psychological, dietary, environmental, as well as somatic causes, results in significant improvement in pelvic pain, when to compared to a standard approach focusing solely on somatic causes [41]. A multidisciplinary approach to chronic pelvic pain in adolescents typically involves medication trials, cognitive-behavioral therapy, physical therapy modalities, and complementary and alternative therapies. A functional approach emphasizes regular school attendance, encourages normal family and school activities, and reduces pain behaviors [40]. Pelvic pain support groups can be helpful for adolescents who have significant school absenteeism and become isolated from peers.

7.1. Pharmacologic Therapies

7.1.1. Antidepressants

On the theory that much pelvic pain springs from hypersensitivity of the peritoneum and contents, often from chemical or inflammatory processes, medicines targeting neuropathic pain are often tried. Due to their neuromodulatory effects and analgesic properties, antidepressants have been used for a variety of chronic pain conditions in adults, including diabetic neuropathy and postherpetic neuralgia; however, there are limited data on efficacy of antidepressants in the treatment of pelvic pain [42, 43]. TCAs are typically chosen for patients who have IC symptoms with urinary frequency or those with diarrhea-predominant irritable bowel symptoms. Patients with poor sleep may benefit from TCAs due to their sedating properties. Because of rare cardiac dysrythmias, a baseline ECG should be considered prior to starting TCAs and if escalating to full antidepressant therapeutic range. A typical starting dose for nortriptyline is 0.2 mg/kg or 10 mg taken at bedtime see (Table 21-2). The dose can be escalated every 4 to 6 days according to pain and side effects until dosing reaches 1 mg/kg/day or 50 mg/day. Plasma concentration and a monitoring ECG should be considered prior to further dose escalation [44]. Selective serotonin reuptake inhibitors are occasionally used for patients who have pain and depressed mood or anxiety, and may be preferred over TCAs in some patients due to less constipating effects.

7.1.2. Anticonvulsants

Another class of medication that can be considered is the anticonvulsants. With little hard data for this group of medications, recommendations are difficult to make, but the low toxicity of several (e.g., gabapentin, pregabalin, oxcarbazepine) make them reasonable options when traditional medications do not help. Dosing is the same as for anticonvulsant purposes (see Chapter 8 for more details).

7.1.3. Tramadol

Tramadol is a centrally acting analgesic that exhibits weak binding to μ opioid receptors and inhibition of serotonin and norepinephrine reuptake. Tramadol is less likely to cause respiratory depression and constipation than pure μ opioid agonists, although risk of respiratory depression is increased when tramadol is combined with other sedating drugs [45]. Tramadol use is less likely to result in analgesic tolerance. Concurrent use of tramadol and tricyclic antidepressants can increase the risk of seizures. Typical adult dosing is 50 to 100 mg orally every 6 hours as needed for pain, with a maximum of 400 mg total dose per day.

7.2. Cognitive-Behavioral Therapy

Many adolescents with chronic pelvic pain experience significant school absenteeism and subsequent isolation from peers. Altered family interactions may serve to reinforce a patient's sick role within

TABLE 21-2. Tricyclic antidepressant and gabapentin titration schedule.

	<50 kg	>50 kg
a. Nortriptyline or amitriptyline	obtain baseline ECG	
Days 1–4	0.2 mg/kg q.h.s.	10 mg q.h.s.
Days 5–8	0.4 mg/kg q.h.s.	20 mg q.h.s.
increase as tolerated every 4 to 6 days until		
i. good analgesia or		
ii. limiting side effects or		
iii. dosing reaches 1 mg/kg/d (<50 kg) or 50 mg (>50 mg)		
iv. if condition iii, consider measuring plasma concentration and ECG before further dose escalation		
b. Gabapentin		
	<50 kg	>50 kg
Days 1–2	2 mg/kg q.h.s.	100 mg q.h.s.
Days 3–4	2 mg/kg b.i.d.	100 mg b.i.d.
Days 4–6	2 mg/kg t.i.d.	100 mg t.i.d.
Days 7–9	2, 2, 4 mg/kg (t.i.d. schedule)	100, 100, 200 mg
increase as tolerated every 3 days (with 50% of daily dose in the evening) until		
i. good analgesia		
ii. limiting side effects		
iii. dosing reaches 60 mg/kg daily (<50 kg) or 3 g daily (>50 kg)		

ECG, electrocardiogram; q.h.s., once daily at bedtime; b.i.d., twice daily; t.i.d., three times daily.
*Adapted with permission from Pain in Infants, Children and Adolescents, 2nd ed. Ed Schechter N, Berde C, Yaster Y. Philadelphia: Lippincott, Williams and Wilkins, 2003.

the family and can foster chronic pain behaviors. Patients with chronic pain are at risk for depression and anxiety which may interfere with their response to treatment. Individual and sometimes family therapy is necessary to improve coping skills and to treat other psychological factors such as depressed mood. Family therapy is aimed at normalizing patient and family interactions and can help reinforce regular school attendance and activities. Through cognitive-behavioral strategies such as self-hypnosis, guided imagery, and progressive muscle relaxation, patients can achieve distraction from pain, learn to greatly reduce muscle tension, and modify their experience of pain [46–48]. Self-hypnosis has been shown to reduce anxiety among adolescents undergoing pelvic examinations [47]. Biofeedback can allow patients to alter their physiologic response to pain; in initial studies thermal biofeedback reduced pain from endometriosis and dysmenorrhea [48, 49].

7.3. Physical Therapy

Limited data suggest that musculoskeletal conditions may play a role in pelvic pain, and that physical therapy may help to reduce pain, but controlled trials are needed to further evaluate efficacy of physical therapy modalities. TENS (transcutaneous electrical nerve stimulation) is often used in the treatment of chronic pain conditions and there is anecdotal evidence for TENS use in treating chronic pelvic pain. Controlled trials have shown mixed results and imply a substantial placebo effect [50]. Nevertheless, the TENS unit is not associated with significant side effects and is generally well tolerated by most adolescents.

7.4. Complementary and Alternative Medicines (CAM)

Acupuncture is one of the most commonly used CAM therapies and there are reports of using acupuncture to treat a variety of obstetrical and gynecologic conditions, including gynecologic cancer pain, pregnancy-related issues, endometriosis, and dysmenorrhea [51, 52]. A retrospective survey among patients of a pediatric pain clinic showed that adolescents with endometriosis frequently used acupuncture, and that 70 percent of patients

found it helpful in reducing pain [53]. Despite the widespread use of other CAM therapies, such as herbal preparations, there are limited data to support their efficacy in the treatment of chronic pelvic pain (see Chapter 16 for general discussion of CAM therapies).

Take-Home Points

• Chronic pelvic pain in adolescents can be a result of gynecologic, as well as non-gynecologic, factors.
• A thorough history and physical exam and systematic approach can help identify etiologies of pain.
• Multidisciplinary approaches combine cognitive-behavioral therapy, physical therapy, medication trials, and CAM therapies; limited evidence supports the effectiveness of a multidisciplinary approach in treating chronic pelvic pain.
• There is a great need for clinical trials examining the efficacy of treatment modalities in adolescents with chronic pelvic pain.

References

1. Klein JR, Litt IF. Epidemiology of adolescent dysmenorrhea. Pediatrics 1981;68:661–664.
2. Howard FM. The role of laparoscopy in chronic pelvic pain: promise and pitfalls. Obstet Gynecol 1993;48:357–387.
3. Jamieson DJ, Steege JF. The prevalence of dysmenorrhea, dyspareunia, pelvic pain, and irritable bowel syndrome in primary care practices. Obstet Gynecol 1996 87:55–58.
4. Laufer MR, Sanfilippo J, Rose G. Adolescent endometriosis: diagnosis and treatment approaches. J Pediatr Adolesc Gynecol. 2003 16:S3–11.
5. Breech LL, Laufer MR. Obstructive anomalies of the female reproductive tract. J Reprod Med 1999;44: 233–240.
6. Andersch B, Milson I. An epidemiologic study of young women with dysmenorrhea. Am J Obstet Gynecol. 1982;144:655–660.
7. Harlow SD, Park M. A longitudinal study of risk factors for the occurrence, duration, and severity of menstrual cramps in a cohort of college women. Br J Obstet Gynecol 1996;103:1134–1142.
8. Schroeder B, Sanfilippo JS. Dysmenorrhea and pelvic pain in adolescents. Pediatr Clin North Am 1999;46:555–571.

9. Marjoribanks J, Proctor ML, Farquhar C. Nonsteroidal anti-inflammatory drugs for primary dysmenorrhoea. Cochrane Database Syst Rev. 2003;4:CD001751.

10. Mehlisch DR. Ketoprofen, ibuprofen, and placebo in the treatment of primary dysmenorrheal: a double-blind crossover comparison. J Clin Pharmacol 1988;28:S29–33.

11. Mehlisch DR. Double-blind crossover comparison of ketoprofen, naproxen, and placebo in patients with primary dysmenorrheal. Clin Ther 1990;12:398–409.

12. Marchini M, Tozzi L, et al. Comparative efficacy of diclofenac dispersible 50 mg and ibuprofen 400 mg in patients with primary dysmenorrhea, a randomized, double-blind within-patient, placebo-controlled study. Int J Clin Pharmacol Ther 1995;33:491–497.

13. Larsson G, Milsom I, Lindstedt G, et al. The influence of a low-dose combined oral contraceptive on menstrual blood loss and iron status. Contraception 1992;46:327–334.

14. Milsom I, Andersch B. Effect of various oral contraceptive combinations on dysmenorrhea. Gynecol Obstet Invest 1984;16:284–292.

15. Vercellini P, Fedele L, Arcaini L, Rognoni MT, Candiani GB. Value of intrauterine device insertion and estrogen administration after hysteroscopic metroplasty. J Reprod Med. 1989;34:447–450.

16. Kontoravdis A, Hassan E, Hassiakos D, et al. Laparoscopic evaluation and management of chronic pelvic pain during adolescence. Clin Exp Obstet Gynecol 1999;26:76–77.

17. Laufer MR, Goitein L, Bush M, Cramer DW, Emans SJ. Prevalence of endometriosis in adolescent girls with chronic pelvic pain not responding to conventional therapy. J Pediatr Adolesc Gynecol. 1997;10:199–202.

18. Fedele L, Parazzini F, Bianchi S, et al. Stage and localization of pelvic endometriosis and pain. Fertil Steril 1990;53:155–158.

19. Parazzini F, Fedele L, Busacca M, et al. Postsurgical medical treatment of advanced endometriosis: results of a randomized clinical trial. Am J Obstet Gynecol 1994;171:1205–1207.

20. Hornstein MD, Hemmings R, Yuzpe AA, Heinrichs WL. Use of nafarelin versus placebo after reductive laparoscopic surgery for endometriosis. Fertil Steril 1997;68:860–864.

21. Vercellini P, Crosignani PG, Fadini R, et al. A gonadotropin-releasing hormone agonist compared with expectant management after conservative therapy for endometriosis. Br J Obstet Gynecol 1999;106:672–677.

22. Gambone JC, Mittman BS, Munro MG, et al. Consensus statement for the management of chronic pelvic pain and endometriosis: Proceedings of an expert-panel consensus process. Fertil Steril 2002;78:961–972.

23. Williams RE, Hartmann KE, Sandler RS, et al. Prevalence and characteristics of irritable bowel syndrome among women with chronic pelvic pain. Obstet Gynecol 2004;104:452–458.

24. Talley NJ. Functional gastrointestinal disorders in 2007 and Rome III: Something new, something borrowed, something objective. Rev Gastroenterol Disord 2007;7:97–105.

25. Van Ginkel R, Voskuijl WP, Benninga MA, Taminiau JA, Boeckxstaens GE. Alterations in rectal sensitivity and motility in childhood irritable bowel syndrome. Gastroenterology. 2001;120:31–38.

26. Lydiard RB. Irritable bowel syndrome, anxiety, and depression: what are the links? J Clin Psychiatry 2001;62:38–45.

27. Kline RM, Kline JJ, Di Palma J, Barbero GJ. Enteric-coated, pH-dependent peppermint oil capsules for the treatment of irritable bowel syndrome in children. J Pediatr 2001;138:125–128.

28. Schroeder B, Sanfilippo JS, Hertweck Sp. Musculoskeletal pelvic pain in a pediatric and adolescent gynecology practice. J Pedatr Adolesc Gynecol 2000;13:90.

29. Tu FF, As-Sanie S, Steege JF. Prevalence of pelvic musculoskeletal disorders in a female chronic pelvic pain clinic. J Reprod Med. 2006;51:185–189.

30. Driscoll AM, Teichman JMH. How do patients with interstitial cystitis present? J Urol 2001;166:2118–2120.

31. Parsons CL, Tatsis V. Prevalence of interstitial cystitis in young women. Urology 2004;64:866–870.

32. Parsons CL, Dell J, Stanford EJ, et al. Increased prevalence of interstitial cystitis: previously unrecognized urologic and gynecologic cases identified using a new symptom questionnaire and intravesical potassium sensitivity. Urology 2002;60:573–578.

33. Parsons CL. Interstitial cystitis: clinical manifestations and diagnostic criteria in over 200 cases. Neurourol Urodyn 1990;9:241–250.

34. Eickson DR, Morgan KC, Ordille S, et al. Nonbladder related symptoms in patients with interstitial cystitis. J Urol 2001;166:557–561.

35. Clemons JL, Arya LA, Myers DL. Diagnosing interstitial cystitis in women with chronic pelvic pain. Obstet Gynecol 2002;100:337–341.

36. Stanford EJ, Koziol J, Feng A. The prevalence of interstitial cystitis, endometriosis, adhesions, and vulvar pain in women with chronic pelvic pain. J Minim Invasive Gynecol 2005;12:43–49.

37. Chung MK, Chung RR, Gordon D, et al. The evil twins of chronic pelvic pain syndrome: Endometriosis and interstitial cystitis. JSLS 2002;6:311–314.

38. Parsons CL. Advances in the treatment of interstitial cystitis. Expert Opin Pharmacother 2006;7:411–419.

39. Weiss JM. Pelvic floor myofascial trigger points: manual therapy for interstitial cystitis and the urgency-frequency syndrome. J Urol 2001;166:2226 -2231.

40. Greco CD. Management of adolescent chronic pelvic pain from endometriosis: a pain center perspective. J Pediatr Adolesc Gynecol 2003;16:S17–19.

41. Peters AA. A randomized clinical trial to compare two different approaches in women with chronic pelvic pain. Obstet Gynecol 1991;77:740–741.

42. Max MB, Culnane M, Schafer SC, et al. Amitriptyline relieves diabetic neuropathy pain in patients with normal or depressed mood. Neurology 1987;37:589–596.

43. Bowsher D. The effects of pre-emptive treatment of postherpetic neuralgia with amitriptyline: A randomized, double-blind, placebo-controlled trial. J Pain Symptom Manage 1997;13:327–331.

44. Berde CB, LeBel AA, Olsson G. Neuropathic pain in children. In: Schechter NL, Berde CB, Yaster M, editors. Pain in Infants, Children, and Adolescents. Philadelphia: Lippincott, Williams & Wilkins, 2003.

45. Sinrup SH. Pharmacologic treatment of pain in polyneuropathy. Neurology 2000;55:915–920.

46. Eller LS. Guided imagery interventions for symptom management. Annu Rev Nurs Res 1999;17:57–84.

47. Rusy LM. Complementary therapies for acute pediatric management. Pediatr Clin North Am 2000;47:589–599.

48. Hawkins RS, Hart AD. The use of thermal biofeedback in the treatment of pain associated with endometriosis: Preliminary findings. Appl Psychophysiol Biofeedback 2003;28:279–289.

49. Kotarinos RK. Pelvic floor physical therapy in urogynecologic disorders. Curr Women's Health Rep. 2003;3:334–339.

50. McQuay HJ, Moore RA, Eccleston C, et al. Systematic review of outpatient services for chronic pain control. Health Technol Assess 1997;1:1–135.

51. Swisher EM, Cohn DE, Goff BA, et al. Use of complementary and alternative medicine among women with gynecologic cancers. Gynecol Oncol 2002;84:363–367.

52. Smith CA, Collins CT, Cyna AM, et al. Complementary and alternative therapies for pain management in labor. Cochrane Database Syst Rev 2006;18:CD003521.

53. Kemper KJ, Sarah R, Silver-Highfield E, et al. On pins and needles? Pediatric pain patients' experience with acupuncture. Pediatrics 2000;105:941–947.

Part V
Special Topics

22
Palliative Care for the Pediatrician

Norbert J. Weidner and Mark J. Meyer

Abstract: A multitude of diagnoses can limit the lives of children. Palliative care represents a branch of care with a distinct, family-centered approach. Symptoms can be far-ranging and include grief, anxiety, and existential concerns, in addition to somatic complaints, such as pain, dyspnea, and nausea. Therefore, a multidisciplinary approach best benefits the family and patient. Despite the varied underlying diagnoses, many of the symptoms will be common and amenable to a thoughtful, basic approach. Key to managing all of the symptoms in the palliative and hospice settings is communication. It is essential to understand the family's goals, fears, and wishes, and to integrate therapy into that superstructure. Fortunately, the primary care physician is in the perfect position to appreciate the basis for the child and family's goals The primary care physician's rapport with the family will facilitate communication and decision-making in what maybe a very stressful journey for the child and family. Palliative and end of life care extend to parents and siblings, who should be monitored for extreme reactions to the death of a loved one and supported as they heal after death has claimed a child.

Key words: Palliative care, hospice, pediatric pain, dying, chronic illness, bereavement.

Introduction

Many enter the practice of pediatric medicine because they have enjoyed the excitement and wonder of participating in the growth and develop-ment of young children and adolescents. Primary care physicians have the opportunity to educate and guide children and their families as they journey to young adulthood. Most often this involves caring for children who are experiencing disease proc-esses for which medical science has been able to provide an answer. However, advances in neonatal and pediatric medicine have converted previously lethal congenital and pediatric illness into chronic life-limiting or life-threatening conditions. Instead of dying at birth or early in childhood, these chil-dren now may live into early adulthood or beyond. This chapter will focus on this group of children with life-threatening conditions and their families, and the role of primary care physicians in partici-pating in or providing palliative care.

1. Epidemiology

Over 50,000 infants, children, and adolescents die in the United States each year, and hundreds of thousands more experience a life-limiting condition [1]. Although the lay press would have one believe that cancer is the leading cause of pediatric deaths, over half of pediatric deaths occur in the first year of life due to congenital malformations, complications of prematurity and low birth weight, sudden infant death syndrome, and the consequences of maternal complications of pregnancy. Older children and adolescents most commonly die from preventable causes such as accidents and homicide [2].

Chris Feudtner further refined our thinking with the chronic complex conditions (CCC) concept, those which are "expected to last at least 12 months

G.A. Walco and K.R. Goldschneider (eds.), *Pain in Children: A Practical Guide for Primary Care.*
© Humana Press, a part of Springer Science + Business Media, 2008

(unless death intervenes) and to involve several different organ systems or one organ system severely enough to require specialty pediatric care and probably some period of hospitalization in a tertiary care center." Such conditions accounted for 21 percent of all pediatric deaths in the United States over a period of two decades, with five percent attributable to cancer CCCs and 16 percent attributable to non-cancer CCCs [3]. Goldman, in Great Britain, has estimated that 50 of 100,000 children were living with life-threatening illness in 1999 and approximately 10 percent of these children die each year [4]. The significance of these numbers is that primary care pediatricians have limited exposure to dying children in their practice. However, it would be anticipated that primary care pediatricians would more routinely care for children experiencing chronic life-threatening illness.

2. Definition of Palliative Care

In 2003 the Institute of Medicine published *When Children Die: Improving Palliative and End of Life Care for Children and Families* [5]. This report presented a call to action to improve the systems of care for children with complex, life-threatening illness and their families. Subsequently, the term "palliative care" has gained increasing prominence in the lexicon of pediatric medicine. However, palliative care has come to mean different things to different people. Too often, palliative care is equated with end-of-life or hospice care. This is easy to understand, when one recognizes that palliative care and hospice or end-of-life care share a similar philosophy. Both wish to address the physical, emotional, and spiritual needs of families and patients facing a life-threatening illness. However, hospice is a managed care benefit, as defined and limited by government regulations, that deals specifically with end-of-life, focusing on an anticipated death. Palliative medicine is a multidisciplinary approach that interacts earlier in the illness trajectory to prevent or relieve symptoms produced by a life-threatening medical condition or its treatment [6]. When palliative care is equated with hospice, palliative practitioners are not invited to the table until the child is close to death. As a result, relationships built on trust (which are central to the provision of palliative care) are not given adequate opportunity to develop.

Others view palliative medicine as an extension of good fundamental medical care; care that not only addresses the disease, but also responds to the psychosocial and spiritual needs of the child and family. If one accepts a broad definition of palliative care as a philosophy of medicine that attempts to fill gaps in care that arise as children and families experience a chronic, life-threatening illness, one can better understand the possibilities of palliative medicine [7]. It is not about dying; rather, care focuses on assisting a child and family to live to the fullest extent possible by enhancing quality of life for the child and family, minimizing suffering, optimizing function, and providing timely and accurate information regarding the disease [8].

2.1. Essential Elements of Pediatric Palliative Care

Palliative care embodies the essence of family-centered care, with the child and family being the unit of care [4]. Palliative care should promote clear and culturally sensitive communication between the child, family, and their primary caregivers that assists the families in understanding the diagnosis, prognosis, and benefits/burdens of treatment options. There is a need to anticipate the illness trajectory and plan for changes in health status. Goals for care, as defined by the child and family, are outlined and communicated across care settings. The child's developmental and decision-making capacity is assessed, and an opportunity exists for the child and family to share in decision-making and care planning. Most importantly, palliative care includes a clearly identified team member responsible for coordinating care and assuring that changing needs and goals of the child and family are met. The hallmark of palliative care has been the management of distressing symptoms, whether they are physical, emotional, or spiritual. Respite and bereavement care round out the remaining elements of palliative care.

3. Identifying Children Who Might Benefit from Palliative Care

Once we understand the components of palliative medicine, we can determine who would benefit from such care. The Association for Children with

TABLE 22-1. Groups of life-threatening diseases in children.

Group	Examples
Disease for which curative treatment may be feasible, but may fail	Cancer Complex congenital or acquired heart disease Cystic fibrosis
Diseases in which premature death is anticipated, but intensive treatment may prolong good quality life	Muscular dystrophy HIV infection and AIDS
Progressive disease for which treatment is exclusively palliative and may extend over many years	Neurodegenerative disease Chromosomal abnormalities
Conditions with severe neurological disability that, although not progressive, lead to vulnerability and complications likely to cause premature death	Cerebral palsy Hypoxic encephalopathy

Life-Threatening or Terminal Conditions and their Families and the Royal College of Paediatrics and Child Health have outlined four broad groups of children living with life-threatening disease who may benefit from palliative services [9].

One can see that the spectrum of life-threatening illness suitable for palliative intervention is quite diverse. It should be noted that all of these conditions place children at risk of a premature death.

4. The Role of the Primary Care Physician

Although the provision of palliative care involves an interdisciplinary team, there is a significant role for the primary care physician. The primary health care team is in a unique position in caring for a child with a chronic life-threatening condition. They have often had the opportunity to develop a relationship with the child, siblings, and other family members during prior care experiences. The primary team will be most familiar with the family's support structure, as well as educational services, and other public and private community services that are important to the welfare of the child and family. Most importantly, the primary team can serve as a compassionate resource during the death of the child and for the bereavement that follows.

In 2002 the American Academy of Pediatrics called for the creation of a medical home for all children with special health care needs. The medical home is more than a central repository for medical information. At the core of the medical home is the concept of family-centered care—which is accessible, continuous, comprehensive, coordinated, compassionate, and culturally effective [10]. These principles are similar to that espoused for palliative care. As outlined in Table 22-1, many of these children with life-threatening illnesses are children with special health care needs.

4.1. Communication

Issues surrounding the communication of information, disease prognosis, and the family's beliefs and traditions are central to parents in evaluating the quality of their child's care [11]. A unique process for improving communication, clinical decision-making and care planning has been developed by the Pediatric Palliative Care Consulting Service at the Children's Hospital and Regional Medical Center in Seattle, Washington [12]. The process is an adaptation of an ethical decision-making model developed by Jonsen, Seigler, and Winslade [13]. The model is widely applicable to different care settings and maintains the child and family at the center of the process. The tool has four domains: 1) medical indications; 2) patient and family preferences; 3) quality of life; and 4) contextual issues. The medical indications domain documents the diagnosis, symptoms, and treatments, including risks and benefits. The patient and family preferences domain considers the developmental stage of the child and the communication style of the child and family. The components of life which give meaning to the child and family are noted in the third domain. Circumstances of the child's life which affect access and delivery of care fall under the contextual domain. An action plan is then formatted and the person responsible for the completion of each item is established. The plan is dynamic and can be altered in response to child or family requests and/or clinical changes in the disease.

4.2. Coordination of Care

A major hurdle for children and families with chronic complex life-threatening illness is coordinating information, subspecialty care, educational services, and other private and community services essential to the health of the child and family. Coordination of care by the primary care group—whether it is by a pediatrician, nurse practitioner, or social worker—along with the development of a written care plan is the cornerstone of palliative care and of the medical home model.

4.3. Respite Care

When care at home is complex and taxing, providing for respite care is a crucial and indispensable form of support. Respite care is an opportunity for caregivers to get a rest from the daily demands of home care which can be associated with caregiver fatigue and burnout [14]. Respite care is provided by another caregiver in the home or an outside facility (nursing home or hospital).

5. End-of-Life Issues

Providing care to children with a life-threatening illness can be a daunting experience. As stated earlier, children with life-threatening illness are at risk for a premature death. For this reason psychosocial, emotional, and spiritual support should ideally be introduced at the time of diagnosis or most certainly during any decline in the illness trajectory.

As death approaches and becomes a more concrete entity, it is crucial to communicate with the family regarding intent of therapy, goals for both life and death, and available options to help the patient and family. Concerns about using analgesics and sedatives need to be addressed, if applicable. Many parents want optimal symptom management, especially of pain and agitation, but have concerns about addiction and hastening their child's death. While opioids or other mediations

can have this effect, it is important to educate the family that the primary goal is comfort, not euthanasia. The Doctrine of Dual Effect suggests that in the terminally and irreversibly ill patient, analgesics that could hasten the demise of the patient can and should be used for their primary function, with a clear conscience. Understanding this concept and meshing it with the goals and wishes of the family as early in the clinical course as is practical will help avoid conflict and frustration for all (see "Total Analgesia" below). Bear in mind that the agreed upon plan can change as the family experiences the child's progression toward death; regular communication is helpful to keep family and caregivers "on the same page."

As the illness or condition progresses, the complexity of the child's illness may result in the primary team feeling less experienced than that of a consultant. Nonetheless, it is important to realize that children with chronic illness rated aspects of interpersonal care as important as the technical competence of physicians when judging the quality of their care [15]. By showing our humanness and compassion, primary care teams can stay connected and vital to children experiencing life-threatening illness and their families [16].

5.1. Grief and Bereavement

The death of child, even when expected, creates a unique loss for which there is no precedent and which challenges our many lifelong assumptions. For grieving parents, the loss of a child's life is a promise not kept—the promise of a full life. Bruce Himelstien described grief as a lifelong process in which parents adjust and integrate the loss into their lives, but they never "get over" the loss [7].

Grief does not begin when death is imminent, but occurs when families experience a new diagnosis or a missed developmental milestone, and persists years beyond the death of the child. Therefore, support should begin at time of diagnosis and continue through bereavement. In the early stages, the role of the primary care physician is to identify this loss and explore the meaning of the new diagnosis. Their role is also to obtain and provide accurate information about the diagnosis to assist parents in developing realistic goals for care. Parents value kind and compassionate caregivers who provide frank information in these instances [17].

Families value home visits tremendously. Such visits can be a powerful way for a health care provider to support the family, as well as gain vast insights into the real life and death issues of terminally ill children and their families. Being physically present relieves the family's sense of abandonment that can come as the end of the child's life draws near, and many care providers have pulled back, either from fear or a feeling they have nothing left to offer. Immediately following death the presence of the physician continues to be important. One need not stay long or "do" anything, either before or immediately after the child's death. A kind word and a held hand are powerful medicines at those times, especially if they come from someone they have bonded with through the course of the disease. Spending time with the child after death is something the family may need permission to do, and giving that permission is a special act that a long-involved physician can perform.

A skilled palliative nurse can help organize the final arrangements, and familiarity will ensure that the family's wishes after death are honored. Efforts to affect a good death through previous funeral planning become apparent at this point. Bereavement care can begin by expressing condolences and helping to assist in the details immediately following death. Funeral attendance is an opportunity to communicate a sincere interest in the family and help with personal healing. A follow-up phone call to the parents following the funeral provides the opportunity to discuss their feelings, and reinforces their understanding of their primary physician's interest to be helpful.

Active grief is a complex reaction to loss with psychological, physical, and behavioral manifestations. Feelings include responsibility, denial, and numbness. Parents and siblings may experience guilt because they believe they did not protect their child from death and suffering. The individual's response to death is variable, but marked by anxiety, crying, and psychological exhaustion. It is common for the bereft to see and hear the child. Somatic complaints such as headaches, back pain, as well as loss of appetite and disrupted sleep are common. The length of active bereavement is individualized, marked by exacerbations of loss, anger, and responsibility. Some suggest that active, uncomplicated grief last 6 months, while other sources suggest bereavement following the death of a child may last many years.

The vast majority of support for the aggrieved will come from family and friends, but the physician has a unique role to play. The primary physician's role is to acknowledge the loss, sadness, and anger of the aggrieved, while identifying those family members who are experiencing complicated grief. Assessment and reassurance of somatic complaints is helpful. The concept that grief follows an organized passage through various stages of psychological adjustment may not be true. Signs of successful adaptation include a sense of meaning for the child's death, a renewed interest in other areas, and hope in the future. More importantly, providers should note how severely the death interferes with daily life as the individual moves through the process. Providers can reach out to bereaved persons by inviting them to discuss what happened, and monitoring for depression, suicidality, sleep disturbances, and social isolation. For families (and physicians) seeking information and support online, Table 22-2 lists some useful web-based resources.

5.2. Complicated Grief

Risks factors for complicated grief include the child's death, sudden and unexpected death, history of psychiatric illness in the bereft, substance abuse, and ambivalent or strained relationships with the deceased [18]. Parents and siblings will not identify themselves as "struggling;" therefore, primary care physicians must take the initiative. Complicated grief can take several forms such as delayed, chronic, masked, or exaggerated grief. Key to all these forms is whether the bereavement is maladaptive. There is a failure to define a new life after the loss. Positive psychological and emotional adaptation to the loss is not made.

All parents of deceased children are at risk for complicated grief. The long-term health effects of the loss of a child indicate that grieving parents have higher mortality from natural and unnatural causes [19]. There is concern that those with complicated grief have higher rates of suicide and substance abuse. The intensity of support and resources necessary to continue adapting to the loss is often beyond the expertise of the pediatrician and requires referral for bereavement services. Many pediatric hospice and palliative care teams include a bereavement coordinator, and interventions include

TABLE 22-2. Web-based resources for physicians and families.

Families:

www.compassionatefriends.org

The mission of The Compassionate Friends is to assist families toward the positive resolution of grief following the death of a child of any age and to provide information to help others be supportive

www.dougy.org

The mission of The Dougy Center for Grieving Children is to provide support for children, teens and their families as they move through their grief process

www.nhpco.org

The National Hospice and Palliative Care Organization provides a web-based resource for families facing serious illness, death and grief

Physicians:

www.chionline.org

The goal of Children's Hospital International is to integrate the hospice concept into pediatrics so that it is an integral part of health care for children and adolescents

www.ippcweb.org

The Initiative for Pediatric Palliative Care (IPPC) is both an education and a quality improvement effort, aimed at enhancing family-centered care for children living with life-threatening conditions

individual and group counseling, including community support groups.

Though poorly explored, the death of a sibling is a catastrophic event. Pediatric assessment of bereaved siblings includes behavioral changes, persistent sadness, social withdrawal, and decreased activity in areas of interest. Providing support to siblings of ill children begins before death and includes honest, age-appropriate language. Siblings should be informed of the severity of the illness, and that death may result, and be invited to ask questions. They should be permitted to say goodbye and be present at the funeral if they choose to be. Children may attend funeral ceremonies under adult supervision. They must know they can leave if they are uncomfortable. Grieving parents may not be able to provide their children with the opportunity to express and discuss their feelings. They may not possess the insight to guide their children through a process in which they are struggling as well. Families may not support expressions of grief and may need outside resources to provide individual attention.

6. Pain and Symptom Management

Children living with life-threatening illness experience numerous symptoms related to their primary disease, as well as side effects from therapy. These symptoms can gravely influence quality of life throughout the course of the disease, and are often exacerbated during the active phase of dying. Patients and their families expect their physicians to provide effective relief from symptoms associated with life-threatening conditions. Effective symptom control is an important physician skill set in palliative care [7]. Though some patients die in the hospital surrounded by teams of specialists, this scenario is more common with cancer diagnoses. Many other patients remain at home with unaddressed symptoms. Children with non-cancer diagnoses, such as complex congenital heart disease, metabolic disorders, chromosomal abnormalities, and neurodegenerative disease suffer from the common symptoms of pain, dyspnea, and anorexia, but often remain at home. In a survey of admissions to Helen House Hospice for Children, of those with neurodegenerative disorders, 38 percent suffered from respiratory problems, with 64 percent of actively dying patients requiring strong opioids for relief of symptoms. Pain in this group was common and more than 80 percent experienced pain in the last month of life [20].

Unfortunately, many physicians feel inadequate treating a child's pain and effective management of symptoms is elusive, even in tertiary oncology centers where advanced care is routine [11]. Assessing symptoms complicates matters as there can be a disparity between parents' and physicians' perceptions of symptoms. Joanne Wolfe in her study of pediatric oncology patients, their parents, and physicians found parents are more likely than physicians to report that their child experienced fatigue, poor appetite, constipation, and diarrhea [17].

Families and patients expect their providers to impart effective insight into the evolution of symptoms as the disease progresses. Though a poor prognosis can represent a failure to providers, skilled management of symptoms and continued care of the patient can eliminate this helplessness. Preparing families for the path ahead is important, including preparative talks to relieve the fear and anxiety of an uncertain future [11]. Families that reported good symptom management also noted effective communication with the medical team, suggesting that good communication with the family facilitates assessment and control of symptoms. Additionally, Mack demonstrated the importance of direct physician communication with the child when developmentally appropriate [21].

6.1. Pain

Even in the setting of life-threatening illness, a basic pain care skill set is sufficient to treat mild and moderate pain. Referral to a pediatric pain specialist should occur when managing pain is expected to be challenging. With the dearth of such specialists, a few general principles can be applied with great benefit.

6.1.1. Initiating Therapy

Therapy is initiated with a thorough assessment of the child followed by a discussion with parents about the parental perceptions of the child's pain, goals of therapy, common side effects, and the expected evaluation and treatment plan if the symptoms continue to evolve. This is an opportunity to address parental concerns regarding addiction and develop a management plan in case symptoms become challenging. Focused discussions build rapport and trust with patients and family members, especially those who are suspicious of opioids. Patients and families are relieved to know their concerns about physical suffering are addressed.

Initiating opioid therapy in the opioid naive patient is done best by starting with low dose, immediate-release medications. Most μ-receptor agonists can be used (see Chapter 8 for details). Note that codeine is not useful for severe pain, and is not effective in 5 to 10 percent of the population [22], so it is not recommended for pain that is projected to escalate. The principle of titration is quite useful in very ill children (see Chapter 8, section 1.2, for details). For example, children with neuromuscular disease and obstructive sleep apnea may not tolerate standard opioid doses and may benefit from smaller doses. Immediate-release opioids should be started at low doses and prescribed every four hours as needed or scheduled. Following assessment, the dose can be increased in increments of 20 percent or more. Analgesics should be administered in a convenient, safe, and effective route. Intramuscular injection is not justified.

Once the pain is under control, twice daily slow-release tablets can supplant the frequent dosing of the immediate-release tablets. For breakthrough pain, rescue doses of immediate-release agents are available to the patient. Increases to the sustained-release opioids are made if more than 4 to 6 doses of immediate-release medication are required in a 24-hour period. Most immediate-release opioids are available as a liquid, making them suitable for delivery to small children, as well as through a variety of enteral devices. For long-acting opioids, enteral methadone and fentanyl transdermal patches are alternatives to the tablets of most extended-release formulations that must be swallowed intact. Both of these therapies should be approached in circumspect fashion, with methadone better left to pain specialists.

6.1.2. Neonates

Misconceptions about neonatal pain are common; most notably that neonates experience pain to a lesser degree than other children, the risk of treating neonates with opioids outweighs the benefits and effective comfort is unlikely to be achieved [23]. Neonates are more susceptible to the respiratory depressant effects of opioids, but effective opioid therapy can be readily initiated in all settings. Starting doses of opioids for children less than 6 months is one-quarter to one-half of the standard starting dose for children. This is followed by careful monitoring and titration to the desired effects as tolerated.

6.2. Opioid Side Effects

Managing opioid-related side effects is important to the child's well-being, and to compliance with therapy. Common side effects are pruritis, constipation, nausea and vomiting, and somnolence. Less common side effects are hallucinations, agitation, myoclonus, and urinary retention. The incidence of opioid-related side effects is dose-dependent. The side effect profiles for μ-receptor agonists are similar, but there is variability among individuals to the various opioids. Some side effects, such as nausea, vomiting, and sedation, can resolve without intervention following initiation of therapy or an increase in dosing. Often this occurs after 2 to 4 days of therapy. However, constipation that will not abate needs to be treated aggressively. Mild side effects are tolerated if effective pain control is achieved. If moderate to severe side effects persist, intervention is required. For symptoms that do not improve with intervention, changing to a different opioid (see "opioid rotation," below) can be effective.

Opioids can have profound effects on the gastrointestinal system: reduction of gastric emptying, inhibition of smooth muscle contractility, and stimulation of the chemoreceptor trigger zone. Nausea and vomiting can occur upon initiation of therapy or following an escalation in dose. Though this will diminish over time, many patients are unwilling to tolerate several days of GI upset. Medications affecting the chemoreceptor trigger zone in the brainstem are useful, such as prochlorperazine and ondansetron.

Pruritis is not generally caused by histamine release, but will sometimes respond to antihistamines, such as diphenhydramine and hydroxyzine. Opioid antagonists, such as low dose naloxone, can reverse many side effects, such as pruritis. Infusions of 0.1 to 0.3 mcg/kg/hour can bring relief, although, for practical reasons, this therapy is limited to patients on continuous intravenous fluids. Opioid agonist-antagonists, when given in small doses, can also relieve opioid-induced pruritis. For instance, nalbuphine at 0.05 mg/kg IV every four hours can be effective. For severe pruritis, opioid rotation may be needed.

Somnolence is a common problem and may be accompanied by respiratory depression. Approaches to remedy this depend upon the severity of symptoms. Naloxone can readily reverse somnolence and respiratory depression when symptoms are severe and life-threatening. Aggressive use of naloxone can reverse analgesic effects. When mild, the offending opioid can be held until somnolence resolves and then restarted at a lower dose, less frequent interval, or both. Reversing excessive sedation should be considered within the context of the goals of care for the patient. Often, somnolence is desirable to assist with disturbed sleep. At bedtime a larger dose of short- or long-acting opioid can be given to provide uninterrupted analgesia and sleep throughout the nighttime hours. An increase of 25 to 100 percent of the usual dose can improve sleep.

6.2.1. Idiosyncratic Reactions

Idiosyncratic reactions to opioids are uncommon, but they can be profound, nonetheless. Idiosyncratic manifestations range from irritability to agitation, delirium, and myoclonus. Younger children are predisposed to these reactions. They occur in the context of continuous infusions and rapidly escalating doses. Idiosyncratic reactions respond well to small doses of benzodiazepines such as lorazepam (0.05 mg/kg), but more severe and persistent reactions require opioid rotation. Methadone has shown to be an effective opioid when idiosyncratic reactions have occurred with multiple opioids.

6.2.2. Opioid Rotation

Though opioids have no ceiling effect, their total daily dose can be limited by side effects and idiosyncratic reactions. Indications for opioid rotation include intolerable side effects even if analgesia has been achieved and in the event of poor analgesia. Additionally, patients who have been receiving the same opioid for a length of time become tolerant to their effects and need a higher dose. By rotating to a new opioid, the individual may have less cross-reactivity to the new agent and also benefit from the same level of analgesia or better, but at a lower equianalgesic dose. Starting dose of the new agent is 50 percent of the equianalgesic dose of the previous opioid.

6.3. Progressing Pain

With progressing pain that follows a period of effective analgesia, increasing the daily dose by 20 percent is often effective. In rapidly advancing pain, the type most often associated with cancer, daily increases can range between 20 and 100 percent of the total daily dose until comfort is achieved. In non-cancer diagnoses, slight increases of 10 to 20 percent of the previous day's dose can provide substantial benefit.

6.3.1. Intractable Pain

While most non-cancer pain is managed by enteral opioids, cancer pain presents challenges to the pediatric practitioner. Pain in cancer is unique in that visceral, neuropathic, and somatic mechanisms of pain are involved. With solid tumor extension, especially with compression of nerve roots or the spinal cord, effective control extends beyond oral medications. Additionally, chemotherapy can result in painful mucositis, bone, joint, and neuropathic pain.

Complex and intractable pain states require aggressive therapy and interventions. Patient controlled analgesic (PCA) pumps are helpful with severe pain and have numerous advantages: they are beneficial with rapidly evolving pain, easy to titrate in small children, suitable for delivery at home (*via* home health care agencies), and are able to deliver opioids, including methadone and opioid agonist-antagonists. Additionally, many of these pumps are portable and can be placed in a back or hip pack. Pumps can operate with an infusion and bolus mode. Subcutaneous infusions can be run through insulin infusion catheters when central intravenous access is not an option. Ketamine, an NMDA-receptor antagonist with analgesic properties, can function as an adjuvant to opioids. Low dose (0.1 to 0.2 mg/kg/hr) or subhypnotic dose intravenous infusions are effective in providing analgesia. Side effects such as sedation and hallucinations develop at higher doses [24, 25].

Continuous neuraxial catheters are indicated for localized pain refractory to aggressive intravenous opioids. Notably in cases where a tumor has directly extended into the spinal cord or nerve roots, intrathecal catheters are uniquely useful. They are infused with a dilute local anesthetic, an opioid, and other adjuvant such as clonidine. These cath-

eters can be tunneled for prolonged use. In these circumstances, pediatric patients are best served by early referral to pediatric pain specialists.

6.3.2. Total Analgesia

Despite all aggressive measures to treat symptoms to achieve comfort, sedation is sometimes necessary. Often this is a subtle threshold that is crossed as analgesics and anxiolytics that possess sedating side effects are titrated to effect pain and agitation. Total analgesia can be an option once all other means to address the symptoms of the child have been exhausted, including consultation with a physician with pediatric palliative care experience. The goal of therapy is to relieve suffering although, in doing so, the patient's level of consciousness may be reduced, and death may be hastened. It is for this reason that total analgesia and its implications should be discussed with the family in advance of initiating therapy. The family needs to consider acceptable levels of consciousness and the risk of hastening their child's demise relative to the relief of suffering. Numerous medications are used to perform total analgesia: opioids, benzodiazepines, ketamine, dexmetomidine, and neuroleptics. Often these are used in combination. The primary medication is selected based upon the symptom causing the greatest suffering and then additional medication can be used to target other sources of suffering.

6.4. Dyspnea

The cause of dyspnea can be attributed to the primary disease, but reversible causes should be investigated. Children with neurodegenerative disease develop progressive dyspnea as a natural consequence. Patients benefit from both pharmacological and nonpharmacological efforts: corticosteroids, bronchodilators, fans, supplemental oxygen, frequent suctioning, positive pressure ventilation, cough assist devices, and good positioning. Antibiotics are often included in palliative care for the treatment of pneumonia. While some would consider these therapeutic measures, they are not inconsistent with palliative concepts in that they contribute to the comfort of the patient. For example, for patients with cystic fibrosis, continuing antibiotics is both therapeutic, but also palliative in that they provide comfort by reducing respiratory distress [26]. Irreversible causes of dyspnea benefit from enteral or intravenous opioids. Nebulized opioids have not been shown to provide any benefit over intravenous opioids. Frequent dose increases may be required in the opioid tolerant patient. Dyspnea is anxiety provoking and benzodiazepines can alleviate the anxiety that accompanies irreversible dyspnea. Promethazine can also be helpful with anxiety in this type of situation.

Families who watch a patient in respiratory distress find it very troubling, even when the patient is no longer responsive. Stridor, deep gasps, rattling secretions, and irregular breathing can cause considerable distress for those present. An infusion or intermittent intravenous injections of glycopyrrolate reduces excessive airway secretions. Frequent suctioning, opioids, and benzodiazepines are helpful, but this must be accompanied by reassurance that the unconscious patient is not suffering.

6.5. Nausea and Vomiting

Nausea and vomiting are common and causes include opioids or other medications, elevated intracranial pressure, bowel obstruction, constipation (opioids), anxiety, and pain. Once the cause has been identified, specific interventions may be invoked, including medications such as metoclopramide, promethazine, prochlorperazine, ondansetron, granisetron, dexamethasone, and scopolamine.

6.6. Seizures

Common causes for new onset seizures at the end of life include infections, metastases, metabolic derangements, and hypoxia. In distinction, patients who have a history of seizure disorder and experience an an increase in seizure activity may, in addition, have an alteration in their longstanding condition. In the latter situation additional investigation may be warranted. New onset seizures may be an indication of rapid disease progression and the active phase of dying has begun. Caregivers should be aware that seizures may result in death. Abortive therapy begins with lorazepam or diazepam. Rectal diazepam or intranasal midazolam are useful for the child at home without intravenous access. For persistent or recurrent seizures, prophylaxis should be initiated.

Take-Home Points

- The child and the family are the unit of care and form the foundation for pediatric palliative care.
- Palliative care should promote clear and culturally sensitive communication between the child, family, and their primary caregivers who assist the family in understanding the diagnosis, prognosis, and the benefits and burdens of treatment options.
- Psychosocial, emotional, and spiritual support should be introduced, ideally, at the time of diagnosis or most certainly during any decline in the illness trajectory.
- It is important to realize that children with chronic illness rated aspects of interpersonal care as important as the technical competence of physicians when judging the quality of their care.
- The vast majority of support for the aggrieved will come from family and friends, but the physician has a unique role to play. The pediatrician's role is to acknowledge the loss, sadness, and anger of the aggrieved while identifying those experiencing complicated grief.
- Patients and their families expect their physicians to provide effective relief from symptoms associated with life-threatening conditions. Effective symptom control is an important physician skill set in palliative care.

References

1. Cancer Pain Relief and Palliative Care. WHO Technical Report Series 804. Geneva: World Health Organization, 1990.
2. Arias E, MacDorman MF, Strobino DM, et al. Annual summary of vital statistics-2002. Pediatrics 2003;112:1215–1230.
3. Feudtner C, Hays RM, Haynes G, Geyer JR, Neff JM, Koepsell TD. Deaths attributed to pediatric complex chronic conditions: National trends and implications for supportive care services. Pediatrics 2001;107: e99–e103.
4. Goldman A. Care of the Dying Child. WHERE?: Oxford University Press, 1999.
5. Field MJ, Behman RE. When children die: Improving palliative and end-of-life care for children and their families. Washington, DC: National Academic Press, 2003.
6. Glazer JP, Hilden JM, Poltorak DY, editors. Pediatric palliative medicine. Child Adolesc Psychiatr Clin N Am 2006;15:xviii.

7. Himelstein B, Hilden JM, Bolt A, Weisman D. Pediatric palliative care. N Engl J Med 2004;350: 1752–1762.

8. National Hospice and Palliative Care Organization: (CHiPPs) Children's Project on Palliative /Hospice Services (e-mail newsletter), July 2003.

9. Goldman A. ABC of palliative care: special problems of children. BMJ 1998;316:49–52.

10. The Medical Home: Medical home initiatives for children with special health care needs project advisory committee. Pediatrics 2002;110:184–186.

11. Contro M, Larson J, Schofield S, Sourkes B, Cohen H. Family perspectives on the quality of pediatric palliative care. Arch Pediatr Adolesc Med 2002;156:14–19.

12. Hayes RM, Haynes G, Geyer JR, Feudtner C. Communication at the end of life. In: Carter B, Levitown M, editors. Palliative Care for Infants, Children, and Adolescents: A Practical Approach. Baltimore, MD: The Johns Hopkins University Press, 2004:112–140.

13. Jonsen A, Seigler M, Winslade W. Clinical Ethics, 6th ed. New York, NY: Macmillan, 2006.

14. Davies B, Steele R, Collins JB, et al. The impact on families of respite care in a children's hospice program. J Palliat Care 2004;20:4.

15. Britto MT, Devellis RF, Hornung RW, et al. Health care preferences and priorities of adolescents with chronic illnesses. Pediatrics 2004;114:1272–1280.

16. Browning DM, Solomon MZ. Relational learning in pediatric palliative care: Transformative education and the culture of medicine. Child Adolesc Psychiatr Clin N Am 2006;15:795–815.

17. Wolfe J, Grier HE, Klar N, et al. Symptoms and suffering at the end of life in children with cancer. New Eng J Med 342:326–333.

18. UNIPAC Two: Alleviating Psychological and Spiritual Pain in the Terminally Ill, 2nd ed. Am Ac of Hosp and Palliative Care 2004;Issue:49.

19. Li J, Precht DH, Mortensen PB, et al. Mortality in parents after death of a child in Denmark: A nationwide follow-up study. The Lancet 2003;361: 363–367.

20. Hunt A, Burne R. Medical and nursing problems of children with neurodegenerative disease. Palliative Medicine 1995;9:19–26.

21. Mack JW, Hilden JM, Watterson J, et al. Parents and physicians perspectives on quality of care at the end of life in children with cancer. J Clin Oncol 2005;23: 9155–9161.

22. Williams DG, Patel A, Howard RF. Pharmacogenetics of codeine metabolism in an urban population of children and its implications for analgesic reliability. Br J Anaesth 2002;89:839–845.

23. Sahler OJ, Frager G, Leveton M, et al. Medical education about end-of-life care in the pediatric setting: Principles, challenges, and opportunities. Pediatrics 2000;105: 575–584.

24. Mercadante S, Arcuri E, Tirelli, et al. Analgesic effect of intravenous ketamine in cancer patients on morphine therapy: a randomized, controlled, double-blind, crossover, double-dose study. J Pain Symptom Manage 2000;20:246–252.

25. Anghelescu DL, Oakes LL. Ketamine use for reduction of opioid tolerance in a 5-year old girl with end-stage abdominal neuroblastoma. J Pain Symptom Manage 2005;30:1–3.

26. Robinson WM, Ravilly S, Berde C, et al. End-of-life care in cystic fibrosis. Pediatrics 1997;100: 205–209.

23
Labeling of Pediatric Pain Medications

Hari Cheryl Sachs, Debbie Avant, and William J. Rodriguez

Abstract: FDA-approved labeling contains a summary of the available and essential scientific information needed for the safe use of a drug for a specific use. With few exceptions, only a limited number of medications frequently used to treat pediatric pain or facilitate analgesia are adequately labeled for pediatric patients. Consequently, most drugs are used off-label in children. Pediatric initiatives have generated more than 300 pediatric studies resulting in new product labeling for over 120 drugs. This chapter reviews several important lessons gleaned from these studies, regulatory highlights of the drug approval process, revisions to product labeling due to the Physician Labeling Rule, and controlled substance regulations as they apply to opioids. Pediatric labeling for drugs commonly used to treat acute and chronic pain, headaches, and muscle spasm is also reviewed, highlighting the significant gaps in labeling which remain, particularly for neonates and young children.

Key words: FDA, Pharmaceuticals, Physician Labeling Rule, DEA.

Introduction

The Food, Drug, and Cosmetic (FD&C) Act requires the United States Food and Drug Administration (FDA) to review and approve all new drugs before they can be marketed in the United States. The FDA evaluates new drugs based upon the scientific evidence obtained from clinical trials, pharmacology and toxicology studies, chemistry and manufacturing data, and proposed packaging and labeling information. Sponsors submit this information to the FDA in a new drug application (NDA). During the review of the NDA, the FDA assesses the safety and efficacy of the drug for its intended use, and determines whether the drug can be marketed in the United States. In the final part of the review process, the FDA and the sponsor negotiate the product's approved labeling.

Before important pediatric legislation was enacted (see Fig. 23-1 below), namely the Food and Drug Modernization Act of 1997 (FDAMA), the Best Pharmaceuticals for Children Act of 2002 (BPCA) and the Pediatric Research Equity Act of 2003 (PREA), many drugs were not approved for use in pediatric patients. In addition, prior to the pediatric legislation and related initiatives, many pharmaceutical manufacturers were reluctant to study drugs in children due to ethical and financial constraints or trial design challenges in studying children [2]. Many physicians erroneously presumed that children with conditions or diseases similar to adults could be treated as "miniature" adults. This assumption, and the lack of adequate pediatric information in labeling, resulted in the empiric use of these medications in children in the absence of evidence-based studies which establish safety and efficacy in the relevant pediatric population.

The number of adequate and well-controlled clinical trials performed in children has increased dramatically in response to these pediatric initiatives. These clinical trials have provided valuable information about the use of drugs in children, including information on efficacy, safety, pharmacokinetics,

G.A. Walco and K.R. Goldschneider (eds.), *Pain in Children: A Practical Guide for Primary Care.*
© Humana Press, a part of Springer Science + Business Media, 2008

Food and Drug Modernization Act of 1997 (FDAMA)

FDAMA created an incentive program known as pediatric exclusivity. Although FDAMA sunset on Jan 1, 2002, the incentive was reauthorized by the Best Pharmaceuticals for Children Act of 2002.

Best Pharmaceuticals for Children Act of 2002 (BPCA): "the carrot"

The pediatric exclusivity incentive reauthorized by BPCA allows the FDA to grant six months of marketing exclusivity to sponsors who complete voluntary pediatric studies in accordance with the written request (WR) issued by the Agency. A WR specifies the conduct of the pediatric studies, including the indication to be studied, pediatric age groups to be included, types of studies (e.g., safety and efficacy, dose ranging PK study, and/or long-term safety) and acceptable study endpoints, as well as the date the studies must be submitted to the Agency. Studies may include indications not approved in adults. Certain biologic agents and antibiotics are ineligible. In order to benefit from pediatric exclusivity, a drug must have existing exclusivity or patent protection. Pediatric exclusivity applies not only to the drug studied in the pediatric population, but also to all the sponsor's formulations, and dosage forms of drug products containing the same active moiety. BPCA also contained important new provisions, such as establishing a six-month review clock for pediatric supplemental new drug applications (sNDAs) and mandating public dissemination of the pediatric information obtained from these studies.

Pediatric Research Equity Act of 2003 (PREA): "the stick"

PREA requires pediatric assessments of new drug and biologic licensing applications (BLAs) for all new active ingredients, indications, dosage forms, dosing regimens, and routes of administration. PREA applies to NDAs and BLAs submitted to the Agency on or after April 1, 1999. PREA works in conjunction with BPCA, but unlike BPCA, PREA applies only to those drugs and biologics developed for diseases and/or conditions that occur in both the adult and pediatric populations. Drugs with Orphan indications are exempt from PREA. The pediatric assessment must be adequate to assess the safety and effectiveness and support dosing of the product for the claimed indications in all relevant pediatric subpopulations. Studies may be deferred if additional safety information is necessary or waived in all or part of the pediatric population if the condition does not occur in children or studies are not feasible. In addition, studies can be waived if evidence suggests that the product would be ineffective, unsafe, or does not represent a meaningful therapeutic benefit over existing therapies and is unlikely to be used in a substantial number of pediatric patients. If a waiver is granted based on evidence that the drug is unsafe or ineffective, this information must appear in the product labeling.

Both BPCA and PREA sunset October 2007. The Food and Drug Administration Amendments Act of 2007, signed into law September 27, 2007, reauthorized BPCA and PREA until October 2012.

FIGURE 23-1. A primer for pediatric legislation [1]

pharmacodynamics, and dosing in the pediatric population. In addition, new age-appropriate pediatric formulations are being developed. The new pediatric information has been incorporated into drug labeling and summaries of these studies are publicly available on the internet (*http://www.fda.gov/cder/pediatric/Summaryreview.htm*). FDAMA and BPCA have generated more than 300 pediatric studies that resulted in new pediatric information in product labeling for over 120 drugs (1997 to 2006). Pediatric studies resulted in approved pediatric pain indications for etodolac, fentanyl, ibuprofen, meloxicam, and oxaprozin, but not for sumatriptan and zolmitriptan. In addition, PREA has resulted in new pediatric information in product labeling for over 50 drugs and biologic products, including the following drug products:, bupivacaine/lidocaine, lidocaine/tetracaine, and epinephrine/lidocaine through December 2006. PREA labeling changes are summarized at *http://www.fda.gov/cder/pediatric/index.htm#prea*.

1. Important Lessons from Pediatric Studies

Several important pharmacokinetic, efficacy, and safety lessons have emerged from the pediatric clinical trials conducted in response to the pediatric initiatives as follows:

1.1. Pharmacokinetics

According to international guidelines, pharmacokinetic studies in the pediatric population should generally be performed in patients with the condition or disease, rather than in healthy children [4]. Pediatric pharmacokinetics, as well as the adult exposure–response relationship of the drug, must be evaluated to identify the appropriate pediatric dose (see Figure 23-2). Pediatric pharmacokinetics can differ from adult pharmacokinetics due to intrinsic factors, such as age, body weight, body surface area, and gender. Due to the complexity of all the factors involved, the pharmacokinetic differences may not be readily apparent or predictable. Growth and developmental changes can also lead to changes in pharmacokinetic parameters. For example, a study of mefenamic acid in 17 preterm infants indicated that the half-life was approximately five times as long as adults, consistent with the low activity of metabolic enzymes in newborn infants [5]. Mefenamic acid has not adequately been investigated in patients less than 14 years of age. Although not all pharmacokinetic differences are clinically significant, clinically significant differences may necessitate a dosing modification. For instance, a population pharmacokinetics study of an etodolac extended-release preparation demonstrated that higher doses, on a milligram per kilogram basis, are recommended in younger children (< 50 kg) with juvenile rheumatoid arthritis (JRA), compared to adults with rheumatoid arthritis [6].

1.2. Efficacy

The appropriate dose for children may be established via pharmacokinetic studies and/or through efficacy trials. For instance, the pediatric efficacy trials of meloxicam using a range of doses comparable to adult exposures demonstrated that the lowest dose (0.125 mg/kg/day) was as effective as higher doses [7]. Not all drugs that are efficacious in adults are shown to be effective in children. Multiple factors may contribute to this disparity, including physiological and pathophysiological differences between adults and children, as well as trial design issues. For example, efficacy has not been established for the use of sumatriptan and zolmitriptan in adolescent migraineurs.

Pharmacokinetics (pk) refers to the way a drug is handled by the body, and includes measures such as area under the curve (AUC) and maximum concentration (Cmax). These and parameters calculated from these measures such as clearance, half-life, and volume of distribution reflect the absorption (A), distribution (D), metabolism (M) and elimination (E). The overall process (ADME) ultimately controls the degree of systemic exposure to a drug and its metabolites after administration. The pharmacokinetic parameters must be considered when establishing the appropriate dose of a drug.

Types of PK studies:

Standard Pk Approach: Single or multiple doses of a drug are administered to a small number of patients (6 to 12) with frequent blood and/or urine collection. Samples are collected over specified intervals and assayed for concentrations of drug and relevant metabolites, if present.

Population Pk Approach: Relies on infrequent (sparse) sampling of blood from a larger population to determine pharmacokinetic measures. In general, 2 to 4 samples are collected per patient. The sampling scheme must be carefully designed in order to estimate population and individual means as well as estimates of intra- and inter-patient variability.

FIGURE 23-2. What is pharmacokinetics? [3]

1.3. Safety

Safety must always be studied in pediatric patients. Pediatric patients may be at a higher risk of serious adverse drug experiences and unexpected adverse drug experiences not typically observed in adults (e.g., Reye's syndrome and aspirin). Furthermore, pediatric patients may be more sensitive than adults to adverse reactions associated with the use of a drug, (e.g., transdermal fentanyl and respiratory depression, prilocaine and methemoglobinemia, nonsteroidal products and Stevens-Johnson syndrome). The effects of a drug on growth and development must also be considered.

2. Regulatory Highlights

FDA approval of a product is based on substantial evidence to establish both safety and efficacy of a drug for a particular use. In general, two adequate and well-controlled studies are necessary to provide independent confirmation of the study results. Thus, two safety and efficacy trials, as well PK studies to establish dosing, are typically necessary for a new indication in children that is different from that in adults (e.g., meloxicam for the treatment of juvenile rheumatoid arthritis). In certain circumstances, the FDA has relied on a large single double-blind, multicenter efficacy and safety study[1] to support approval of a new indication (e.g., celecoxib for treatment of the signs and symptoms of JRA). In this instance, confirmatory evidence from a long-term open-label tolerability and safety extension study and pharmacokinetic studies were also required.

For many products approved in adults, extrapolating efficacy in children may be permissible. Extrapolation is permitted when the pathophysiology of the disease and the effect(s) of the drug, both beneficial and adverse, in children are similar to those in adults. Additional pediatric pharmacokinetics and/or safety information is required to establish safety and appropriate dosing (21 CFR 314.55). The extrapolation of efficacy has been permitted for drugs such as ibuprofen (nonprescription use: fever, minor aches and pain, cold symptoms), fentanyl (management of chronic pain) and oxaprozin (treatment of the signs and symptoms of JRA). In these cases at least one pediatric safety trial was required in combination with pediatric pharmacokinetic data. For ibuprofen, the age range was extended down to 6 months from 2 years based on a large safety database of greater than 41,000 patients. The safety of transdermal fentanyl was established in three open-label trials in 291 patients, ages 2 to 18 years of age. Extrapolation of efficacy for oxaprozin in children ages 6 to 16 years of age with JRA is supported by evidence from adequate and well-controlled studies in adult rheumatoid arthritis patients and is based on the similarity in the course of the disease and the drug's mechanism of action in these two patient populations. A randomized, open-label, 2-week study in pediatric patients with JRA (≥6 years, n = 44) to evaluate pharmacokinetics and safety was also performed.

3. FDA-Approved Labeling

Under the FD&C Act, FDA-approved labeling, also known as the package insert, includes only those drug uses approved by the FDA based upon information submitted by the sponsor as part of a New Drug Application (NDA) or subsequent application, known as a supplemental NDA. Frequently, health care professionals are unaware of the significant differences between FDA-approved labeling and drug information resources such as the Physicians' Desk Reference (PDR) and ASHP Drug Information monographs. These resources and other pediatric drug handbooks or electronic references may also contain off-label uses and other information based upon the medical literature and expert recommendations not found in the

---

[1] Section 115 of FDAMA amended the definition of substantial evidence in section 505(d) of the Federal Food, Drug, and Cosmetic Act (the FD&C Act) (21 U.S.C. 355(d)) to clarify that FDA, at its discretion, may make exception to the general requirement that there must be more than one adequate and well-controlled investigation to support an effectiveness determination. Section 115 of the Modernization Act provides in relevant part that "[i]f the [agency] determines, based on relevant science, that data from one adequate and well-controlled clinical investigation and confirmatory evidence (obtained prior to or after such investigation) are sufficient to establish effectiveness, the [agency] may consider such data and evidence to constitute substantial evidence [of effectiveness]."

FDA-approved labeling. Uses of a drug product in a manner not contained in labeling (e.g., new or modified uses, new dosage regimens, new routes of administration, or use in additional patient populations) are known as off-label uses. The FD&C Act does not limit the manner in which a physician may use an approved drug. A physician may choose to prescribe a drug for conditions or in treatment regimens or patient populations that are not included in approved labeling. Off-label uses are especially common in pediatrics, oncology, and rare diseases. New or modified uses, as well as new dosage regimens, new routes of administration, or additional patient populations may be added to drug labeling after initial drug approval. The sponsor must submit a supplemental NDA, containing new clinical studies and additional information outlined in 21 CFR 314.50 to the FDA for review. The Agency will review the supplemental application to determine if there is sufficient evidence to establish effectiveness to revise product labeling.

Labeling contains a summary of the essential scientific information needed for the safe use of a drug for a particular use. Effective June 30, 2006, pursuant to the enactment of the Physician Labeling Rule, the FDA instituted major revisions to product labeling to provide health care professionals with clear and concise prescribing information.[2] In an effort to manage the risks of medication use and reduce medical errors, the newly designed labeling is intended to present the most up-to-date information in an easy-to-read format that draws physician and patient attention to the most important pieces of drug information before a product is prescribed. The new format will also facilitate the use of electronic prescribing tools and other electronic information resources. Detailed information regarding the new format can be found at *http://www.fda.gov/cder/regulatory/ physLabel/default.htm*. The new labeling format includes new sections such as Highlights and Table of Contents. The Highlights section for a fictitious product appears in Figure 23-3.

The Highlights section of the labeling includes an approximately half-page summary which provides immediate access to the most important or commonly referred to information (e.g., Boxed Warning, Indications and Usage, Dosage and Administration, Dosage Forms and Strengths). The initial United States approval date and revision date, if any, are also included. In addition, to alert practitioners and patients to important changes or additions to labeling, a list of substantive changes to Boxed Warnings, Indications and Usage, Dosage and Administration, Contraindications, and Warnings and Precautions will be included in a section entitled, "Recent Major Changes." Contact information to report an adverse drug reaction will be easily accessible at the end of the Highlights section. The Table of Contents will serve as a navigational tool and will reference the full prescribing information by sections and subsections.

Certain sections of labeling have also been restructured. In the new format, information from the old Warnings section and old Precautions section is combined into a single new Warnings and Precautions section. This section will be followed by the Adverse Reactions section, consolidating risk information in one location. Several new sections have been added: 1) Use in Special Populations– pediatrics, geriatrics; 2) Drug Interactions (which has been separated from Precautions); and 3) Patient Counseling Information. FDA-approved patient package information, if any, must be reprinted at the end. In addition to the new sections, new information has also been added to product labeling. Clinical studies and non-clinical toxicology information are now required for all products. Changes in labeling such as a new dosage form and medication strength will be highlighted. The established pharmacologic class for the drug product must now appear in the Indications and Usage section.

The new requirements only apply to drugs that were approved on or after June 30, 2006, drugs that have been approved in the five years prior to June 30, 2006, and older drugs for which there is a major change in the prescribing information (e.g., approval of a new use). Older approved drug products can voluntarily revise their prescribing information. Labeling for applications submitted on or after June 30, 2006 must be submitted in the new format. The implementation of the new

---

[2] Final Rule: Requirements on the Content and Format of Labeling for Human Prescription Drug and Biological Products, January 24, 2006. Effective June 30, 2006.

HIGHLIGHTS OF PRESCRIBING INFORMATION
These highlights do not include all the information needed to use Imdicon
safely and effectively. See full prescribing information for Imdicon.

IMDICON® (cholinasol) CAPSULES
Initial U.S. Approval: 200X

**WARNING: LIFE-THREATENING HEMATOLOGICAL ADVERSE
REACTIONS**

See full prescribing information for complete boxed warning.
**Monitor for hematological adverse reactions every 2 weeks for first 3
months of treatment (5.2). Discontinue Imdicon immediately if any of the
following occur:**
- **Neutropenia/agranulocytosis (5.1)**
- **Thrombotic thrombocytopenic purpura (5.1)**
- **Aplastic anemia (5.1)**

-----------------------RECENT MAJOR CHANGES-----------------

Indications and Usage, Coronary Stenting (1.2)	2/200X
Dosage and Administration, Coronary Stenting (2.2)	2/200X

-----------------------INDICATIONS AND USAGE-----------------
Imdicon is an adenosine diphosphate (ADP) antagonist platelet aggregation
inhibitor indicated for:
- Reducing the risk of thrombotic stroke in patients who have experienced
  stroke precursors or who have had a completed thrombotic stroke (1.1)
- Reducing the incidence of subacute coronary stent thrombosis, when
  used with aspirin (1.2)
Important limitations:
- For stroke, Imdicon should be reserved for patients who are intolerant of
  or allergic to aspirin or who have failed aspirin therapy (1.1)

-----------------------DOSAGE AND ADMINISTRATION-----------------
- Stroke: 50 mg once daily with food. (2.1)
- Coronary Stenting: 50 mg once daily with food, with antiplatelet doses
  of aspirin, for up to 30 days following stent implantation (2.2)
Discontinue in renally impaired patients if hemorrhagic or hematopoietic
problems are encountered (2.3, 8.6, 12.3)

-----------------------DOSAGE FORMS AND STRENGTHS-----------------
Capsules: 50 mg (3)

-----------------------CONTRAINDICATIONS-----------------
- Hematopoietic disorders or a history of TTP or aplastic anemia (4)
- Hemostatic disorder or active bleeding (4)
- Severe hepatic impairment (4, 8.7)

-----------------------WARNINGS AND PRECAUTIONS-----------------
- Neutropenia (2.4% incidence; may occur suddenly; typically resolves
  within 1-2 weeks of discontinuation), thrombotic thrombocytopenic
  purpura (TTP), aplastic anemia, agranulocytosis, pancytopenia,
  leukemia, and thrombocytopenia can occur (5.1)
- Monitor for hematological adverse reactions every 2 weeks through the
  third month of treatment (5.2)

-----------------------ADVERSE REACTIONS-----------------
Most common adverse reactions (incidence >2%) are diarrhea, nausea,
dyspepsia, rash, gastrointestinal pain, neutropenia, and purpura (6.1).

**To report SUSPECTED ADVERSE REACTIONS, contact
(manufacturer) at (phone # and Web address) or FDA at 1-800-FDA-1088
or *www.fda.gov/medwatch.***

-----------------------DRUG INTERACTIONS-----------------
- Anticoagulants: Discontinue prior to switching to Imdicon (5.3, 7.1)
- Phenytoin: Elevated phenytoin levels have been reported. Monitor
  levels. (7.2)

-----------------------USE IN SPECIFIC POPULATIONS-----------------
- Hepatic impairment: Dose may need adjustment. Contraindicated in
  severe hepatic disease (4, 8.7, 12.3)
- Renal impairment: Dose may need adjustment (2.3, 8.6, 12.3)

**See 17 for PATIENT COUNSELING INFORMATION and FDA-
approved patient labeling**

Revised: 5/200X

FULL PRESCRIBING INFORMATION: CONTENTS*

FIGURE 23-3. Highlights of prescribing information for a fictitious product [8]

---

content and format revisions to labeling for applications approved in the five years prior to June 30, 2006 will be gradual. Electronic product labeling is accessible at "DailyMed," an interagency online clearinghouse maintained by the FDA and the National Library of Medicine. The link for "DailyMed" is *http://dailymed.nlm.nih.gov*. Drug approval history as well as drug labeling can also be found at "Drugs@FDA" *http://www.access-data.fda.gov/scripts/cder/drugsatfda/index.cfm*.

4. Special Topics: DEA Regulations

Labeling for substances such as opioids and their antagonists includes information on the potential for abuse, misuse, and diversion. The Controlled Substances Act (CSA) governs the legal distribution and use of most substances with significant abuse potential. The Drug Enforcement Agency is the primary federal agency charged with enforcing these regulations. The DEA schedules (see Table 23-1) are ranked from I (highest abuse potential) to V (least abuse potential). Schedule II to V substances have approved medical uses. The DEA regulates the prescription requirements for controlled substances, including the manner in which a prescription can be communicated to the pharmacist (oral, facsimile, written), the life of the prescription, and the number of refills permitted. In addition, physicians should be familiar with specific state regulations since some states have regulations that are stricter than the federal requirements. When state and federal regulations differ, the stricter requirement takes precedence.

TABLE 23-1. DEA schedules: selected pain-related examples of drugs from each schedule.

Schedule	Accepted Medical Use	Selected Examples	Prescription Requirement	Refills
Schedule I	No	Marijuana, THC, LSD, mescaline, MDMA, peyote, heroin	N/A	N/A
Schedule II	Yes	Alfentanil, dihydrocodeine, codeine, hydrocodone, fentanyl, levorphanol, meperidine, methadone, morphine, oxycodone, oxymorphone	Written prescription required, verbal order only in emergency (written prescription must be presented to pharmacist within seven days)	Prohibited
Schedule III	Yes	Codeine combination products, dihydrocodeine combination products, hydrocodone combination products, ketamine, paregoric and anabolic steroids	Written, facsimile, verbal order	Five refills or 6 months, whichever occurs first
Schedule IV	Yes	Butorphanol, propoxyphene combinations including propoxyphene/APAP, pentazocine combinations including pentazocine/naloxone	Written, facsimile, verbal order	Five refills or 6 months, whichever occurs first
Schedule V	Yes	Products containing limited quantities of: codeine (not more than 200 mg /100 mL or per 100 g) dihydrocodeine (100 mg /100 mL or per 100 g)	Written, facsimile, verbal order	As authorized by practitioner

See 21 CFR 1308.11–1308.15 for the complete list of Schedules of Controlled Substances [9, 10].

5. Pediatric Labeling for Drugs Commonly Used For Analgesia or Anesthesia as of December 2006

The following section describes general indications (e.g., acute pain, chronic pain, headache, and muscle relaxants) for pain medications commonly used in children. Details regarding FDA-approved indications related to pain can be found in Table 23-2 (Pediatric Labeling of Drugs Commonly Used for Analgesia or Anesthesia) and Table 23-3 (FDA-Approved Indications for Drugs Approved to Treat Pain in Adults only).

5.1. Acute Pain

5.1.1. Acetaminophen, Aspirin, and Nonsteroidal Agents

To treat minor aches and pain, acetaminophen and ibuprofen (2 years and older) and naproxen (for adolescents) are available over-the-counter (OTC).

Prescription ibuprofen suspension labeling contains dosing information for children 6 months to 2 years of age. Acetaminophen and ibuprofen are common components in combination products for the relief of moderate to severe pain, although many are not approved in children (see Table 23-2 and 23-3 for the specific products which are approved in children). Combination products such as acetaminophen and pentazocine, as well as naloxone and pentazocine, are approved for use in adolescents (see Opioids section, below).

A single dose of ketorolac (IV or IM) is indicated for the short-term treatment of severe, acute pain requiring analgesia at the opioid level for children 2 years and older. Oral agents such as mefenamic acid and diflunisal may be used in adolescents. Mefenamic acid is indicated for the short-term treatment (less than 1 week) of mild to moderate pain or primary dysmenorrhea in adolescents 14 years of age and older. Diflunisal is approved for the treatment of mild to moderate pain in adolescents 12 years of age and older.

TABLE 23-2. Pediatric labeling of drugs commonly used for analgesia or anesthesia. FDA-approved indications and dosing for commonly utilized pain medications (based on package insert as of Feb 2007).

Drug	Trade Name	Formulation	Indication in Adults	Indication in Children by Age	Pediatric Dosing	Maximum Dose	Comments
Acetaminophen, aspirin and NSAIDs							
Acetaminophen	Tylenol	Tablet, chewable, sprinkle capsule, suspension, elixir, rectal suppository	Fever, Minor aches and pains	≥ 2 years	24–35 lbs: 160 mg 36–47 lbs: 240 mg 48–59 lbs: 320 mg 60–71 lbs: 400 mg 72–95 lbs: 480 mg	5 doses/day	Manufacturer suggested dosing regimens in younger children are NOT FDA-approved
Aspirin	Various	Chewable tablet, tablet, caplet	Minor aches and pains	The CFR permits aspirin to be used in children 3 years and older, but most manufacturers have chosen only to market aspirin for 12 years and older due to the concern of Reye's syndrome	≥ 12 years: 325 to 650 mg q 4 hrs Professional labeling for JRA: 90 to 130 mg/kg/day (21 CFR 343.80)	3,900 mg/day	Per 21 CFR 201.314, aspirin and other salicylates must have special warnings for use in children including Reye's syndrome warning. Retail containers of 1¼ grain (pediatric) containing more than 36 tablets aspirin tablets cannot be distributed
Celecoxib	Celebrex	Oral capsule	Acute pain, dysmenorrhea, OA, RA, ankylosing spondylitis	JRA ≥ 2 years	≥10 to ≤25kg: 50 mg BID >25Kg: 100mg BID	Adults: 200 mg BID, not longer than 24 weeks	Use lowest effective dose for shortest duration consistent with individual treatment goals Celecoxib should be used only with caution in patients with systemic onset JRA
Diflunisal	Generic	Oral tablet	Mild to moderate pain, OA, RA	≥ 12 years	1,000 mg initally, 500 mg q 8 to 12 hr	1,500 mg	Lower doses appropriate depending on pain severity, patient response, and weight Precautions: Reye's syndrome

	Generic			JRA ≥ 6 years		20 mg/kg (1,000 mg)	Balance risk/benefit, use lowest effective dose
Etodolac XL		Extended-release tablet	Acute pain, OA, RA	JRA ≥ 6 years	20 to 30 kg: 400 mg 31 to 45 kg: 600 mg 46 to 60 kg: 800 mg > 60 kg: 1000 mg	20 mg/kg (1,000 mg)	Balance risk/benefit, use lowest effective dose
Ibuprofen	Advil, Motrin, generic	Oral suspension, chewable tablet, capsule, liquigel	Rx: Mild to moderate pain, OA, RA, dysmenorrhea OTC: Minor aches and pain, fever	Rx: Mild to moderate pain, OA, RA, dysmenorrhea 6mo to 2 years JRA, fever OTC: ≥ 2 years	Fever: 5 to 10 mg/kg q 6 to 8h Pain: 10 mg/kg q 6 to 8h JRA: 30 to 40 mg/kg/day divided TID to QID	40 mg/kg/day (pain and fever) 50 mg/kg/day (JRA)	Monitor liver function at doses > 30 mg/kg/day
Indomethacin	Indocin, Indocin SR	Oral suspension, extended release capsule, rectal suppository	Moderate to severe RA, OA, gouty arthritis, ankylosing spondylitis; acute shoulder bursitis or tendinitis	≥ 14 years (Dose is suggested for patients 2 years and older)	starting dose: 1 to 2 mg/kg in divided doses	4 mg/kg/day (150 to 200 mg)	Intravenous forms not indicated for pain (indicated for PDA closure) If use in children ≥ 2 years, monitor closely including period assessment of liver function
Ketorolac	Toradol	Injectable	Short term (5 days) moderate to severe acute pain at opioid level	≥ 2 years: Single dose therapy only	Single dose therapy 1 mg/kg IM 0.5 mg/kg IV	Single dose therapy IM: 30 mg IV: 15 mg	Oral forms not approved in children
Mefenamic acid	Ponstel	Oral capsule	Short term (7 days) mild to moderate pain, dysmenorrhea	≥ 14 years	500 mg initially, 250 mg q 6hr prm	One week	Use lowest effective dose for the shortest duration consistent with individual patient goals
Meloxicam	Mobic	Oral tablet, suspension	OA, RA	JRA ≥ 2 years	0.125 mg/kg	7.5 mg	Use lowest dose available for shortest duration
Naproxen	Naproxyn, EC Naproxen, Anaprox, Anaprox DS	Oral Tablet, delayed release tablet, suspension	Pain, RA, OA, ankylosing spondylitis, tendonitis, bursitis, gout, dysmenorrhea	JRA ≥ 2 years	5 mg/kg BID	15 mg/kg/day	Nonprescription dosing ≥ 12 years as pain reliever/fever reducer: 200 mg naproxen (220 mg naproxen sodium) po BID

(continued)

TABLE 23-2. (continued)

Drug	Trade Name	Formulation	Indication in Adults	Indication in Children by Age	Pediatric Dosing	Maximum Dose	Comments
Oxaprozin	Daypro	Oral tablet	OA, RA	JRA ≥ 6 years	22 to 31 kg: 600 mg 32 to 54 kg: 900 mg ≥ 55 kg: 1,200 mg	1,200 mg	Individualize doses
Tolmetin	Tolectin, Tolectin DS	Tablet, capsules	OA, RA (acute flares and long-term management)	JRA ≥ 2 years	20 mg/kg/day divided TID or QID Maintenance 15 to 30 mg/kg/day	30 mg/kg/day	Use lowest effective dose for the shortest duration
Amide anesthetics							
Articaine	Septocaine	Injectable	Dental and periodontal procedures	≥ 4 years	Dosages should be reduced commensurate with age, body weight and physical condition	7 mg/kg	Contains sodium metabisulfite
Bupivacaine hydrochloride and lidocaine hydrochloride	Duocaine	Injectable	Ophthalmologic surgery (parabulbar, retrobulbar or facial block)	≥ 12 years	Usual dose: Retrobulbar: 2 to 5 mL Peribulbar: 6 to 12 mL	0.18 mL/kg (12 mL or 120 mg lidocaine and 45 mg bupivacaine)	Adjust dose if contains epinephrine Not approved for spinal in children
Chloroprocaine (1 and 2%)	Nesacaine 1 and 2%	Injectable	Local anesthesia (infiltration, peripheral) Not lumbar or caudal	All ages	0.5 to 1.0% suggested for infiltration, 1.0 to 1.5% nerve block	Difficult to recommend maximum, dose varies with weight and age and should not exceed	Contains PABA
Chloroprocaine 2 and 3%	Nesacaine-MPF 2 and 3%	Injectable	Local anesthesia (infiltration, peripheral and central nerve block, including lumbar and caudal epidural)	All ages	Determined by weight and age, lowest effective dose	11 mg/kg	
Clonidine hydrochloride	Duraclon	Injectable	Severe pain in cancer patients in combination with opiates	Restricted to severe intractable pain unresponsive to conventional analgesic techniques	0.5 ug/kg/hr via continuous epidural infusion	30 ug/hr (experience in adults above 40 ug/hr is limited)	

Lidocaine hydrochloride (0.5, 1 and 1.5%)	Xylocaine	Injectable	Local or regional anesthesia (peripheral nerve, caudal and lumbar epidural blocks)	All ages	Reduce dose commensurate with body weight and age	4 mg/kg	
Lidocaine hydrochloride (2%)	Anestacon, Xylocaine	Topical jelly, oral solution	Topical anesthesia of mucus membranes in mouth, reducing gagging during dental X-rays or impressions	All ages	Reduce dose commensurate with body weight and age	4.5 mg/kg	
Lidocaine hydrochloride (4%)	Laryng-O-Jet Kit	Topical	Topical anesthesia of mucous membranes in respiratory tract (endoscopy, bronchoscopy, endotracheal intubation)	All ages	0.6 to 3 mg/kg	4.5 mg/kg or 300 mg	
Lidocaine and epinephrine bitartrate	Lignospan	Injectable	Local anesthesia (peripheral nerve block or infiltration)	All ages	Reduce dose commensurate with body weight and age	4 mg/kg	May contain sodium bisulfite
Mepivacaine (1, 1.5 and 2%)	Carbocaine, Polocaine	Injectable	Local or regional analgesia, Anesthesia by infiltration, peripheral and central block	All ages	Dose carefully, measure as a percentage of adult dose based on weight	5 to 6 mg/kg	< 3 years or 30 lbs: use concentrations < 2%
Mepivacaine hydrochloride with or without levonordefrin	Carbocaine 3% and Carbocaine 2% with Neo-Cobefrin	Injectable	Local anesthesia for dental procedures	All ages	Lowest dose necessary	2%: 3 mg/lb (180 mg) 3%: 3 mg/lb (270 mg)	May contain sodium sulfite
Prilocaine hydrochloride	Citanest Plain	Injectable	Local anesthesia for dental procedures	All ages	< 10 years: usually one half cartridge (40 mg)	8 mg/kg if < 70 kg	May contain sodium metabisulfite

(continued)

TABLE 23-2. (continued)

Drug	Trade Name	Formulation	Indication in Adults	Indication in Children by Age	Pediatric Dosing	Maximum Dose	Comments
Opioids							
Buprenorphine injectable	Buprenex	Injectable	Moderate to severe pain	≥ 2 years	≥ 13 year: 0.3 mg IM or slow IV q 6hr 2 to 6 mcg/kg q 4 to 6 hr	One time (single) dose in adults 0.6mg	
Fentanyl citrate	Sublimaze	Injectable	Analgesia, Anesthesia	≥ 2 years	low dose: 1 to 3 mcg/kg [higher doses are approved for anesthesia/monitored settings]	adults 50 to 100 mcg	rare cases of methemoglobinemia in preterm neonates (combined use of other agents); direct cause and effect relationship not established
Fentanyl	Duragesic	Transdermal patch	Persistent, moderate to severe pain, requiring continuous, around the clock opioid administration and cannot be managed by other means	≥ 2 years opioid tolerant	Individually titrated, starting doses of 25 mcg/h and higher were used in clinical trials	Not specified Maximum starting dose adults: 100 mcg/h	NOT intended for acute postoperative pain (e.g., tonsillectomy)
Meperidine	Demerol	Injectable	Moderate to moderately severe pain	All ages	0.5 to 1 mg/lb IM or SQ q 3 to 4 h prn	50 to 150 mg	Neonates and preterm infants more susceptible to adverse events, such as respiratory suppression PCA pump not recommended < 19 years
Meperidine hydrochloride	Demerol	Oral solution, tablet	Moderate to severe pain	All ages	1.1 mg/kg to 1.8 mg/kg po, q 3 to 4 h prn	50 to 150 mg	

Generic	Brand	Formulation	Indication	Age	Dosage	Maximum	Comments
Naloxone hydrochloride	Narcan	Injection	Complete or partial reversal of narcotic depression, including respiratory depression	All ages	Narcotic overdose: 0.01 mg/kg initially, repeat 0.1 mg/kg Postoperative: 0.005 to 0.01 mg IV q 2 to 3 minutes until reversal Neonates: 0.01 mg/kg	Initial dose up to 2 mg Question diagnosis if no response after 10 mg	May administer IV, IM or subcutaneously (AAP does not endorse SC or IM in opiate intoxication due to erratic or delayed absorption)

Combination products

Generic	Brand	Formulation	Indication	Age	Dosage	Maximum	Comments
Acetaminophen and butalbital	Bucet, Butapap, Tencon	Oral tablet	Acute tension (muscle contraction) Headache	≥ 12 years	1 or 2 tablets every 4 hrs (50 mg butalbital and 325 mg acetaminophen) or 1 tablet q 4 hours (50 mg butalbital and 650 mg acetaminophen)	6 tablets/day (300 mg butalbital)	
Acetaminophen and codeine phosphate	Codrix Generic	Oral tablet, suspension	Mild to moderately severe pain	≥ 3 years (suspension only)	0.5 mg/kg codeine phosphate (120 mg acetaminophen and 12 mg codeine phosphate/5 mL)	Adult 15 mL q 4 hr prn 7 to 12 year 10 mL TID or QID 3 to 6 year: 6 mL TID to QID	Contains sodium metabisulfite
Acetaminophen butalbital and caffeine	Esgic-Plus, Fioricet	Oral capsules	Tension (muscle contraction) Headache	≥ 12 years	1 capsule q 4hr (each capsule contains 50 mg butalbital, 325 or 500 mg acetaminophen and 40 mg caffeine)	6 capsules/day	
Acetaminophen and hydrocodone bitartrate	Lortab	Oral solution, syrup, and elixir	Moderate to moderately severe pain	≥ 2 years	*(see dosing table below)*	*(see dosing table below)*	Not all formulations approved for children
Acetaminophen and pentazocine	Talacen	Oral tablet	Mild to moderate pain	≥ 12 years	1 tablet q 4 hr prn	6 tablets/day	

Acetaminophen and hydrocodone bitartrate dosing:

Weight (kg)	Age (years)	Dose (q 4 to 6h)	Maximum total daily dose (6 doses/day)
12 to 15	2 to 3	3.75 mL	22.5 mL
16 to 22	4 to 6	5 mL	30 mL
23 to 31	7 to 9	7.5 mL	45 mL
23 to 45	10 to 13	10 mL	60 mL
≥ 46 kg	≥ 14	15 mL	120 mL

(continued)

TABLE 23-2. (continued)

Drug	Trade Name	Formulation	Indication in Adults	Indication in Children by Age	Pediatric Dosing	Maximum Dose	Comments
Aspirin, caffeine and dihydrocodeine bitartrate	Synalgos-DC	Oral capsule	Moderate to moderately severe pain	≥ 12 years	2 capsules q 4hr prn	Not specified	
Aspirin, butalbital, caffeine and codeine phosphate	Generic form	Oral capsule	Muscle contraction (tension) headache	≥ 12 years	1–2 capsules q 4hr prn (each capsule contains 50mg butalbital, 325mg aspirin, 40mg caffeine and 30mg codeine phosphate	6 capsules	
Ibuprofen and oxycodone	Combunox	Oral tablet	Short-term (7 days) acute, moderate to severe pain	≥ 14 years	1 tablet (5 mg oxycodone/ 400mg ibuprofen)	4 tablets per 24 hours, 7 days total	Studied in children for dental surgery
Naloxone hydrochloride and pentazocine hydrochloride	Talwin NX	Oral tablet	Moderate to severe pain	≥ 12 years	1 to 2 tablets q 3 to 4hr (each tablet equivalent to 50mg base pentazocine and 0.5mg base naloxone)	12 tablets/day	Lethal reactions when injected
Carisoprodol, aspirin and codeine	Soma compound with codeine	Oral tablet	Acute, painful, musculoskeletal conditions when codeine desired	≥ 12 years	1 or 2 tablets QID	None listed	Adjunct to rest, PT and other measures
Muscle Relaxants							
Baclofen	Kemstro	Tablets, orally disintegrating	Spasticity from multiple sclerosis or spinal cord injury/ disease	≥ 12 years	Dose titration: 5 mg TID × 3 days, 10mg TID × 3 days, 15mg TID × 3 days, 20mg TID × 3 days	80mg (20mg QID)	Not indicated for skeletal muscle spasm from rheumatic disorder or cerebral palsy
Baclofen intrathecal	Lioresal	Injectable, Intrathecal	Severe spasticity of spinal cord or cerebral origin	≥ 4 years and sufficient mass to accommodate pump	Individually titrated based on screening dose: Initial screening dose 25 to 50 mcg, titrate by 5 to 15% increments	Screening dose: 100mcg Range for maintenance 24 to 1,199 mcg/day in children < 12 years	Not recommended IV, IM, SC or epidural Must respond to screening dose

246

Carisoprodol	Soma	Oral tablet	Acute painful, musculoskeletal conditions	≥ 12 years	350 mg TID and qhs	Not specified	Adjunct to rest, PT and other measures
Cyclobenzaprine	Flexeril	Oral tablet	Short term (2 to 3 weeks) Muscle spasm	≥ 15 years	5 mg TID	10 mg TID, no more than 2 to 3 weeks	Not effective in cerebral palsy
Dantrolene sodium	Dantrium	Oral capsule	Chronic spasticity (upper motor neuron, spinal cord injury, cerebral palsy or multiple sclerosis)	≥ 5 years	Titration: 0.5 mg/kg qd × 7 days, TID × 7days, 1 mg/kg TID for 7 days, 2 mg/kg TID based on response	100 mg QID	IV formulation, as well as oral approved for management and prevention of malignant hyperthermia
Metaxalone	Skelaxin	Oral tablet	Acute, painful musculoskeletal conditions	≥ 12 years	800 mg TID	800 mg QID	Adjunctive to rest, PT, and other measures

Topical

Lidocaine hydrochloride and epinephrine topical iontophoretic patch	LidoSite Topical System Kit	Topical system	Local analgesia (intact skin) for superficial dermatologic procedures (venipuncture, intravenous cannulation, and laser ablation of superficial skin lesions)	≥ 5 years	One patch	New patch may be applied to different site after 30 minutes	Contains sodium metabisulfite

Lidocaine and prilocaine (2.5% each)	EMLA	Topical	Local analgesia (intact skin), genital mucous membranes for minor surgery or pretreatment for infiltration	Neonates (≥ 37 weeks) and older				Monitor neonates (methemoglobinemia) Maximum doses are broad guidelines and apply to patients with normal intact skin and normal renal and hepatic function Controlled studies in children < 7 years have shown less overall benefit than older children or adults

Age/Weight	Maximum Dose (g)	Maximum Area (cm²)	Maximum Application Time (hr)
0 up to 3 mo or < 5 kg	1	10	1
3 up to 12 mo or > 5 kg	2	20	4
1 to 6 y and > 10 kg	10	100	4
7 to 12 years and > 20 kg	20	200	4

(continued)

TABLE 23-2. (continued)

Drug	Trade Name	Formulation	Indication in Adults	Indication in Children by Age	Pediatric Dosing	Maximum Dose	Comments
Lidocaine and tetracaine (70 mg each)	Synera	Transdermal patch	Local dermal analgesia for superficial venous access and dermatologic procedures	≥ 3 years	Apply 20 to 30 min before venipuncture or 30 min before superficial dermatologic procedure	May repeat one time in another site for venous access	Safe use in infants 4 to 6 months of age documented in one study S-Caine™ Peel (Lidocaine and Tetracaine 7%/7% Cream) is intended for adults only
Miscellaneous							
Etomidate	Amidate	Injectable	Induction of anesthesia	≥ 10 years	0.2 to 0.6 mg/kg		Not recommended in patients below age 10 years

RA- Rheumatoid arthritis
OA- Osteoarthritis
JRA- Juvenile Rheumatoid Arthritis
Note: Pediatric indications are the same as adults unless specified. Labeling may have been updated since Feb 2007. See current package insert for full prescribing information. Labeling for products listed as indicated for "all ages" includes labeling for all pediatric age groups and in some instances includes general weight-based dosing. Trade names are given as examples, and do not imply brand preference. Generic preparations are available for many medications.

TABLE 23-3. FDA-approved indications for drugs approved to treat pain in adults only (based on package insert as of Feb 2007).

Active ingredient (Trade Name)	Adult Indication (Pain related)	Comments
NSAIDs		
Diclofenac (Voltaran)	Arthritis (OA, RA), ankylosing spondylitis	
Diclofenac potassium (Cataflam)	Mild to moderate pain, arthritis (OA, RA), dysmenorrhea	
Diclofenac sodium/misoprostol (Arthrotec)	Arthritis (OA, RA) in patients with high risk of NSAID-induced gastric or duodenal ulcers	
Fenoprofen (Nalfon, Nalfon 200)	Mild to moderate pain, Arthritis (RA, OA)	
Flurbiprofen (Ansaid)	Arthritis (RA, OA)	
Ketoprofen (Orudis, Oruvail)	Arthritis (RA, OA)	Extended release not recommended for acute pain
	Acute pain, dysmenorrhea	
Nabumetone (generic forms)	Arthritis (RA, OA)	
Piroxicam (Feldene)	Arthritis (RA, OA)	
Sulindac (Clinoril)	Arthritis (RA, OA, gouty), ankylosing spondylitis, subacromial bursitis/ supraspinatus tendinitis	
Opioid Analgesics		
Butorphanol tartrate (Stadol)	Pain, anesthesia	
Fentanyl citrate (Actiq, Fentora)	Breakthrough cancer pain in opioid-tolerant patients	Clinical study of 15 children too small to permit conclusions regarding safety and efficacy
Fentanyl hydrochloride (Ionsys)	Short-term management of acute, postoperative pain	Iontophoresis system
		Preliminary pediatric studies suggest pediatric patients more vulnerable to application site reactions, which were more severe than adults
Hydromorphone hydrochloride (Dilaudad HP)	Moderate to severe pain in opioid tolerant patients, requiring larger than usual doses of opioids to provide pain relief	
Hydromorphone hydrochloride (Dilaudad)	Pain	
Levorphanol tartrate (Levo Dromoran)	Moderate to severe pain, Preoperative medication	
Methadone hydrochloride injectable (Dolophine)	Moderate to severe pain, Opioid Addiction	Not all dosage forms approved for pain
Morphine sulfate injectable (Astramorph PF, Duramorph PF, Infumorph)	Analgesia (IV, epidural, intrathecal)	Provides pain relief without loss of motor, sensory or sympathetic function
Morphine sulfate oral (Kadian, MS Contin, Oramorph SR)	Moderate to severe pain when continuous, around-the-clock opioid analgesic is needed for an extended period	Prolonged elimination half-life and decreased clearance in neonates
Nalbuphine hydrochloride (Nubain)	Moderate to severe pain	
	Anesthesia, preoperative, postoperative and obstetric analgesia	
Oxycodone hydrochloride (Oxycontin, Roxicodone)	Moderate to severe pain when continuous, around-the-clock opioid analgesia is needed	Not intended for prn use
Oxymorphone (injectable)	Moderate to severe pain	
(Numorphan)	Anesthesia, obstetric analgesia	

(continued)

TABLE 23-3. (continued)

Active ingredient (Trade Name)	Adult Indication (Pain related)	Comments
Oxymorphone (oral) (Opana, Opana ER)	Moderate to severe pain	Extended-release forms for adult patients requiring continuous opioid treatment, not intended as a prn analgesic or postoperative use
Pentazocine lactate (Talwin)	Moderate to severe pain, anesthesia	Approved as preoperative or preanesthetic agent in children ≥ 1 year, not for pain
Propoxyphene hydrochloride (Darvon)	Mild to moderate pain	
Propoxyphene napsylate (Darvon-N)	Mild to moderate pain	
Tramadol hydrochloride (Ultram)	Mild to moderately severe pain	
Combination therapies		
Acetaminophen and hydrocodone bitartrate (Lortab, Vicodin and Vicodin ES)	Moderate to moderately severe pain	
Acetaminophen and oxycodone hydrochloride (Percocet, Oxycet, Percocet, Roxicet, Roxilox, Tylox)	Moderate to moderately severe pain	
Acetaminophen and propoxyphene hydrochloride (Wygesic)	Mild to Moderate severe pain	
Acetaminophen and propoxyphene napsylate (Darvecet-N 50, Darvocet A500)	Mild to moderate pain, with or without fever	
Acetaminophen and tramadol hydrochloride (Ultracet)	Short-term (< 5 days) management of acute pain	
Aspirin, caffeine, ophenadrine citrate (Norgesic)	Mild to moderate pain of acute musculoskeletal disorders	Warnings: Reye's syndrome
		Orphenadrine component indicated as adjunct therapy to rest, physical therapy and other measures
Aspirin, caffeine, propoxyphene hydrochloride oral capsule (Darvon Compound-65)	Relief of mild to moderate pain, with or without fever	Warnings: Reye's syndrome
Aspirin and oxycondone hydrochloride (Percodan)	Moderate to moderately severe pain	Contraindicated in children due to Reyes's syndrome
Ibuprofen and hydrocodone (Vicoprofen)	Short-term (< 10 days) management of acute pain	
Epidural		
Bupivacaine hydrochloride (Marcaine)	Spinal anesthesia	Combination product (with lidocaine) approved for ophthalmologic surgery in children
Ropivacaine hydrochloride monohydrate (Naropin)	Acute pain management (including epidural block and continuous epidural), local or regional anesthesia	
Local anesthetic		
Lidocaine 2.5%/ prilocaine periodontal gel (Oraqix)	Localized anesthesia in periodontal pockets	Very young children more susceptible to methemoglobinemia
Migraine		
Selective 5-hydroxytryptamine receptor subtype agonist		
Almotriptan (Axert)	Acute migraine only	Postmarketing experience from other triptans have shown clinically significant pediatric AE similar to adult
Eletriptan (Relpax)	Acute migraine only	Pediatric trial did not establish efficacy of tablets. Postmarketing experience from other triptans have shown clinically significant pediatric adverse events (AE) similar to those reported in adults

(continued)

TABLE 23-3. (continued)

Active ingredient (Trade Name)	Adult Indication (Pain related)	Comments
Frovatriptan (Frova)	Acute migraine only	Postmarketing experience from other triptans have shown clinically significant pediatric AE similar to those reported in adults
Naratriptan (Amerge)	Acute migraine only	Pediatric trial did not establish efficacy of tablets. AEs similar to those reported in adult clinical trials
Rizatriptan (Maxalt, Maxalt-MLT)	Acute migraine only	Pediatric trials did not establish efficacy of tablets. Postmarketing experience from other triptans have shown clinically significant pediatric AE similar to those reported in adults
Sumatiptan (Imitrex, Imetrex Statdose)	Acute migraine and cluster HA, not hemiplegic or basilar	Pediatric trials did not establish efficacy of either nasal spray or oral form. Postmarketing experience documents that serious AEs rarely reported in adults, including stroke, visual loss, and death have occurred in the pediatric population after use of subcutaneous, oral, and/ or nasal sumatriptan
Zolmitriptan (Zomig, Zomig-ZMT)	Acute migraine only	Pediatric trials did not establish efficacy of tablets. Postmarketing experience from other triptans have shown clinically significant pediatric AE similar to those reported in adults
Other		
Acetaminophen, butalbital, caffeine and codeine (Fioricet with codeine)	Muscle contraction (tension) Headache	
Aspirin, butalbal and caffeine (Fiorinal)	Muscle contraction (tension) Headache	Warnings: Reye's syndrome
Aspirin, butalbital, caffeine and codeine (Fiorinal with codeine)	Muscle contraction (tension) HA	Warnings: Reye's syndrome
Dihydroergotamine mesylate nasal spray (Migranal)	Acute Migraine HA	
Divalproex sodium (Depakote)	Migraine HA prophylaxis	In children, approved for Epilepsy $\geq$ 2 years, not migraine
Ergotamine tartrate with or without caffeine (Cafergot)	Abort or prevent vascular headache	
Propranolol hydrochloride (Inderal)	Migraine prophylaxis	High levels noted in patients with Trisomy 21, suggesting bioavailablity may be increased
Topiramate (Topamax)	Migraine prophylaxis	In children, approved for Epilepsy (adjunctive $\geq$ 2 years, monotherapy $\geq$ 10 years), not migraine
Muscle Relaxants		
Chlorzoxazone (Parafon forte)	Acute muscle spasm (adjunct to rest, physical therapy (PT), etc.)	
Methocarbamol (Robaxin)	Acute muscle spasm (adjunct to rest, PT, etc.)	In children, approved for tetanus
Orphenadrine citrate (Norflex)	Acute muscle spasm (adjunct to rest, PT, etc)	
Tizanidine (Zanaflex) Neuropathy	Spasticity	Short-acting

(continued)

TABLE 23-3. (continued)

Active ingredient (Trade Name)	Adult Indication (Pain related)	Comments
Duloxetine (Cymbalta)	Diabetic peripheral neuropathic pain	Boxed warning: suicidality in children and adolescents
Gabapentin (Neurontin)	Postherpetic neuralgia	In children, approved for Epilepsy ≥ 3 years, not neuralgia
Pregabalin (Lyrica)	Diabetic neuropathy, Postherpetic neuralgia	
Carbamezepine (Carbatrol)	Trigeminal neuralgia	In children, approved for epilepsy
Miscellaneous		
Dexmedetomidine (Precedex)	Sedation in initially intubated and mechanically ventilated patients in an intensive care setting	Continuous infusion, not to exceed 24 hr
Ketamine hydrochloride (Ketalar)	Anesthesia	
Ziconotide (Prialt)	Severe, chronic pain where intrathecal therapy is warranted	

Note: consult current package insert for full prescribing information. Trade names are given as examples, and do not imply brand preference. Generic preparations are available for many medications.

Several NSAIDs are approved for the treatment of JRA. Celecoxib, ibuprofen, meloxicam, naproxen, and tolmetin are approved for use in children 2 years of age and older. Aspirin carries professional labeling for patients with JRA on an mg/kg basis. Etodolac and oxaprozin are approved for use in children 6 years of age and older. Indomethacin is indicated for use in adolescents older than 14 years of age. However, other nonsteroidal agents such as diclofenac, ketoprofen, nabumetone, piroxicam, and sulindac are not approved for use in children. Medication Guides are required for selected products that pose a significant public health risk, including prescription NSAIDs. Medication Guides provide useful information so that patients can use their medications safety and effectively. The Medication Guide must be provided to the patient at the time the prescription is dispensed.

5.1.2. Opioids

A limited number of intravenous and oral opioid products are approved for pediatric use. Intravenous meperidine is approved for the relief of moderate to severe pain in pediatric patients of all ages. Since preterm infants and neonates may be more susceptible to adverse effects such as respiratory depression, meperidine should be used with caution in this age group. In children older than 2 years of age, buprenorphine (IV) is indicated for the treatment of moderate to severe pain. Fentanyl citrate is also approved for surgical analgesia in this age group. Rare cases of

clinically significant methemoglobinemia have been reported in preterm neonates undergoing anesthesia with fentanyl, pancuronium, and atropine. Other intravenous products commonly used in children such as morphine sulfate, methadone, hydromorphone, and butorphanol have not been approved for use in children.

Oral opioids that are approved for use in children are limited to codeine, hydrocodone, and meperidine. Codeine and acetaminophen oral solution is approved for use in children older than 3 years with mild-to-moderate pain. Hydrocodone and acetaminophen oral solution is also indicated for the same use in children 2 years of age and older. Meperidine syrup or tablets, as age appropriate, may be used to relieve moderate or severe pain in children of all ages, although preterm infants and neonates may be more susceptible to adverse effects. In contrast, morphine sulfate has not been systemically evaluated in children, although pharmacokinetic information is available in labeling for Kadian, a sustained release formulation of morphine sulfate. Hydromorphone and oxycodone are not indicated for use in children.

5.1.3. Epidurals

Several agents are approved for epidural anesthesia in pediatric patients, including chloroprocaine, lidocaine, and mepivicane. However, bupivacaine as a single agent is not recommended for use in pediatric spinal anesthesia, and intrathecal clonidine is restricted to use in pediatric patients with severe, intractable pain from malignancy. Thus, agents such as bupivacaine, clonidine, fentanyl, ketamine, and ropivacaine are used off-label for epidural anesthesia.

5.1.4. Local Anesthesia

Chloroprocaine, lidocaine, and mepivacaine may be used for local anesthesia (infiltration, peripheral or central nerve block). The combination of lidocaine and bupivacaine is approved for use in patients older than 12 years of age requiring parabulbar, retrobulbar, or facial nerve blocks. Articaine (in pediatric patients greater than 4 years of age) and mepivacaine (all ages) may be used for nerve blocks in dental and periodontal procedures.

5.1.5. Topical Anesthesia

Specific concentrations of external analgesics are approved via over-the-counter drug monographs. OTC drug monographs specify the active ingredients that are generally recognized as safe and effective (GRASE). These ingredients may be included in a drug product for a specific therapeutic class. Active ingredients used for topical anesthesia include benzocaine (5 to 20%), butamben picrate (1%), dibucaine (0.25 to 1%), dyclonine hydrochloride (0.25 to 1%), lidocaine (0.5 to 4%), lidocaine hydrochloride (0.5 to 1%), pramoxine hydrochloride (0.5 to 1%), and tetracaine (1 to 2%). Prescription products containing tetracaine and lidocaine (7% each), lidocaine and prilocaine (2.5% each), and 2 percent lidocaine are approved for one-time use in children.

5.2. Chronic Pain

Although available, most transdermal, buccal, or nasal opioids are not approved for pediatric patients; only fentanyl transdermal system is approved in *opioid-tolerant* pediatric patients older than 2 years of age for the management of persistent, moderate to severe pain that requires continuous, around-the-clock opioid administration for an extended period of time and cannot be managed by other measures. Due to the potential for serious or life-threatening hypoventilation, fentanyl transdermal system is contraindicated in patients who are not opioid-tolerant in the management of acute, mild, or intermittent pain or in patients who require opioid analgesia for a short period of time and in the management of postoperative pain. Intrathecal

clonidine is restricted for use in pediatric patients with intractable cancer pain that is not responsive to more conventional analgesic techniques.

Several agents used to treat chronic pain are approved in adults, but not in the pediatric population. For instance, duloxetine and pregabalin are approved for adults with diabetic peripheral neuropathy. Similarly, gabapentin, pregabalin, and 5 percent lidocaine patches are approved for the treatment of postherpetic neuralgia in adults only. In addition, carbamezepine is approved for the treatment of trigeminal neuralgia in adults only. Several other antidepressants or anticonvulsants, although used for the treatment of chronic pain, are not approved for this purpose in either adults or children.

5.3. Headaches

Acetaminophen, butalbital, and caffeine are indicated to relieve tension or muscle contraction headaches in adolescents. Although eletriptan, naratriptan, rizatriptan, sumatriptan, and zolmitriptan have been studied in adolescent migraineurs, efficacy has not been established in children. The remaining triptans have not been studied in children. Similarly, while divalproex sodium, propranolol, and topiramate are approved for migraine prophylaxis in adults, these products are not approved for this use in children. Dihydroergotamine and ergotamine are also not approved for use in children.

5.4. Muscle Relaxants

Carisoprodol, cyclobenzapine, and metaxalone are approved as adjuncts to rest and physical therapy for relief of muscle spasm in adolescents. A combination product containing carisoprodol, aspirin, and codeine phosphate is approved in adolescents as adjunctive therapy to rest and physical therapy and other measures for the relief of pain, muscle spasm, and limited mobility associated with acute, painful musculoskeletal injuries. Dantrolene is indicated for the treatment of chronic spasticity in children ≥ 5 years of age, including spasticity due to cerebral palsy. Intrathecal baclofen is approved for severe spasticity in patients 4 years of age and older who have sufficient body mass to tolerate the implantable pump. Oral baclofen is approved only to alleviate signs and symptoms of spasticity from multiple sclerosis and spinal cord injury and other spinal disorders in children ≥ 12 years of age. Note that the efficacy of oral baclofen for the treatment of cerebral palsy has not been established. Therefore, this is an unapproved indication.

6. Gaps in Labeling

Gaps in labeling are greatest for neonates, followed closely by children less than 2 years of age. The only intravenous and oral formulation for relief of pain which has dosing for neonates is meperidine. Recommendations state that meperidine should be used with caution in this age group since preterm infants and neonates may be more susceptible to adverse events such as respiratory depression. Pharmacokinetic parameters are available in neonates for oral morphine sulfate, although this product is not approved for children of any age. Limited pharmacokinetic information on mefenamic acid in premature infants indicates that half-life is prolonged (approximately five times as long as adults) although safety and effectiveness have not been established in patients below the age of 14 years. Lidocaine hydrochloride and mepivacaine are approved for local or regional anesthesia in neonates and older children, although close monitoring is suggested. Topical lidocaine/prilocaine and certain lidocaine/tetracaine products are approved in children, but a dosage adjustment is recommended in younger children. Close monitoring of children less than 3 months is suggested since risks include methemoglobinemia.

Take-Home Points

- In order for a drug to receive FDA approval, safety and efficacy for its intended use must be established.

  - Two adequate and well-controlled trials are required for most new indications.
  - For drugs approved in adults, extrapolation of efficacy in children may be permissible in certain circumstances.
  - Extrapolation is appropriate when the FDA concludes that the pathophysiology of disease and the effect of the drug (both beneficial and adverse) are similar in adults and children.
  - Pharmacokinetic information to establish dosing and safety data must be obtained when efficacy is extrapolated.

  - Safety must always be studied in pediatric patients. Pediatric patients may be at a higher risk of serious adverse drug experiences and unexpected adverse drug experiences not typically observed in adults

- A new labeling content and format, specified by the Physician Labeling Rule, is intended to provide the most up-to-date information in an easy-to-read format and reduce medication errors related to misunderstood or incorrectly applied drug information.

  - Prescribing information contains a summary of the most important and frequently referenced information (Highlights) and a Table of Contents.
  - Risk information (Contraindications, Warnings and Precautions, and Adverse Reactions) has been consolidated into one location.
  - Recent major changes to the labeling are more easily identified.

- With the exception of local (infiltrative) or topical anesthesia, only a limited number of medications frequently used to treat pediatric pain or facilitate analgesia are adequately labeled for pediatric patients.

- Children older than 6 months of age:

  - Oral: ibuprofen (pain and fever)

- Children older than two years of age:

  - Oral: acetaminophen, aspirin (> 3 years), celecoxib (JRA), meperidine, meloxicam (JRA), naproxen (JRA), hydrocodone, tolmetin; combination products: acetaminophen and codeine (> 3 years)
  - Intravenous agents: buprenorphine, meperidine, and fentanyl citrate
  - Epidural: chloroprocaine, lidocaine and mepivicane
  - Continuous epidural: clonidine (intractable cancer pain)
  - Transdermal fentanyl (opioid-tolerant patients only)

- Children older than 6 years of age:

  - Oral: etodolac and oxaprozin (JRA)

- Adolescents only:

  - Oral: diflunisal, indomethacin, mefenamic acid, combination products containing acetaminophen, butalbital and caffeine, acetaminophen and pentazocine, ibuprofen and oxycodone, naloxone and

pentazocine, cyclobenzaprine and metaxalone, carisoprodol, aspirin and codeine phosphate
- Epidural: bupivacaine/lidocaine

- Pediatric initiatives such as FDAMA, BPCA and PREA have facilitated studies in pediatric patients (through December 2006)

  - More than 300 pediatric studies and 120 labeling changes related to BPCA
  - More than 50 labeling changes related to PREA
- Most pain therapies still need to be studied in pediatric patients since pharmacokinetics, dosing, efficacy, and safety may differ from that in adults.

Resources

DailyMed: *http://dailymed.nlm.nih.gov.*
Drugs@FDA: *http://www.accessdata.fda.gov/scripts/cder/drugsatfda/index.cfm*
Summaries of medical and clinical pharmacology reviews of pediatric studies: *http://www.fda.gov/cder/pediatric/Summaryreview.htm*
PREA Labeling changes: *http://www.fda.gov/cder/pediatric/index.htm#prea*
Medwatch: *http://www.fda.gov/medwatch/index.html*
New Requirements for Prescribing Information: *http://www.fda.gov/cder/regulatory/physLabel/default.htm*

The views expressed are those of the authors. No official support or endorsements by the United States Food and Drug Administration is provided or should be inferred. No commercial interest or other conflict of interest exists between the authors and the pharmaceutical companies.

References

1. Draft Guidance: How to comply with the Pediatric Research Equity Act: *http://www.fda.gov.cder/guidance/6215dft.pdf.*
2. Roberts R, Rodriguez W, Murphy D, et al. Pediatric drug labeling: Improving the safety and efficacy of pediatric therapies. JAMA 2003;290:905–911.
3. Draft Guidance: General considerations for pediatric pharmacokinetic studies for drugs and biologic products: *www.fda.gov/cder/guidance/1970dft.pdf.*
4. Guidance for Industry: ICH E11 Clinical investigation of medicinal products in the pediatric population. 2000.
5. Ponstel [package insert] Alpharetta, GA: First Horizon Pharmaceutical Corp; 2005.
6. Pediatric Exclusivity Labeling Changes (etodolac): *http://www.fda.gov/cder/pediatric/labelchange.htm.*
7. Summaries of medical and clinical pharmacology reviews of pediatric studies. Meloxicam: *http://www.fda.gov/cder/pediatric/Summaryreview.htm.*
8. New requirements for prescribing information: *http://www.fda.gov/cder/regulatory/physLabel/default.htm.*
9. 21 USC 812 Schedules of controlled substances: *http://www.dea.gov/pubs/csa/812.htm.*
10. 21 USC 829 Prescriptions: *http://www.dea.gov/pubs/csa/829.htm.*

24
Pediatrician as Advocate

Carol Schadelbauer

Abstract: Advocating for improvements in the treatment and care of children in pain is often left to the pediatric pain specialists who spend their lives focused on the topic. Yet, so much of children's pain is first seen and heard during the commonplace pediatric visit. From the time they are born, children are faced with pain in the form of needle sticks for blood draws and vaccines, to chronic headaches and bellyaches of later childhood and adolescence. Are primary care physicians doing all they can to advocate for good pain care in their own offices, with colleagues, and the public? The art of advocating isn't rocket science. It includes developing a message—choosing memorable words to say, telling stories that will bring life and clarity to the message, and taking time to develop a plan to become a better advocate. Parents and children seek the trusted advice of pediatricians, and if the doctor's message is memorable and empathetic, they will depend on it more than most information they are bombarded with in the media and online. Primary care physicians are in the right position to advocate for better care of children's pain.

Key words: Pain advocate, communications strategy, storytelling, messages, barriers to advocacy, media interviews, working with policymakers.

Introduction

My oldest son Alec was soon to enter kindergarten, and I knew he was going to receive a shot or two at his 5-year wellness check-up. In the examination room, Alec bounced around the room as usual, riding the doctor's stool with wheels like it was an amusement park ride. He liked his doctor. He looked forward to the cool sticker he would receive at the end of the exam.

Then the nurse came in and said it was time for shots. "Mom, hold your child in your lap," she said. She proceeded to give him five shots with large needles, one after the other. One in each leg. Another in an arm. Two more in the other arm. The "Scooby-Doo" band-aids she put on each shot site did nothing to calm the screams, the crying and the terror in my son's eyes.

The shots lasted 30 seconds in all. But the pain and memory will last a lifetime for my son.

Each year, after his 5-year-old experience, a month before his annual check up, he would beg that I call the doctor's office to confirm that there will be no shot. To keep him calm, I called every time even though we both knew his next shot wouldn't be administered until he was entering middle school.

A week before his 11-year-old check up, he started having nightmares and couldn't sleep. He was sweating just thinking about it.

Let me explain that I'm not one of those intense, demanding moms. My mother was a doctor who told me on a regular basis to "suck it up" and deal with minor pain or when I got a fever. But I'm also a communications strategist and, for several years, I have been working with pediatric pain experts, coaching them about how to clearly communicate important issues about pain to Americans. From them I've learned that there is an anesthetic cream

G.A. Walco and K.R. Goldschneider (eds.), *Pain in Children: A Practical Guide for Primary Care.*
© Humana Press, a part of Springer Science + Business Media, 2008

that can be applied before a shot to numb the area and reduce the pain. From them, I've learned that distraction—blowing bubbles, listening to music—is a scientifically proven method to reduce the physical and mental distress of pain.

To my surprise, I learned that recent research (see Chapter 2 for discussion) is showing that the intensity of pain we feel as children can have a life-long effect on the pain we feel as adults. I've also learned that damage to pain receptors in infancy or childhood will cause us pain as adults. Do pediatricians know this? Do orthopedic surgeons who deal with the broken bones of childhood know this? Do neonatologists who give sick infants dozens of shots in a day know this?

Back to my son's story. I called the pediatrician to tell him of my son's fear and asked if he could prescribe the anesthetic cream. "That cream takes forever to work," the nurse said. "The shot lasts a second, and he'll be fine. You don't need it." Not the answer I was looking for. Thank goodness, my neighbor is a nurse in the pediatric intensive care unit at a local hospital. She had a tube of the cream. She said she uses it on her children all the time before she goes to check-ups, and it works. I took it. So, armed with the cream on and Alec's iPod blaring in his ears, I took my son, trembling and sweating, to his 11-year-old check-up. As expected, the shot took a second and Alec survived this encounter. He now has the strength to face pain head on—knowing he has the right tools to do it. He just got a flu shot without a hitch.

I know pediatricians and their staff are advocates for my children and all the children they serve. They are kind-hearted, intelligent, wonderful people. They are there at all hours of the day and night, and there aren't other professionals who give as much to their patients and families as pediatricians and medical professionals who serve children. Then, why shouldn't pediatricians advocate for one of the most common ailments they see every day—acute and chronic pain?

My story describes acute pain that may have longer term effects than we ever thought. But what about the pre-teen bellyaches that don't go away or the chronic headaches that are written off as stress-induced? Are we taking care of children's pain so they can be productive and happy kids? If pediatricians are savvy enough to ask our children if they eat their vegetables and wear their bike helmets, isn't it reasonable to ask children if they feel any repetitive pain? If they feel stressed out? One pediatrician at a busy Washington, D.C.-area practice says she adds stress-related questions to her standard list of queries to seek out any chronic pain issues that children may be unwilling to discuss. She asks, "Do you think there is anything in your life that needs to change? Are things going on at home or at school that are stressors?" She says taking the time to add a couple of questions like this opens up doors with her patients.

The American Academy of Pediatrics is taking into account the new research on long-term effects of pain felt in childhood—and asking pediatricians to take more notice. Their policies clearly discuss this new research, and they ask neonatologists who manage acute pain in newborns on a regular basis to have an "effective pain-prevention program" in place [1]. They offer scientifically-based advice for dealing with children's acute pain [2]. While the research and policy exist, they do not always readily translate into practice, and there may be room for a major shift among pediatricians to better manage children's pain.

1. Barriers to Pain Advocacy in Primary Care

Dr. Paul Norton, a pediatrician in Milwaukee for 25 years, tells me what I think most pediatricians would say. His number one goal is to help the patient get the right care, but so often barriers get in the way. Those barriers are "economics, time, and lack of knowledge." He also said one of the biggest barriers is parents who desire a "quick fix" rather than a thoughtful plan for pain treatment. These barriers were so confining for Dr. Norton that after 25 years as a general pediatrician, he has become a developmental and behavioral pediatrician, allowing him 45 minutes—instead of 15—with each patient, and he's taken a pay cut to do it.

Dr. Norton says that efforts to implement good pain practices such as use of anesthetic cream and stocking sterile sucrose to apply to a baby's pacifier during circumcision, and even taking a few extra minutes to talk with an adolescent about chronic pain, meet resistance from staff because not every patient needs this time or these preventive strategies.

Insurance companies don't pay for extra talk time. One pediatric gastroenterologist in Columbus, Ohio, says he often treats basic constipation in a specialist setting that could or should be easily treated in the pediatrician's office. He says that, under the system of a 15-minute visit, pediatricians don't have enough time to be assured that it isn't something more than constipation, or they can't convince the anxious parent that it truly is just constipation.

One pediatrician in the Washington, D.C.-area says, "I don't know what others do, but I don't look at reimbursement issues. Certainly, procedures make me more money than counseling, but counseling can open doors for kids that have never been opened. A lot of pediatricians think they shouldn't do lots of counseling, but we do." She says it results in better care of their patients, with only one side effect, longer waits in the waiting room which she says her families don't mind.

Then there is the "lack of knowledge." Pediatric pain experts tell me that pediatricians and family practitioners are not treating pain as well as they could because pain is not a "hallmark event" like diabetes or cancer. It is, instead, a symptom of these conditions. Pediatricians are trained to use pain as an indicator for the diagnosis. In other words, masking the pain with strong medications or other treatments may cover up an important diagnosis. This may mean unrelieved pain will last longer. Pain management isn't clear cut medicine, and sometimes the line between physical and mental treatment is blurred. Pain is often considered a side effect of a disease or procedure or acute injury. But when the statistics show that pain is the number one reason people seek medical care in the United States, [3] and untreated pain can destroy a life, it should be part of regular care.

Some physicians say they are afraid to deal with pain treatment. They don't want to get involved in prescribing high potency pain medications, fearing prosecution by federal agents who are cracking down on physicians they claim are over-prescribing narcotics.

Other pediatricians observe that much chronic pain is not "organic," as they say, but functional. In other words, the pain is related to stress, and only specialists can take care of the patient. They may think it is all psychological, and refer to a therapist.

These barriers are real, but in many cases, can be overcome. Dr. Norton says, "Trying to advocate for good pain care doesn't always work well. It isn't easy." But, an advocate dedicated to making change will keep trying.

2. Physician as Advocate

Primary care physicians are the best messengers, and the best advocates for children's pain. Advocating takes many forms—and it isn't restricted to the exam room with the child and his parent. There are endless opportunities for child advocates to share a message locally, regionally and nationally. Pediatricians can serve as spokespeople with television, print, and radio reporters who, through their stories, reach millions of parents, children, and even peers who may not know what you now know about pain in children. Advocates are needed to influence insurance company executives to reimburse pain care, and meet with state and federal policymakers who hold many of the regulatory keys for improving the health care system.

What does it mean to be an advocate? The effective advocate should focus on:

• Memorable messages
• Stories
• A goal and plan of action

The first two work anywhere. The third is worth pursuing if you intend to reach out beyond the exam room to become an advocate for pain in children among your peers, or with health leaders locally and nationally.

3. The Importance of the Message

Andy Goodman is one of the nation's leading public relations experts who specializes in social change campaigns. His counsel: recognize that "truth is only half the battle." Telling kids "it will only hurt for a second" may be the truth, but how is that truth understood? What are the long-term effects of those words?

I am fascinated by how pharmaceutical companies deliver messages. Their advertisements are effective because they are engaging, and strike a cord with so many people. A recent one for the antidepressant *Cymbalta*®, a product of Eli Lilly and Company (a product that does not have an indication for use in pediatrics), uses the phrase "Depression hurts emotionally and physically. But you don't have to." Making the connection to the real physical pains of depression is a new angle. Consumers viewing the advertisement may realize for the first time that the aches and pains they are feeling may not be "just about getting old," but may be something treatable—something that, if treated, could change their lives.

Advertising agencies know how to "message." But what pediatricians have that advertising executives don't is a medical degree, as well as an office full of patients who trust their advice, perhaps more than anything they hear, read, or see. Your words are powerful, even in a world of a million messages delivered in dozens of mediums today. The average youth today multitasks with the television, iPods, radio, instant messaging, and the Internet to pack 8.5 hours of media exposure into 6.5 hours each day, 7 days per week (see Figure 24-1), according to a report from the Henry J. Kaiser Family Foundation [4]. And the depth of detail of the messages they are receiving has shrunk. The average length of a television sound bite has shrunk from 42 seconds in 1968, to 7.3 seconds in 2000 [5]. It may be closer to five seconds now.

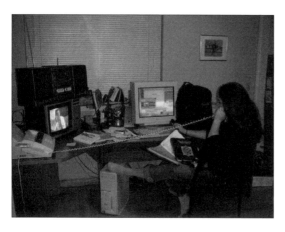

FIGURE 24-1. Jessica Altman, daughter of Drew Altman, PhD, president and chief executive officer of the Henry J. Kaiser Family Foundation, is part of a new generation that multitasks to pack 8.5 hours of media exposure into 6.5 hours each day, 7 days per week. ("Generation M: Media in the Lives of Children, 2005: Henry J. Kaiser Family Foundation)

In contrast, most pediatric office well-visits are around 15 minutes, an eternity to a child and a parent in today's world. This time is a chance to slow down, listen, and organize your own messages, including those about pain management. In order to break through the media clutter, you need to speak in memorable ways.

4. Developing Your Message

So much of good messaging is just being an empathetic person. What will sound best to this child? What will be honest, but clear? What does the parent need from me right now?

Health advocates and others can improve their messages with some simple steps:

- Develop a message that "speaks in headlines" and has vivid images. Your words are competing against millions of sound bites out there.
- Avoid jargon that an average patient or parent won't understand. For example, instead of saying "opioids" say "strong pain medications."
- Use carefully chosen national and local statistics to reinforce your points. Parents like statistics if they are clear. Instead of saying "75 percent of children have side effects…" say "three out of four children…"
- Use succinct "real life" examples to add texture to your comments. Personal experiences and stories resonate with everyone.
- Narrow your message to no more than three points. Our short-attention-span society cannot handle much more.

These tips apply in whatever setting you're in —in the exam room with a child, in a board room with insurance executives, at the annual pediatric meeting when you're giving a speech, or with a policymaker. The messenger is as important as the message—and pediatricians, trustworthy and comforting, are in the best position to do it.

5. Story Telling

Most Americans get their information from local television news (see Table 24-1) [6]. This may be because today's world gives us very little time to

TABLE 24-1. "Seven in 10 U.S. adults say they watch broadcast news at least several times per week."

	Daily/ Several times a week	Daily	Several times a week	Several times a month/ year	Several times a month	Several times a year	Never
	Media usage						
	"How often do you do any of the following?" (Data reflect percent of respondents endorsing)						
Base: All adults							
Watch local broadcast news	77	54	22	17	10	7	6
Watch network broadcast or cable news	71	49	22	21	13	9	8
Read a local daily newspaper	63	41	22	28	16	12	9
Go online to get news	64	40	24	26	15	11	11
Listen to radio news broadcasts	54	32	21	26	13	13	20
Listen to talk radio stations	37	22	15	30	12	17	34
Read a national newspaper (The Wall Street Journal, USA Today, The New York Times, etc.)	18	10	8	40	14	27	41
Listen to satellite radio programming	19	12	7	13	6	7	68

Note: Percentages may not add up to 100 percent due to rounding

consume information. Newspapers that require more time than a quick television story are at the bottom of the list as sources of information. It also may be because local television news often tells stories first. Their news stories—usually one minute to 90-seconds long—use a simple formula in this order:

- A patient or victim tells his or her own story,
- A leading authority or expert is interviewed, and
- The interviews are interspersed with plenty of background video of the patient and/or the expert in real-life situations.

Local television epitomizes the way the average American likes to receive information. For this reason, in the communications field, we teach people to tell stories. They are engaging. You want to know the punch line. And there is always a punch line or a lesson to be learned. If I led this chapter with the statement that too many pediatricians are not advocating for children's pain, you most likely would have turned to the next chapter. Leading with what is hopefully an engaging story is a great entrance into the research or the solution or the concept you want to get across. The art of story-telling can be seen all around us. Communicators

will tell you that stories are the framework for remembering facts—they mirror everyday life and are easy to understand. For example, consider "old wives tales"; whether factual or not, these brief, colorful vignettes transmit information very effectively.

Telling parents and their children your own experiences with other patients (anonymously, of course) or even about your own childhood experiences with getting shots for the first time may be a calming way to begin a discussion. Funny stories are even better to break up a tough conversation or prepare a child for an injection.

Pediatricians have told me that there is some risk to telling too many of your own personal stories —mainly because it may reduce your credibility as an expert. But communicators will argue that point. Anything that humanizes an expert or makes them less academic makes them more trusted. Stories have that power.

The Washington, D.C.-area pediatrician was examining an 11-year-old boy about to enter middle school. She told him that he will grow a lot in the next year or two, and that he may feel irritable, grumpy or angry sometimes. She shared a story about her own son's pre-adolescent experience. They discovered that so many times when he was irritable, he was simply hungry—he was a growing boy! So she reminded her patient to stop and think about having some healthy food instead of getting angry with his little brother or parents. Now he has learned to stop, think, and eat first—a valuable lesson well taught with a simple story.

6. Goal and a Plan of Action: Advocating for Kids' Pain Outside of the Exam Room

Advocates aren't just born. They prepare themselves by developing messages, taking action, making the right moves and by becoming students of communications strategy. Advocating outside of the exam room takes time. With that in mind, developing a goal for the next 6 months or 1 year is a good first step. The goal needs to be realistic. Trying to change reimbursement standards to include more time for counseling may be more than you can pull off alone, especially if you are in a busy private practice. But committing to speak publicly when you can about children's pain in local media interviews, or starting a "pain group" at your affiliated hospital, or joining an AAP committee focused on the issue of chronic pain in adolescents are doable goals.

If you are dedicated to speaking out about the problem of children's acute and chronic pain, and about your solutions to the problem, here are some ideas for advocating that you can include in a personalized advocacy plan:

- **Develop messages.** What do you want to say about pain in children? What messages will resonate with each audience—children, parents, peers, reporters, or legislators?
- **Train staff on common messages.** Physicians, nurses, front office staff, and anyone working in your office should understand the messages you use to communicate about children's pain. Train them on the key messages you develop. You should all be speaking from the same page.
- **Organize like-minded experts.** Organize a group of pediatricians and family practitioners in your area to discuss what can be done to improve

pain care. Invite pediatric pain experts to join in. Include specialists who treat children's pain —orthopedists, neonatologists, oncologists, etc.
- **Accept speaking invitations, or ask to speak.** Local women's or men's groups, health fairs, PTA and school board meetings, foundations, corporations…look for opportunities to get your message out.
- **Write opinion editorials.** To reach the public, consider drafting an opinion editorial for your local newspaper as opportunities arise. For example, one pediatrician told me that parents are afraid to give their children strong pain medications for fear of addiction, even when the pediatrician believes, for the short-term, that these medications are warranted. An opinion editorial written and placed in the local newspaper by a respected pediatrician can go a long way in educating parents about pain treatment. In today's world, your opinion will be shared with more parents than you can imagine. Once something of interest is published, it is often sent nationally and even internationally by parents who use the Internet and blogging to share important messages.
- **Accept media opportunities.** If the local or national television producer calls you to be interviewed about anything from recommendations about the flu shot to chronic headaches, take the opportunity! You will reach thousands, perhaps millions, of parents who are eager for information about their children.

The goal and the plan are a great start, but the last ingredient is critical—the courage to do it. If you want to educate, motivate, or change behavior or policy, it takes time and commitment.

June Dahl, PhD, professor of pharmacology at the University of Wisconsin School of Medicine and Public Health, and recognized for her leadership in promoting cancer pain relief in the United States, had a goal: to integrate pain management into all patient care. She is one reason medical professionals in hospitals are now required to ask all patients about their pain.

In 1997, Dahl approached the Joint Commission on Accreditation of Healthcare Organizations, the principal organization responsible for accrediting health care organizations in the United States, and proposed that patients' pain assessment be required for hospitals seeking accreditation. It took several committee meetings, securing grant money from a foundation to pursue this effort, and the nerve to face a series of rejections and keep on trying. In just a few years, the pain standards were approved and became effective in January 2001. Dr. Dahl's efforts led to a sea of change in understanding and incorporating good pain care into every practice and every hospital.

Very few people have the time to take on such a challenge, but even the smallest effort to educate the public about the importance of managing children's pain can be significant.

Take-Home Points

- Primary care physicians are the best messengers, and the best advocates for managing children's pain.
- Barriers exist for becoming an advocate for kids' pain care, but most can be overcome.
- There are three steps for advocating: 1) developing memorable messages, 2) telling engaging stories, and 3) developing a goal and a plan of action.
- Pediatricians' messages need to "speak in headlines," be jargon-free, and feel human.

- Being an advocate outside of the exam room means taking opportunities to speak in public and with peers about the importance of good pain care.

References

1. AAP Policy Statement. Prevention and management of pain in the neonate: an update. Pediatrics 2006;118:2231–2241.
2. AAP Policy Statement. The assessment and management of acute pain in infants, children, and adolescents. Pediatrics 2001;108:793–797.
3. Pain Facts from the American Pain Foundation. *www.painfoundation.org.*
4. Roberts DF, Foehr UG, Rideout V. Generation M: Media in the lives of 8-18 year-olds. Report to the Henry J. Kaiser Family Foundation, 2005. Accessed at *www.kff.org/entmedia/upload/Generation-M-Media-in-the-Lives-of-8-18-Year-olds-Report.pdf.*
5. "The Shrinking Soundbite: Network Election News Study Finds Decline in Candidate News Time" Center for Media and Public Affairs Election Watch Report, September 28, 2000.
6. Seven in Ten U.S. Adults Say They Watch Broadcast News at Least Several Times a Week. The Harris Poll® #20, February 24, 2006. *http://www.harrisinteractive.com/harris_poll/index.asp?PID=644.*

25
Conclusion

What to Do When There is Nothing to Do

Kenneth R. Goldschneider

Referral note: "16 y.o. with back pain, depression,"
missing school, headaches, [other issues] multiple
therapies tried…"good luck"
Good luck, indeed. It was not the first time those
words appeared on a referral form. The sound of
heads banging against walls resounded through
those two words. They virtually guaranteed that the
patient, the family, and her physician had run out
of things to do, the frustration level would be high
and the optimism for help low. What was there to
offer her?

Introduction

Pain is an entity as complex as it is pervasive;
its assessment and treatment can be vexing and
frustrating. Yet, its treatment can be effective, and
bringing relief to or preventing physical discomfort and mental/emotional suffering is satisfying.
A number of specialists from many fields of pain
management have come together between the cov-
ers of this book to share both knowledge and
practical tips on how to assist pediatric patients
who are at risk for pain, be it acute or chronic, or
who present to the primary care office with long-term
pain. There were gaps, though. There were gaps
in knowledge, gaps in FDA-approved medication
suggestions, gaps in the understanding of physiology
and psychology.

Evidence-based medicine has become the rightful
watchword of our practices, and we all strive to
use the best available data and evidence to guide
our evaluations and treatments. But the field of
pain management is fraught with places where

the evidence is sparse, even absent. That condition is not unique to the practice of pain medicine.
The combination of oft-times challenging pain
assessment, off-label use of medications, the risks
—perceived and real—of using opioids, difficulty
in eliciting mechanisms through history and physical exams, and the pressure from families to "do
something…no child should have to suffer pain
like this" is daunting. It is this situation to which
this chapter is devoted.

1. There is Always Something to Offer

"You're the only one who believes me," said a
young lady, whose pain had brought her from
out-of-state to one of our clinics. "No one at home
does; they say I'm just trying to get attention." It
did not take a huge effort to help her. It started with
a sympathetic ear, one that was not interrupted by a
mouth too quick to say "but…" or "the X-rays are
normal…" or "you're just under a lot of stress…"
Validation of her feelings, of her fears, of her pain
was enough to bring her at least partial relief. That
is something that primary health care providers,
who already know the patient, can bring to the
table at least as well as specialists. As we all know,
pain can be nebulous and is entirely subjective.
There is no harm in confirming the patient's experience. It does not encourage poor coping, it does
not reduce function, and it does not differentiate
between somatic and psychological mechanisms.
It maintains a dialogue. If a patient says they are
afraid of needles, then one should address the fear,

not try to talk the patient out of it. If headaches are causing the patient to miss school, then a dialogue will permit a fuller history, and build a trusting rapport that can lead to full use of the biopsychosocial model of treatment.

A common theme among patients referred to specialty pain clinics is that the trust and dialogue has been broken, or is in great need of repair. The patients in that situation come in expecting to be disbelieved and often wonder why they are bothering to see "another thousand doctors" who "won't know what to do, either." Another common sticking point is when psychology is held out as a last resort, thus implying that the search for a "real" cause has failed, and that the patient must, therefore, have a mental illness or be malingering.

Early and straightforward discussion of all evaluation and treatment options can reduce pejorative feelings about care, and prime the patient and family for full participation in a multidisciplinary program (see Fig. 25-1 for a typical care plan, which introduces all specialties as equal). Similarly, introducing the family to palliative care weeks or months before death becomes a certain endpoint can provide the family with services early enough to allow greater quality of life for a longer time. In a sense, these are examples of anticipatory guidance, which can be done so much better in the primary care setting than in the tertiary one.

2. There is Always Something to Do (at Least by the Patient)

As the examples above suggest, the biopsychosocial model of pain care flows naturally from tenets of primary care. Establishing an ongoing relationship with a child as a developing, biological organism in the context of a family structure and social functioning is common to both approaches. It makes sense that so many of the guidelines for evaluating and treating pain can fit almost seamlessly into primary practice. Some adjustments in expectations are needed, though. "Cure" in the typical medical sense may not apply. It is as much a goal of pain management to maximize function as it is to provide comfort, and when pain cannot be eradicated, it may become the primary goal. This is true for acute, chronic, and palliative care realms. Seeing their physicians as healers, families

often expect doctors to make pain go away, and not "just" manage it. Often patients take on a very passive role, allowing the all-knowing doctor to make them better, or to prevent pain or alleviate the suffering…and it is our calling and training to do so. But even in the acute setting, the more active a role the patient can take, the better.

As a pediatric anesthesiologist induces anesthesia, it is usual to involve the child in guided imagery, hypnosis, storytelling, or simply actively holding the mask or injecting the IV medication. Having taken an active role, the children are less fearful of the masks that settle over their faces, or of seeing the lights and equipment in the operating room. A little premedication can help the process along, too. Similarly, distraction, hypnosis, or active involvement can reduce the distress of immunizations or blood draws. Add to that the simple, but effective topical anesthetics and there is quite a bit to offer. Even for the more complex chronic pain conditions, or the palliative care situations, there is much to offer that requires more creativity and compassion than technology or training. The continuity of care, the understanding of development and the established trusting relationship between doctor and patient give primary practitioners potent tools with which to guide patients into the role of a successfully active participant in their own treatment.

3. FDA Approval and Medication Use

Medications play a large role in the treatment of both acute and chronic pain. As described in some chapters, the range of medications is large. The use of a given medicine can be surprising to practitioners and parents, and the FDA has labeled only a fraction of the medications we use for the age group in question. So, what does one do when the medication is "off-label" for the intended use? How does one explain to families that anticonvulsants or antidepressants will be prescribed, when there is no depression or seizure in sight? Further, as we all move toward evidence-based practice, what does one do when there are no randomized-controlled trials for using a medication in a particular case? As seen in Fig. 25-1, a typical care map for back pain, the medications considered have modest

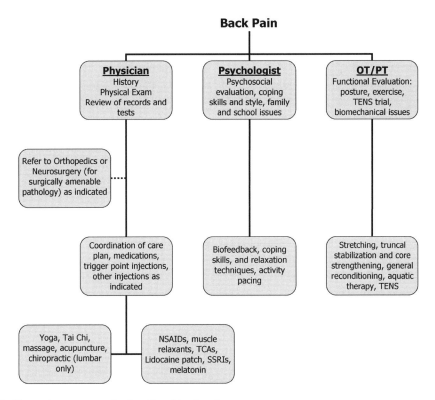

FIGURE 25-1. Illustrative care map for functional back pain.

scientific literature to support their use, and do not have FDA indications for back pain.

In the medical treatment pathway, drug options include several products for which there is no specific FDA indication for back pain, yet they are efficacious, and find their way into treatment algorithms. Two things are worth considering in this instance. First, when randomized-controlled trials are lacking, a drug should be chosen based on all available data, thoughtful consideration, presumed mechanism, pharmacology, and expert consensus.

Second, by knowing basic mechanisms behind a pain problem, one can proceed on the basis of theory. If hypersensitivity is seen, then a medication that calms irritable nerves is worth trying. How one explains the off-label use of a medicine to a family varies on personal preference, but a couple of example explanations follow. Anticonvulsants can be explained by describing that "seizures are misfiring nerves in the brain, and visceral hyperalgesia, CRPS and such states are misfiring nerves outside the brain. The medications that calm the irritable nerves in the brain can do something similar for the other

nerves, and reduce the pain." Descending inhibitory pathways in the brain and spinal cord involve similar neurochemistry to the chemistry of depression, and that relationship can be used to explain why antidepressants can be used for certain types of pain. In the end, use of off-label medications becomes a necessity when research cannot keep up with the varying potential uses of a drug, and the market share is too small to attract the attention of the pharmaceutical industry. This makes medicating pain in children as much a piece of the art of medicine as developing a good bedside manner.

Opioids bring up a separate set of issues. In the setting of acute pain treatment, parents often fear that their child may overdose or become addicted. Knowledge of proper dosing, use of titration, and the use of protocols with monitoring and rescue mechanisms are very important, and such can be communicated to the families to reassure that their child's safety is being attended to along with their pain. The risk of addiction is low, but the media attention is high. Children who present with no history of addiction or psychiatric disease that are given opioids for acute purposes will not leave the acute setting addicted. However, those patients requiring opioids for over one week or so will become tolerant, and the differences should be explained to the families up front. One can use the preoperative office visit to educate the parents about the likely use of opioids for postoperative pain, and to empower the parent to ask the surgeon or acute pain team member how pain will be taken care of, and how medications will be administered safely.

In the chronic setting, opioids are more rarely used, and the potential for misuse is greater. It is reasonable to screen for risk factors for misuse, including family history of misuse, alcoholism, and personal history of psychiatric or substance use problems. Controlled substance contracts are useful to clearly communicate the terms of use of these medications, and specify the circumstances of refills, use of drug testing, arrangements for replacement of lost of stolen medications and so on. Drug testing is useful to screen for diversion, and concomitant use of undesirable substances. By proceeding in a careful manner, the goal of analgesia and improved function can be accomplished with opioids, as a limited and structured part of a multidisciplinary care plan.

4. Looking Ahead

Advocating on behalf of your patients to your partners, affiliated hospitals, elected officials, insurance companies, and to the public as to what can and should be done for pain can expand the field of pain care for children in concrete and productive ways. Reinforcing the plan established by a multidisciplinary pain clinic, and helping guide the family toward greater functioning and away from fruitless "diagnostic" testing likewise advances pain care in ways that the tertiary centers could never do.

The expansion of pain care as well as the provision of good palliative services rests in large part on the shoulders of primary care physicians. As described earlier in this book, resources and financial considerations limit the number and regional distribution of comprehensive pain centers, and will for many years. Primary care physicians will always have more contact points with children in

pain and, therefore, can have the greatest impact in improving their care.

Expansion of interactive websites and advances in telemedicine may have great impact on the ability of primary and tertiary care providers to join forces. Existing and developing websites will focus more on providing access to resources, and directing physicians and families to expert care and advice in proximity to the patient. The ever-expanding ability to share information quickly via the internet will also become a routine way in which we all will be able to join efforts to provide optimal pain care, education, and advocacy.

Beyond the clinical realm, primary care workers can speak for the children in many forums. Advocacy for pain care can be a powerful way to provide children the care they need. Pediatricians, family practitioners, and general practice physicians can provide a powerful voice.

5. "Good Luck"

Our young lady presented at the outset of the chapter easily met the referral criteria suggested in Table 25-1, but her treatment plan followed a multidisciplinary care plan (Fig. 25-1). We established rapport and validated her experience, while confirming that her primary doctor was on the right track with many of his thoughts and suggestions. We confirmed that proper tests had been done, and that no "red flags" signaled danger. The concept of pain as a primary disorder was presented, along with

---

TABLE 25-1. Referral criteria for the Pediatric Complex Pain Clinic at the Alberta Children's Hospital.

1. Pain is characterized as chronic, complex, and difficult to manage, for whom no other service has been effective
2. Lack of a diagnosis and no clear treatment plan
3. Pain management cannot be achieved by family or community physician or another appropriate clinic (e.g., rheumatology, gastrointestinal, neurology)
4. Children demonstrate one or more of the following: pain resulting in uncontrollable, frightening or adverse experiences; pain leading to chronic physical disability, high anxiety, major sleep disturbance, frequent school absence, social withdrawal, parenting distress, family dysfunction, depression or feelings of hopelessness

(Used with permission of and gratitude to our colleagues at Alberta Children's Hospital)

the relationship with depression. A plan was made: a slowly progressive return to function, as coping and anxiety and depression management skills were applied. Her medications were optimized (an antidepressant, a muscle relaxant, and melatonin). Physical therapy and an exercise plan were tied to attaining functional goals that she valued. She was both empowered and given responsibility for her own care at a level she could handle. Passive modalities such as chiropractic and massage were limited to assisting with flare-up management, as she made the transition to active involvement in her own therapy. Her parents were involved in the educational aspects and taught ways to be helpful, but not too helpful. While the plan worked, it took several months for her to feel better, with greater function, less depression, and less pain.

The elements of the young lady's care have been wonderfully laid out in the text that precedes this chapter. Each pain practitioner who contributed to this book is an excellent clinician, as well as knowledgeable authority, and for those times when a little extra help would be useful, the author list is a wonderful resource by which to find assistance.

Final Take-Home Points

- Primary care practitioners have the greatest potential for impact in pediatric pain management.
- A significant impact can be made on acute pain, whether in the office or after referral to a hospital or emergency department.
- Continuity of care, trust, rapport, and communication are critical to helping a family through a complex, chronic pain problem or palliative care situation.
- Choice of medication often comes down to thoughtful application of theory, presumed mechanism of pain, expert consensus, and empiric trial. Reassessment at regular intervals can makes this process a safe one.
- Primary caregivers can be powerful advocates to families, other health care providers, and sociopolitical entities on behalf of their patients.
- Whether in the acute, chronic, or palliative care realms, patients benefit most when multiple modalities are used.
- Psychology is not just for the mentally ill any more than physical therapy is only for the disabled; families need to know this up front.

Index

Printed in the United States of America